Beauty
in a
Box

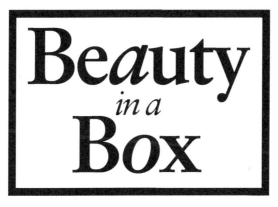

Beauty *in a* Box

DETANGLING THE ROOTS OF CANADA'S BLACK BEAUTY CULTURE

CHERYL THOMPSON

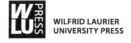

WILFRID LAURIER
UNIVERSITY PRESS

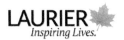

This book has been published with the help of a grant from the Canadian Federation for the Humanities and Social Sciences, through the Awards to Scholarly Publications Program, using funds provided by the Social Sciences and Humanities Research Council of Canada. Wilfrid Laurier University Press acknowledges the support of the Canada Council for the Arts for our publishing program. We acknowledge the financial support of the Government of Canada through the Canada Book Fund for our publishing activities. This work was supported by the Research Support Fund.

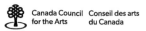
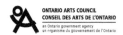

Library and Archives Canada Cataloguing in Publication

Thompson, Cheryl, 1977–, author
    Beauty in a box : detangling the roots of Canada's black beauty culture / Cheryl Thompson.

Includes bibliographical references and index.
Issued in print and electronic formats.
ISBN 978-1-77112-358-7 (softcover).—ISBN 978-1-77112-360-0 (EPUB).—
ISBN 978-1-77112-359-4 (PDF)

    1. Black Canadian women—Health and hygiene—History—20th century. 2. Beauty, Personal—Canada—History—20th century. 3. Beauty, Personal—Social aspects—Canada—History—20th century. 4. Beauty culture—Social aspects—Canada—History—20th century. 5. Black Canadian women—Social conditions—20th century. 6. African-American women—Race identity. 7. African-Americans—Race identity. 8. Hair—Social aspects—United States. 9. Beauty, Personal—United States. I. Title.

HQ1220.C3T46 2019   391.0089'96071   C2018-904624-4
                                                    C2018-904625-2

Cover and text design by Chris Rowat Design.

© 2019 Wilfrid Laurier University Press
Waterloo, Ontario, Canada
www.wlupress.wlu.ca

This book is printed on FSC® certified paper and is certified Ecologo. It contains post-consumer fibre, is processed chlorine free, and is manufactured using biogas energy.

Printed in Canada

Every reasonable effort has been made to acquire permission for copyright material used in this text, and to acknowledge all such indebtedness accurately. Any errors and omissions called to the publisher's attention will be corrected in future printings.

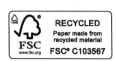

CONTENTS

INTRODUCTION

This book is about black beauty culture in Canada. Historically, the topic has received little scholarly attention in terms of Canadian history, advertising history, media studies, and histories of race and racism. This book aims to fill in this gap. *Beauty in a Box* is one of the first book-length projects to explore not only the discursive politics attached to black women's hair and skin but also the historical, transnational flow of products, beauty imagery, and services between the United States and Canada since the nineteenth century. One of the reasons why this topic has not received much attention until now is that the task of locating black voices in the Canadian historical record has been and remains a difficult challenge. There is also a general lack of cultural awareness about black Canadian women's consumer practices.

In *No Burden to Carry* (1991), for example, Dionne Brand observed of black women in Ontario that "these black women could talk about black women's lives in the 1920s, 1930s, 1940s, and 1950s, decades which seem to be missing in the historical record of black life in Canada."[1] The dearth of information about, and references to, black women led Brand to employ oral history as a method of inquiry. By recuperating textual histories along with records of a visual, ephemeral black culture, *Beauty in a Box* fills a gap in the historical record about black Canadian women not only in the period between the two world wars but in the post-1960s period, when a black immigration wave fundamentally changed black communities and the nation. This book argues that black beauty culture is an important aspect of the Canadian narrative that deserves not only critical intervention but also inclusion in wider conversations about race, capitalism, black feminism, retail consumerism, media, and advertising.

This book is also a transnational study. As a theoretical frame, transnationalism is often used to explore two separate issues. In the first instance, the conceptual framework of transnationalism describes large-scale processes, movements, and migrations that cross national borders, as well as the transformation of the everyday lives of people whose practices and social locations are restructured in, and through, their entanglements with, and within, multiple sites of diaspora.[2] In Canada, much of the scholarship on transnationalism as it relates to race has focused on this definition, as well as migrations and movements away from and back to the Caribbean. As D. Alissa Trotz observes, "[This scholarship] ... (the vast bulk of which addresses itself to the post-1960s period) has tended to frame the debate in terms of settlement, assimilation, incorporation, adjustment and marginalization."[3] Such scholarship has also placed heightened importance on the border and on discourses of belonging and *not* belonging to the nation, as well as emphasizing the experiences of Caribbean diasporas in Toronto and Montreal. *Beauty in a Box* engages in a similar transnational discussion, primarily in the first three chapters, where I chart not only the movement of black people into Canada and between provinces but also the strategies used by Caribbean and African American immigrants in the first half of the twentieth century to build community, establish diasporic networks, and redefine themselves amid a dominant culture rife with anti-black and anti-immigration sentiment.

In the second instance, this book uses a definition of transnationalism that describes the movement of consumer capitalism into Canada and the convergence between local media and global advertising. It aims to explore the circulation of media, goods, and products from the United States and Canada, and how that circulation has been shaped by a globalizing American culture, especially in the post-1970s era, when black consumer and aesthetic practices reflected an *Americanized* form of blackness. Stated otherwise, as images crossed the border, ideologies and aesthetic practices also entered Canada, which led to a standard of beauty that more resembles an African American standard than one said to "represent" a black Canadian standard.

In her examination of the circulation and travel of Indian citizens between India and the United States at the end of the twentieth century, Interpal Grewal found that "Americanness was produced transnationally by cultural, political and economic practices, so that becoming American did not always or necessarily connote full participation or belonging to a nation-state."[4] Consumer culture, she explains further, "produced other transnational identifications and subjects where desires and fantasies crossed national borders but also remained tied to national imaginaries."[5] I argue that, while black Canadians did not necessarily travel to and from the United States as in the Indian context, similarly, there were cultural and economic practices that were co-produced through the circulation of "African Americanness" via local black media throughout the twentieth century. Canada's consumer culture also co-produced transnational identifications and subjects. As a result, African American images, products, and ideologies crossed the border as desires and fantasies via advertising and, later, television and film.

This book articulates a spatial understanding of how the transnational—as movements/migrations and as desires/fantasies—has shaped black Canadian culture. *Beauty in a Box* probes the distance between black communities across the country, both geographic and symbolic, but it also considers their proximity to African American communities, especially regarding cultural, aesthetic, and consumer practices. Importantly, Robin Winks's *The Blacks in Canada: A History* (1971) was the first book to provide a comprehensive early history of black people in Canada. In it, Winks, a white author and history scholar who taught at Yale University, acknowledged the role black people played in Canadian history, especially regarding community-building and resistance to anti-black racism, but he also downplayed the importance of the advertising pages of the black press, among other things. Many of these publications were short-lived, and even though they may have contributed to a sense of racial pride among African Canadians, Winks opined that the papers "performed a temporarily useful supplemental function while generally avoiding controversial themes."[6] Second, he argued that these newspapers carried more advertising than news, and that the advertisements often were of a "dubious nature," emphasizing hairpieces, cosmetics, and funeral parlours, together with references to butchers, dairies, restaurants, plumbers, and laundries that would accept black customers.[7]

Winks, who was writing at a time of social unrest in America, stripped away the myth of Canada as a place where black people were welcomed with open arms, but he still did not allow African Americans and black Canadians much agency.[8] As Martin Berger observes of civil rights images in the 1960s, their success was hinged on "focusing attention on acts of violence and away from historically rooted injustices in public accommodation, voting rights, housing policies, and labor practices." The photographs of racial violence, he writes further, "read in isolation illustrated racism as an interpersonal problem . . . and this obscured the structural inequalities that benefited whites in the South as well as the North."[9] Many white critics and scholars alike who were supportive of civil rights in the 1960s still tended to view black people through a lens of passivity, regarding them as hapless martyrs or unfairly attacked victims.[10] Thus, it is through the writings of African American historians, cultural critics, and visual scholars that we can locate a perspective on the black experience that is not obscured by the black victim/white saviour binary that permeated many of the works produced in the late 1960s and early 1970s by white scholars such as Winks about the black experience in Canada and the United States.

When researching the first chapter of this book (which covers the time between the two world wars) there were many instances when finding African Canadian voices in the historical record proved a nearly impossible task. For this reason, *Beauty in a Box* focuses on black newspaper discourse to elucidate the gap in the Canadian historical record regarding black Canada before the 1960s. Rather than employ oral history, I performed textual, visual, and discourse analyses of black Canadian newspapers in the provinces of Ontario and Nova Scotia to trace a history of black aesthetics and consumer practices. The discursive and visual histories of African Americans and Afro-Caribbean people who lived and built communities from Windsor to Owen Sound in Ontario, African Nova Scotians who settled in some of the oldest communities in that province, African Americans who migrated to Toronto and Montreal in the early twentieth century, Caribbean immigrants to both those cities in the post-1960s, and black communities in Calgary and Edmonton are the primary focus of this book.

Significantly, the literature on African American photographic history, beauty and hair practices, and cultural history has been widely explored; by comparison, there is significantly less material and fewer aesthetic artifacts in the Canadian record that I could use to reliably speak to the African Canadian experience with respect to these topics prior to the 1970s. What I have done in these instances is rely on the advertising and editorial matter in black Canadian newspapers. In writing a book about black beauty culture, I faced the issue of trying to understand the centuries-long positioning of white womanhood as superior to black womanhood, and the binaries of difference—beautiful/ugly, feminine/masculine, demure/hypersexual—that have delineated the boundaries of beauty—socially, culturally, and visually. I then had to consider how and why these binaries continue to circulate today. Further, I had to understand the commercialization and systemization of beauty, as a consumer commodity, that developed over the course of the nineteenth and twentieth centuries, which added further levels of signification to black beauty aesthetic practices, as well as gendered and racialized binaries of difference. Given that Canadian media have, historically, relied upon American cultural and economic imports, I had to probe how, and to what extent, black communities have relied on African American imports—media, products, and in some ways, cultural identities.

This book also privileges English-speaking Canada for several reasons. Most notably, consumer culture has, historically, been driven by anglophone companies. In her examination of the history of department stores in Canada, Donica Belisle found that between 1890 and 1940, department stores became powerful agents of Canadian modernization. Companies such as Eaton's, Simpson's, and the Hudson's Bay Company (or the HBC, commonly known as The Bay) "helped revolutionize the ways Canadians thought about and experienced shopping, living standards, and goods."[11] These retailers also played a pivotal role in the construction of an anglophone beauty culture in Canada; each company was owned and managed by anglophones, and while they served customers of varying ethnic and linguistic backgrounds, English Canadian forms of retail and consumerism became the dominant forms in the country. As a result, English Canadian culture also became "quintessential Canadian culture."[12] The Hudson's Bay Company was established in the seventeenth century as a North American fur-trading venture backed by British financiers; in 1670, the company was granted by King Charles II of England exclusive trading rights to the territory.[13] Simpson's was founded by Robert Simpson in 1858, and Eaton's was founded in 1869 by Timothy Eaton. A francophone culture did develop around retail and consumerism; most notably, the largest francophone store, Dupuis Frères, which was founded by Nazaire Dupuis in 1868 in the east end of Montreal, became a model for francophone consumer culture.[14] The French Canadian origins of the owner, his links with the clergy, and the placement of the store in the city's east end, at a time when most department stores in Montreal were located further west, made the store extremely popular with its essentially French-speaking customers.[15] By and large, however, English Canadian retailers have created and disseminated consumer culture on a national level.

Importantly, the transnational links between black Canada and black America with respect to migration and the growth of urban centres across the country can be traced back to the first decades of the twentieth century. In 1921, Canada's population was just under 8.8 million, and its largest cities, Toronto and Montreal, had populations of about 521,000 and 639,000, respectively.[16] Comparatively, the growth of the American population, which had reached over 100 million by 1920, combined with its higher per capita income compared to Europe, gave the American market a unique status following World War I,[17] one which helped to foster a consumer culture that Canada could not reproduce. Thus, throughout the 1920s there existed a reliance upon the United States for cultural production and popular culture such as radio, a dependency that by 1949 led to the establishment of the Royal Commission on the Development of Arts and Letters, known as "the Massey Commission," and the subsequent Massey Report (1951), which resulted in the development of the Canadian Broadcasting Corporation (CBC), the National Library, and the establishment of the Canada Council for the Arts in an effort to promote, preserve, and protect Canadian culture. While these developments have been widely explored, there is little scholarship that has contended with how the encroachment of African American cultural production and popular culture has affected black Canadian culture. This book represents one of the first attempts to explore the impact of African American images, products, and ideologies on black Canada.

As in the United States, black communities in Canada were built and thrived in the country's largest cities—Toronto and Montreal. Black beauty culture businesses also thrived there even though these cities had relatively small populations compared to cities such as New York, Chicago, and Philadelphia. During what became known as "The Great Migration," roughly from 1915 to 1940 (the time span is sometimes cited as 1915 to 1960), large numbers of African Americans left the rural South and moved to the urban North, resulting in a steady rise in the proportion of African Americans living in cities. The urban population of African Americans went from 27 percent in 1916 to 35 percent in 1920 and 44 percent in 1930; by 1940, nearly half of all African Americans were urban.[18] Similarly, many black immigrants to Canada during the same period settled in cities and the level of black urbanization rose to 11 percent above the national average;[19] overall, however, growth of the black population remained fairly stagnant. While the Afro-Caribbean enclaves that characterized New York City neighbourhoods in the early twentieth century were largely absent from Toronto until midcentury, the two cities were intimately connected through diaspora. As Jared Toney notes, "West Indians arriving from Halifax, Montreal, New York, Central and South America, and directly from the Caribbean found a small but growing black population in Toronto (West Indian, African, American, and Canadian)."[20] The 1921 census data also shows about 1,200 black people living in that city (a number that remained relatively flat until the 1961 census) and the black population in Canada as just over 18,000, of whom approximately 7,200 were living in Ontario.[21] In Montreal, by the time of the 1941 census, the black population numbered just under 1,800.[22]

Thus, even as black people were increasingly living in Canadian cites, until the 1970s, there was no substantive public discourse about urbanization or interregional and intraregional migration that considered their experiences. As early as the 1920s, there were transnational connections between diasporic black populations in Toronto, New York, and Montreal. There were also interregional connections between Toronto and Nova Scotia, such as in the case of Daniel Braithwaite, born in Sydney in 1919 to Barbadian parents who had left the Caribbean for the promise of work and a better life and who settled in Toronto in 1927.[23] In the 1950s, Braithwaite was part of a group of activists in Toronto who launched a campaign that successfully rid the city's public schools of *Little Black Sambo*, a children's book that depicted black people in a derogatory manner. In his study of Toronto's Afro-Caribbean immigrant population in the 1920s, Toney addressed the ways in which "the local" and "the global" might be analyzed and "understood as cultural categories implicated in the production" of identity.[24] He also considered the local resonances of global diasporic processes and practices, identifying how borders shaped the contours of transnational communities in the first decades of the twentieth century. Similarly, I probe the development and circulation of black beauty ephemera within "local" black communities in relation to "global" (in this case, America's) beauty industries and imagery. *Beauty in a Box* does not ignore the cultural influence of African Americans in the twentieth century, but concerted effort is made to not let that narrative deny the existence and experiences of African Canadians, even as there are fewer examples to draw from in the years between the two world wars. Significantly, because there is such a concentrated focus on advertising throughout this book, it is important to situate its historical development in the context of Canada, as well.

Advertising initially developed during the eighteenth century when credit emerged. Prior to 1850, advertising was not widespread in newspapers in Europe and North America. By the late nineteenth century, however, newspapers and magazines had expanded their operations to accommodate advertisers' demand for space and to realize the revenue that advertisers and advertising represented; this convergence between print and advertising marked a turning point in Western media culture.[25]

It allowed for the creation and marketing of new kinds of products, and advertising thus made consumer products as much a part of people's lives as more familiar "natural commodities."[26] The movement of American advertising agencies into Canada began in the early twentieth century as British investment in the country began to decrease and American interests increased their investments. Magazines first took advertisers at the turn of the twentieth century, and by the 1910s their style had settled into what Naomi Wolf has called "cozy, relaxed, and intimate."[27] Between 1900 and 1930, in an effort to create a dependency on consumer goods, department store advertisements portrayed consumerism as "natural," a portrayal that indicated to Canadians that they were consumerist and that Canada was a modern consumer nation.[28] Shawn Michelle Smith aptly notes that, in this milieu, "popular women's magazines targeted white middle-class women as the engineers of the mechanical reproduction of the white middle-class family."[29] The dominant culture viewed black women through the lens of abstraction, ultimately removing them from the visual landscape of consumer modernity.

Canadian art historian Charmaine Nelson opines that the colonial origins of modernism must be examined within the context of *negrophilia*, the social and cultural phenomenon through which blackness, as supposedly primitive, was revealed and celebrated. "We must scrutinize it as a generative force and interrogate it as the very process through which Africanness and blackness were othered and the white body/self located as 'civilized,' beautiful, rational, and intelligent,"[30] she writes. The *primitive*, as Petrine Archer-Straw argues, "represented the process through which Europeans suggested their own superiority by placing inferior status on others. This process was entirely one-sided: it was simply a way for Europeans to project their fear of difference onto other races."[31] In the nineteenth century, advertising incorporated black imagery into product promotion by pairing the "exotic" *otherness* of blackness, typically stereotypes that portrayed blacks negatively as maids, menials, and hypersexualized primitives, with humour and attractive packaging. The Canada that women's magazines, department stores, and advertisers helped to build was based on class and race privileges rooted in the social relations of the *primitive*. Modernity's gaze depicted black people as forming part of a world that was modern, but they were not viewed as born *of* that world. In the emergent advertising and women's magazine industries of modern North America, the exclusion of black women helped to further entrench the belief that the panorama of modernity was for, and *of*, white women.

Modernity, a time and concept, is often articulated as being a moment of paradox; a moment marked by many contradictions. Modernity describes the paradoxical effects of an urban, capitalist order—its rationalized work, bureaucracy, and efficiency beginning in the late nineteenth century on the one hand, but its fleeting encounters, self-consciousness, and continuous novelty through the first decades of the twentieth century on the other.[32] While modernity is a slippery concept that does not have one singular definition, Liz Conor observes that the modern vision helped to condition women's self-perception as modern, which meant that gendered representations became embodied. "If modernization has been defined by changing modes and relations of production—new commodity markets and the expansion of cultural consumption, urbanization, migration, democratization, and technology and its popularization in leisure forms—the visual realm was constituted through these changes and became a primary site for contesting the significance of these innovations for identity,"[33] she writes.

One of the key aspects of modern womanhood, Conor asserts, is that "appearing" described how the changed conditions of feminine visibility in modernity invited a practice of the self which was centred on one's visual status and effects. "'Feminine visibility,'" she explains further, "refers to the entire range of women's capacity to be seen: from self-apprehension in a mirror, to being seen in public space, to becoming an image through industrialized visual technologies such as the camera."[34] As Sarah-Jane Mathieu asserts, "Canada's enrapture with modernity—overwhelmingly defined as railway technology during the late nineteenth century—was predicated upon the racialized and gendered constructions that enabled that technology in the first place."[35] "Just as Canadians celebrated their newfound status as an Anglo-Saxon modern nation-state in the first decades of the twentieth century, they made deliberate racialized and gendered decisions—codified into law and institutional practices—about what the nation-state would be, who would belong to it, and who would not,"[36] Mathieu writes further. Throughout this modern period (1860s to 1960s), racist ideologies, in addition to consumerist and patriotic ideologies, formed part of Canadian advertising but also department store visual culture.

In *Retail Nation: Department Stores and the Making of Modern Canada* (2011), Belisle asserts that between 1890 and 1940, Eaton's, Simpson's, and the HBC portrayed First Nations peoples as pre-modern and Africans and Asians as labourers, while white Canadians were always shown as consumers. "Department stores suggested how mass merchandising helped to establish modern European civilization," she writes, and at the centre of this political economy were the imperialist legacies of racial hierarchies.[37] For example, in its 1933 Christmas catalogue, Simpson's offered "Happy Topsy": the only black doll among a dozen white dolls. She is described as "a real lovable pickaninny" with a "roguish smile."[38] The pickaninny, like the mammy and the Jezebel, were stereotypes of black children and women that were created under chattel slavery but became popularized in nineteenth-century sentimental literature, then spread to blackface minstrel stage productions, and eventually were embedded into modern advertising imagery. The characteristics of the pickaninny included dark or sometimes jet-black skin, and exaggerated eyes and mouth; pickaninnies also often wore ragged clothes (to suggest parental neglect) and were sometimes partially or fully naked.[39] When *Chatelaine* magazine appeared in 1928, it also perpetuated stereotypes about black women and children. While it was not the first women's magazine in Canada, by the 1950s it had become the most influential. Before it, the *Canadian Home Journal* (1905–59) contained recipes, dress patterns, behavioural advice, and short stories, and other magazines soon followed, such as *Everywoman's World* (1914–22), *Canadian Homes and Gardens* (1924–62), and *Mayfair* (1927–59), published by the Maclean Publishing Company.[40] By the 1930s, *Mayfair* was a high-fashion magazine catering to upper-class Canadian women; it had modelled itself very much on the style of American *Vogue*.[41]

Chatelaine modelled itself after *Ladies' Home Journal* and *Better Homes and Gardens* with its advice columns, non-fiction, women's biographies, poetry, and articles on fashion and beauty; it also targeted the modern middle-class Anglo-Saxon housewife.[42] *Chatelaine*'s female editors from 1928 through the 1950s conscientiously organized the magazine to both reflect and help shape modern, middle-class Canadian womanhood.[43] An immigrant woman to Canada from Eastern Europe in the 1930s with no access to a radio and a limited knowledge of English, for example, would have looked to *Chatelaine* to provide a visual and textual guide for attaining the modern ideal of Canadian womanhood. The magazine was thus an active disseminator of Canadian nationalism and modern standards of beauty.

Like department store catalogues, women's magazines and advertisements in the first decades of the twentieth century perpetuated theories of the racial superiority of the white, Anglo-Saxon race by reinforcing such beliefs in the cultivation of a personal beauty. An advertisement for a "Just Grown Up" Topsy doll, for instance, appearing in the September 1937 issue of *Chatelaine* magazine, read, "You just can't help liking this happy-go-lucky, fat, colored baby doll."[44] The stereotype of Topsy, from a character introduced in Harriet Beecher Stowe's 1852 novel *Uncle Tom's Cabin*, was a "pickaninny" characterization of black childhood. When Topsy is introduced in the novel, Stowe describes her as "one of the blackest of her race; and her round shining eyes, glittering as glass beads, moved with quick and restless glances over everything in the room.... Her woolly hair was braided in sundry little tails, which stuck out in every direction."[45] "Mammy" images also occupied more than their share of space in the United States' cultural imagination and in the editorial content and advertising imagery of mainstream periodicals like the *Ladies' Home Journal*[46]— but were also to be found in the pages of *Chatelaine*.

As Kimberly Wallace-Sanders writes, "'Mammy' is part of the lexicon of antebellum mythology.... [Her] stereotypical attributes—her deeply sonorous and effortlessly soothing voice, her infinite patience, her raucous laugh, her self-deprecating wit, her implicit understanding and acceptance of her inferiority and her devotion to whites—all point to a long-lasting and troubled marriage of racial and gender essentialism, mythology, and southern nostalgia."[47] In the December 1936 issue of *Chatelaine*, for example, a "Mammy [Memo] Pad," was presented as "a useful and amusing novelty for the kitchen."[48] The presence of such advertising points to how ubiquitous the circulated image of a pre-modern, *primitive* black womanhood was in Canada and that, in the interwar years, the notion of modern femininity excluded black women.

Importantly, the arrival of Afro-Caribbean people and non-English-speaking Europeans in the early twentieth century created an impetus among white Anglo-Saxon, English-speaking Canadians to make as their main goal the assimilation of newcomers into Anglo-conformity. Many English Canadians, however, still believed that "white Anglo-Saxons were racially superior and immigrants were welcomed according to the degree to which they approached this ideal."[49] Immigrants were ranked on a sliding scale—white British and Americans first, northern and western Europeans next, after them the central and eastern Europeans (including Jews), and last of all Asians and black people. The 1950s marked a period when some articles in *Chatelaine* began to explore issues of race and ethnicity. These editorials tended to be sympathetic to new immigrants to the country, often celebrating highlights (particularly cuisine and household customs), and, as evidenced by Jeannine Locke's 1957 piece "Can the Hungarians Fit In?" these articles were often "how-to" pieces on assimilating into Canadian society.[50] Eastern or northern European immigrants were able to use these images and editorials to acquire the tools to approximate Anglo-Saxon values, and, because they were close(r) in proximity to whiteness, they attained citizenship rights and cultural acceptance sooner and with less resistance than did black people, Asians, and South Asians, who ranked least on the nation's priority scale, and who were typically not interpolated into the dominant media culture.

Department store catalogues and women's magazines similarly adhered to a racialized sliding scale in their representation of non-white Canadians. In Eaton's catalogues, for instance, Belisle found that "people of African and Asian descent were never depicted in catalogues as wearers of department store clothing, users of department store furniture, or readers of department store books. Instead their representation supplemented the value of goods for sale."[51] Stated otherwise, black people and Asians were exotic additions, not consumers of Eaton's products. Valerie Korinek, in *Roughing It in the Suburbs: Reading* Chatelaine *Magazine in the Fifties and Sixties* (2000), notes that, racially, "the people depicted in [*Chatelaine*] advertisements continued to be very homogeneous (96 percent were white); only a handful of ads in either decade featured people of colour, and then they were usually trademarked product icons, such as Aunt Jemima."[52] Importantly, while Korinek's and Belisle's work has broadened our understanding of retail consumerism and women's magazine culture, both failed to locate a black consumer and print culture as existing in its own right not singularly as represented within and through the dominant Canadian retail sector and pages of women's magazines and store catalogues.

One of the aims of this book is to explain why, over the course of the twentieth century, Canadian women's magazines, advertisers, and retailers went from excluding black women from product and retail merchandising, beauty advertising, and editorials to incorporating black women, products, and images into their retail displays, advertising, and editorial content. In addition, it probes how black community newspapers promoted black beauty culture, linking black Canada in a transnational, diasporic network between "the local" and "the global." *Beauty in a Box* takes as a starting point that black Canadian newspapers played an important and undeniable role in documenting black life, speaking on behalf of and for black Canadians, and espousing black beauty culture ideologies, practices, and imagery. Since the early twentieth centuries, these newspapers have curated a textual and visual record of black life in Canada. Without these newspapers, writing this book would have been virtually impossible. As Noliwe Rooks observed, the importance of African American women's magazines "lies in their asking us to think more deeply about or, in some instances, rethink what we are sure we know about relationships between groups of African Americans in different regions, and to listen in on intra-racial conversations from a number of historical periods and geographic locales."[53] By exploring the contents of black Canadian newspapers, this book asks us to think more deeply about Canadian media history, and to rethink what we think we know about black beauty culture across historical periods, geographic space, time, and place.

The *Canadian Observer* (1914–19), published out of Toronto and edited by Joseph R. B. Whitney, was the first black Canadian newspaper to reach a national audience. The *Atlantic Advocate*, a monthly journal out of Halifax, Nova Scotia, circulated for a few years during the First World War, as well. The *Canadian Observer* helped to give black Canadians a platform not only to challenge the Canadian government's anti-black sentiments and policies of the period but also to shed light on the accomplishments of black Canadians during the Great War. In her analysis of the *Canadian Observer*'s pages, Melissa Shaw added to the story of the all-black No. 2 Construction Battalion's full inclusion in the Canadian Expeditionary Forces during World War I, and, in so doing, her work furthered the initial efforts of Calvin Ruck's *Canada's Black Battalion: No. 2 Construction 1916–1920* (1986).

Shaw underscored the vital role that editorials in the *Canadian Observer* played in articulating a uniquely black Canadian point of view during a time when black people had virtually no outlet within the dominant public sphere to espouse their opinions. "A wide variety of military documents located in the Library and Archives of Canada (LAC) allow a rare glimpse into how anti-Black racism was expressed through both state and society apparatuses," she writes, adding that, as a result, "the *Canadian Observer* is a key and hitherto underutilized source that lends historically rich insights to my analysis."[54] Thus, the *Canadian Observer* stands as an important historical artifact that provides us with a deeper understanding of black life and resistance to anti-black racism in the early twentieth century, but it also contains some of the earliest evidence of a local and transnational black beauty culture.

In a front-page editorial on July 31, 1915, titled "An Open Letter to the Colored Race in Canada," for example, Joseph Whitney wrote, "I think you will agree that, as a race, we are not, in Canada, making the progress we should be making. Population considered, we are not a factor in the national life of this country."[55] The letter was a call to action to the newspaper's readers to provide some possible explanations for why black Canadians had yet to establish themselves within the dominant public sphere as African Americans had begun to do stateside. Black women entrepreneurs also advertised their services in the newspaper from the outset. These advertisements were not only for beauty culture but also for black women-operated businesses that welcomed black patronage. For instance, on April 15, 1916, Mary E. Henderson, superintendent of Toronto's Young Women's Christian Association (YWCA), located on Ontario Street near the intersections of Bloor and Sherbourne Streets (present-day St. James Town), posted an advertisement in the newspaper that read, "[The YWCA] offers to colored young women safe, comfortable, reasonable accommodation, pleasant parlors, in which to entertain company, social evenings; song service on Sunday afternoons."[56] In June that same year, a beauty advertisement in the newspaper asked, "Do you want a wealth of soft lubricant hair?"[57] The hair restoration product was offered for sale by mail order from an A. W. Hackley, but Madam R. D. Jones, who resided in Windsor, Ontario, sold it for fifty cents per box. In chapter 1, I explain how, in the first decades of the twentieth century, it was common practice for black women to sell from their homes products that were imported from the United States.

Importantly, there has been little scholarly inquiry into black Canadian newspapers, and those who have written about them, such as Winks, have tended to minimize their importance and that of the beauty culture and the black-owned businesses that advertised in their pages. It is within these pages that we can gain a deeper sense of how, as Toney points out, "local entrepreneurs and spiritual leaders galvanized and solidified the immigrant population while also functioning as important links to the Caribbean and black diasporas."[58] The three segments of Toronto's black community in the early twentieth century—Afro-Caribbeans, African Americans, and African Nova Scotians—all made use of the *Canadian Observer* to promote community developments. Thus, the existence of a black consumer culture, as evidenced by newspaper advertisements and some editorial content, helps elucidate similarities between, and differences among, this diverse population. Further, downplaying black community newspapers because of their content, or measuring their size against the dominant newspapers, such as the *Toronto Daily Star*, which by 1929 had a circulation of 175,000, becoming the largest circulation newspaper in Canada,[59] only serves to malign their importance. The mere presence of these newspapers, advertisements, and editorials stand on their own as forming part of an early black Canadian media and consumer culture that cannot be located elsewhere.

When the *Dawn of Tomorrow* (1923–71) appeared in London, Ontario, the weekly newspaper, which dubbed itself as "Devoted to the Interests of the Darker Races," became a paper of record for not only localized and diasporic black community news, but also news on the black church, anti-black racism in Canadian society, and, most importantly, beauty culture. London proved an ideal place to launch a newspaper because it was a chief metropolitan centre for black people between Toronto and Windsor. Many African Americans had also been present in the corridor between Windsor, Hamilton, London, and Toronto since the nineteenth century. The *Dawn*'s editor, James F. Jenkins, was an African American who had moved to London in the early twentieth century. In "Cultivating Narratives of Race, Faith, and Community: *The Dawn of Tomorrow*, 1923–1971," I undertook one of the first comprehensive readings of the newspaper, noting that Jenkins paid closed attention to diasporic connections between Canada and America while simultaneously acknowledging the realities of black life north of the border, an action that mirrored those of Whitney's *Canadian Observer*.

Images of black women that appeared in the *Dawn* suggest that the paper was an extension of Jenkins' Canadian League for the Advancement of Colored People (CLACP), formally chartered in 1925 as the Canadian equivalent to the National Association for the Advancement of Colored People (NAACP). Though the CLACP never achieved national status, it had mirrored some of its editorial practices after the African American press and the NAACP. For instance, when Jenkins's wife Christina Elizabeth, who also served as advertising manager, gave birth to twins in November 1926, a photograph of her wearing a white hat and a pearl necklace appeared on the newspaper's front page.[60] As Deborah Willis and Carla Williams aptly note, the ideal of family and by extension the black community was an essential element in positive representations of African American women: "Images of black women ... with their own children attest to the significance of the familial bond and family pride that sitters sought to record for posterity."[61] The photographs of black Canadian women also stand as proof that racial uplift sentiments also circulated in Canada.

While the photographs and advertisements for hair and cosmetic products that lined the *Dawn*'s pages from the 1920s to the 1950s might seem trivial for a newspaper by today's standards, black newspapers understood that black women, as consumers and producers of beauty products, held the power to change the naturalized representations of the *primitive* that had socially and sexually debased them. By the time *The Clarion* appeared in 1940s Nova Scotia, and later, the *West Indian News Observer, Contrast,* and *Share* magazine in 1960s and 1970s Toronto, we have the existence of a decades-long black Canadian media that from today's vantage point must be understood as invaluable to recuperating the lives and experiences of black communities that, in many instances, cannot be located through other texts, and that is significantly missing from the dominant Canadian historical record.

Ultimately, *Beauty in a Box* aims to foster transnational conversations across time, space, and place by locating black Canadian print media—and the promotion, cultivation, growth, and development of black beauty culture within their pages—at the centre. Whereas in her book *Hope in a Jar: The Making of America's Beauty Culture* (1998) historian Kathy Peiss focused primarily on early beauty culture in America and the ways that a system of mass production, distribution, marketing, and advertising transformed cosmetic and hair firms into global enterprises, which led to the creation of a mass consumer market for beauty culture, I contend that similar systems of mass production, distribution, marketing, and advertising developed in Canada. I also assert that wider socio-cultural African American developments that coincided with the Great Migration, such as the "New Negro" and "New Negro Woman," made their way into Canada in the early twentieth century via newspaper editorials and aesthetic practices.

In the first decades of the twentieth century, within African American communities, black women faced internal pressures to "uplift" the race via their appearance. In the *Crisis,* for instance, the official magazine of the NAACP founded in 1910 by W. E. B. Du Bois, editorials about how the New Negro should be portrayed ran alongside images of neatly dressed African American women. Such images implicitly signalled how the New Negro Woman should also "appear" through her clothing and beauty practices to cultivate a visible black femininity.[62] The Great Migration had led to a "newness" that could be seen in the emergence of the cultural movement known as the Harlem Renaissance and cultural practices such as the embrace of photographic portraiture in the African American photography studios that arose in the first decades of the new century. From the 1920s onward, the concept of "newness" was also visible in the pages of black Canadian media in ways that spoke to the transnational adoption of an *Americanized* New Negro identity but also to a localized *new* African Canadian identity and forms of cultural production.

It is also important to understand the development of black beauty culture in Canada in relation to two conflicting yet concurrent shifts that took place over the course of the twentieth century. The first, marked by exclusionary socio-cultural practices and policies, spans from approximately 1911 to 1951, and the second, marked by anti-discrimination legislation and immigration policy changes, spans 1954 to the present. During the first phase, black Canadians were excluded from public acts of citizenship, such as military service. Racist immigration policies also restricted the growth of the black population. As Mathieu observes, "In 1922, Canada's leading news periodical, *Maclean's*, ran a special exposé on immigration and conceded, 'If our history is one of immigration our problems have been, are, and will continue to be problems of race.' Consequently, throughout the Jim Crow era...Canadians—bureaucrats, employers, and citizens alike—saw blacks as an immigrant problem."[63] Canada's Jim Crow segregation was not a system of de jure policies like in the United States (1877–1954) but during the same period, a de facto colour line—enforced socially, culturally, institutionally, and via the dominant media—existed from coast to coast. "Canadians crafted their own Jim Crow model, producing their own distinct language and rationalizations when propping up white supremacist ideology and practices,"[64] Mathieu writes further.

Over the last ten years, numerous scholars have begun to unpack the racialized and gendered narratives that circulated in pre-1960s Canada. Graham Reynolds's *Viola Desmond's Canada: A History of Blacks and Racial Segregation in the Promised Land* (2016), for example, shed light on the pervasiveness of Jim Crow segregation in Nova Scotia. His work reveals how discriminatory social practices, at a local level, were enforced and sanctioned. Reynolds also points to the life of Viola Desmond, who (as is discussed chapter 2) was a beautician and entrepreneur who became a champion of integration—by accident—when she refused to move from a "whites only" seating section to a "coloured" one in a New Glasgow, Nova Scotia, cinema in 1946. After she was selected in 2016 to appear on the revised Canadian ten-dollar bill, Desmond became a national figure, and yet the conditions under which she lived in 1940s Halifax are scarcely remembered across the country. As Reynolds poignantly writes, "The Viola Desmond incident is not an isolated example of our national ignorance regarding racial segregation and the struggle for racial equity in Canada."[65] On the contrary, "Over the long course of Canadian history, there has been a strong undercurrent of racial discrimination toward Blacks."[66] In *Policing Black Lives: State Violence in Canada from Slavery to the Present* (2017), Robyn Maynard echoed Reynolds's account by rooting histories of racial prejudice and discrimination in Canadian slavery through Jim Crow to the contemporary realities of state-sanctioned violence against black men and women. Maynard's discussion of the repositioning of Canada's national myth in the mid-twentieth century towards an embrace of multicultural-ism marks the second period in the twentieth century that is of importance to this book.

During the second phase, beginning in the mid-twentieth century, black community was still marked by socio-cultural exclusion from the dominant culture, but post-1960s Canadian society transformed from an overtly racist and anti-black nation to one *becoming* culturally diverse and "multicultural," in part because of social policy. It is important that I locate my own personal narrative in this milieu, as it helps to connect me to the topic on a personal level, not merely as an academic. In the late 1960s, my parents immigrated to Canada from Jamaica. By 1972, they had left downtown Toronto for the suburbs of Scarborough, located east of the downtown core. Changes to Canadian immigration policy during the decade meant that black people, like my parents, were encouraged to come to Canada. The opening of Canadian immigration offices in Jamaica and Trinidad and Tobago in 1967, and later in other predominantly black nations such as Haiti, Barbados, Kenya, and Côte d'Ivoire were another significant impetus for the immigration of blacks from the Caribbean to Canada.[67] The Caribbean-born population more than doubled from 1962 to 1967, and it had tripled by the mid-1970s.[68] Like my parents, many of these immigrants moved out to the suburbs and elsewhere during the 1970s and 1980s, becoming part of an emergent middle class that would help to transform Canada's mostly white (and British) suburbs of the 1950s and 1960s into the racially and ethnically diverse communities that many of them are today. Since the late 1960s, "diversity," as both an ethos and a brand, has also become part of what it means to be Canadian. Some of these Caribbean immigrants to Toronto in the 1960s through the 1980s opened beauty salons, barbershops, and beauty product stores, and some launched local community newspapers. These newspapers would serve as counter-hegemonic spaces where news about "the local" and "the global" diaspora could be shared and black beauty culture could be promoted. Advertisements and editorials from local hair salons and barbershops, beauty product shops, and department stores and drugstores that, in the post-1967 "multicultural" era began to solicit black consumers, all relied upon these newly formed West Indian-operated newspapers—*West Indian News Observer, Contrast,* and *Share*—to promote their businesses and to reach black women consumers. This wave of black newspapers, appearing in the late 1960s and 1970s, also reflected the shifting Canadian identity with respect to race and cultural diversity.

In October 1971, when Prime Minister Pierre Trudeau proclaimed in Parliament that Canada would adopt a policy of "official multiculturalism" and that the state would recognize cultural diversity as a national value, the idea was that such a proclamation would help to inspire confidence in what it meant to be Canadian.[69] One of the consequences of this act was that histories of racial oppression such as anti-black immigration policies, discrimination in housing and employment, and racist advertising imagery were simultaneously erased from the public memory. In its stead was a new version of Canada—an inclusive, diverse, multicultural nation. Trudeau's statement, along with a policy that followed in 1988, became a symbolic form of erasure for black communities. While these concepts formed part of the dominant hegemony, they became emblematic of the tension that comes with being both black *and* Canadian. As Barrington Walker notes, while Canada is a country that celebrates "diversity" and "multiculturalism" as important elements of our national character, "our relationship with these much-celebrated values is complex and fraught" as far as black Canadians and other racialized groups are concerned.[70] Maynard similarly writes that "for most Black people residing in Canada, neither racial equity, nor to use Trudeau's words, 'inclusion' or 'liberty' have been achieved. Instead…economic, social and political subjugation remain a definitive fact of Black life in Canada."[71] This shift toward Canadian "diversity" was most visible in Toronto, which during this time became the largest city in Canada, surpassing Montreal by the mid-1970s.

Growing up in Scarborough, I witnessed the borough become more culturally diverse. There were many instances in the early 1980s, however, when I was reminded that while the city's demographics were changing, there was not necessarily increased levels of cultural awareness about difference, especially black hair. At one point during my childhood there was an outbreak of head lice across Toronto's public schools. Back then, in-house nurses would use little wooden sticks to check students' hair for head lice. I vividly remember the day a nurse checked my hair. It was one of the first times that I realized that my hair's coarse texture meant that I was different from the others. If a nurse combed through my neatly braided hair, I thought the other kids at school would surely make fun of me; before this incident, other kids had often teased my twin sister and me because of our elaborate African-inspired hairstyles, which my mother meticulously created every other week. To my fellow students, our hair creations were "odd," and some even wondered aloud why our hair texture was different to theirs. As I entered the room to have my head examined, I gazed up at three white nurses peering down at me with curious eyes. I remember thinking the situation was not going to end very well. At that moment, one of them looked at me, then across to her colleagues, and then in a hushed tone she whispered, "I don't know what to do with this." By "this" she meant my hair. For her, tightly coiled black hair was something she never had to (and did not want to) think about. Thirty years later, when I was one of three black women asked to appear on *Canada A.M.*, a morning show that aired on CTV, a Canadian English-language television network, I was reminded of how far the black hair conversation had come. Alongside playwright Trey Anthony, creator of the play and short-lived sitcom, *'Da Kink in My Hair* (discussed in chapter 5) and Janet Campbell, owner of a natural hair studio in Toronto, we were there to talk about black hair.

The segment, hosted by Marci Ien, who is also black, marked one of the first televised discussions of black beauty on Canadian television. We spoke of family pressures to straighten our hair with chemical "relaxers" so that we "look professional" at work and school, and how in the media, beauty is often narrowly defined by white standards such that many black women feel pressure to straighten their hair and/or wear hair weaves (real or synthetic hair added to one's natural hair for length and/or fullness) so that our hair is soft and flowing, like that of other women. Anthony also pointed out that one of the myths about women who wear their hair "natural" (i.e., not chemically straightened or covered under a hair weave), both within and outside black communities, is that they are political and are more "connected to their roots" (i.e., Africa) than women who "relax" their hair or wear weaves, but this is not always the case. After the segment I thought to myself, black hair really is a complicated subject. On the one hand, for many black women it conjures up painful childhood memories of being teased by others and having their hair combed and, in some cases, permanently damaged by poor hair care techniques. On the other hand, on a cultural level, our hair is imbued with dual and sometimes conflicting meanings that are downright confusing and that have often left me unable to get to the root of why that is. While natural hairstyles like Afros, dreadlocks, or cornrows (tightly braided rows of hair) might denote a black woman's politics, they can also be just a hairstyle or her preference, with no political meaning whatsoever. Similarly, the topic of black women's skin is also complicated.

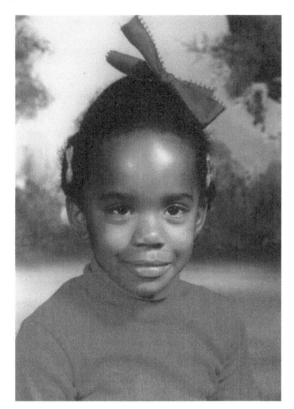

Figure 1. My childhood school picture, Scarborough,
Ontario, early 1980s.

In *The Color Complex* (1992), Kathy Russell, Midge Wilson, and Ronald Hall observed of African American communities, "Beneath a surface appearance of Black solidarity lies a matrix of attitudes about skin color and features in which color, not character, establishes friendships; degree of lightness, not expertise, influences hiring; and complexion, not talent, dictates casting for television and film."[72] While some black women believe that lighter skin enables more opportunities in terms of career or relationships than darker skin, light-skinned women's racial solidarity might be called into question as being "not black enough," denying these women the right to participate in discussions around hair and skin, which are at the core of many black women's identities. Thus, black beauty is not just about hairstyles or skin tones but is always-already about the tension between collective black identity and a black woman's individual choices. At the centre of this juxtaposition are ideologies and narratives about cultural identity, black representation in advertising and media industries, and solidarity—both within the local context but also transnationally and in relation to other sites of black diaspora.

Even though, as black Canadians, we have our own unique histories, experiences, and relationship with the state, African American histories, experiences, and cultural products have always influenced and shaped black Canadians, especially in terms of the fashion and modelling industries. In the National Film Board film *The Colour of Beauty* (2010), for instance, Elizabeth St. Philip followed black Canadian model Renee Thompson (no relation) as she tried to make it as a top fashion model in New York. The film exposed the fact that black models, irrespective of citizenship, still struggle in an American-dominated industry where white women continue to represent the standard of beauty. The film captured how modelling agencies rarely hire black models, and when they do, they want them to look, as one New York casting director admitted, "like a white girl dipped in chocolate." Thompson recounted hearing comments like "No black girls allowed on casting calls" or "We're not looking for black girls, only brunette white girls." Her agent, Justin Peery, also admitted that the fashion world seems interested only in the different skin pigment of black women; those "lucky few girls" with white features (a straight nose, lips that are not *too* big) are the ones considered beautiful.

A 2017 survey of spring runway season revealed that for the first time in recent history, more than 25 percent of the model castings were non-white; still, this meant that 74.6 percent of the models cast were white, and only 25.4 percent were racialized women, of which 10.3 percent were black.[73] Lisa Tant, editor-in-chief of the Canadian women's magazine *Flare*, and Jeanne Beker, host of *Fashion Television*, were reluctant to call such discrepancies racist, but both openly admit that from the designer through to the magazine editors, there is a lack of interest in black models. Significantly, both Tant and Beker made no mention of how or why black women are excluded from Canada's beauty industry, though they could openly point to, and tried to give reasons for, such exclusion/absences in America. It is clear, however, from the promotional practices of Canada's largest retailers that black women are not on their priority lists.

In September 2011, for instance, Hudson's Bay launched a new digital beauty magazine that mixed editorial content with e-commerce. The *National Post* described the new flipbook-style magazine as giving customers the ability to flip, click, and buy any of the products on the virtual page. "Everything from NARS lip pencils and Shiseido's latest eye shadow palettes to Marc Jacobs Lola perfume (more proof that the department store's cosmetics division, under Shelley Rozenwald's direction, is getting serious about online beauty retailing in Canada)," the article noted.[74] The monthly edition of *Beauty: The Guide*, edited by former *Cosmetics* magazine editor Dave Lackie, includes regular updates and instructional videos by The Bay's national makeup artist Dino Dilio. It went completely unnoticed by media outlets and consumer critics that, as a "guide to beauty," it features almost exclusively white women. In December 2016, Liberian model and blogger Deddeh Howard took to the Internet to express her frustration with seeing the same (white) faces dominating billboards and fashion glossies while racially diverse models are overlooked.[75] "Even though I was told by agencies that I have an amazing look and [they] wish they could represent me, they already have a black model. Besides having an abundance of white models. It seemed as if one or two black models on the roster are enough to represent us all. When you are told that, trust me, it feels bizarre," the model lamented on her blog.[76] Just as Canada's modelling and fashion worlds have refused to incorporate black women into their ranks, black Canadian women, like African American women, have also encountered discrimination because of their natural hair at school and at places of employment.

In 2016, *NBCNews.com* reported on a case in the 11th US Circuit Court of Appeals that ruled against a lawsuit filed by the Equal Employment Opportunity Commission (EEOC) against Catastrophe Management Solutions (CMS) for firing a black woman because she wore her hair in dreadlocks.[77] The lawsuit, filed by EEOC on behalf of Chastity Jones, marked thirty-five years since the landmark black hair case, *Rogers v. American Airlines* (1981), discussed in chapter 3, which set a legal precedent that gave employers a right to discriminate against black women because of their hair. Like Renee Rogers, a ticket agent for American Airlines who, after being fired for wearing her hair in cornrows, filed suit against the airline carrier, claiming that its grooming policy violated the Civil Rights Act of 1964, EEOC also claimed that Jones's termination was in violation of the Civil Rights Act. According to the news report, the court of appeals ruled that CMS's "race-neutral grooming policy" was not discriminatory because while hairstyles are "culturally associated with race" they are "not immutable physical characteristics." Stated otherwise, the court ruled that a hairstyle might be closely associated with one's culture but because it is changeable, it is not protectable under the law and an employer is within its rights to use it as a reason to deny employment.

In 2015, a black Grade 8 student at Amesbury Middle School in north Toronto was allegedly asked to leave school early because of her crochet braids (a combination of cornrows and hair extensions). In an interview with the *Toronto Star*, the child's mother, Terressa Sutherland, said that the principal of the school, who is also a black woman, approached her daughter several times about her hair and that the principal had brought her daughter to her office because of it.[78] "She basically told me that my daughter's hair is not professional and...that as a parent from the Caribbean, my daughter should not have her hair open," said Sutherland. A few months later, Akua Agyemfra, a black waitress at Jack Astor's Bar and Grill in Toronto, was sent home during her shift because her hair was in a bun. In an interview with *CBC News*, she said that on her third day of training at the restaurant the assistant manager sat her down and said, "I'm sorry to have to let you go home" because "a lot of the [non-black] girls [are] talking about [your] hair and that it was in a bun and theirs isn't."[79] In both cases, people in positions of power felt that black hair was not "professional."

In April 2016, Cree Ballah, an employee at a Zara clothing store in Toronto's east end told *CBC News* that she would likely quit her job and file a complaint with the Ontario Human Rights Commission after managers gave her a hard time about her hair, which was in box braids and gathered in the back.[80] In a written statement, Zara said the company is "diverse and multicultural" and does not tolerate any form of discrimination, and that it had "no formal policy" regarding employees' hairstyles, just that they "look professional." These discrimination headlines made me recall my own hair experiences growing up in Scarborough. The fact that hair cases and discrimination incidents continue to appear in the twenty-first century points to why black beauty matters not only as a study of inquiry but also as a window into the continued politics attached to black women's bodies and aesthetics, which are, in some cases, just as salient today as they were two centuries ago.

Significantly, I could not have endeavoured to tackle this subject were it not for the numerous African American writers, historians, black feminists, and cultural theorists who were the first to write the history of black beauty culture in the United States. The politicization of black women's beauty, particularly hair, has been the subject of several scholarly works for nearly twenty years. Ayana Byrd and Lori Tharps's *Hair Story: Untangling the Roots of Black Hair in America* (2001) provided one of the most in-depth examinations of black hair, from slavery to the rise of African American beauty entrepreneurs such as Madam C. J. Walker (the first woman millionaire), whose "shampoo-press-and-curl" method of hair care revolu-tionized the black beauty business. Byrd and Tharps explained why the black hair care business was at the centre of African American communi-ties amid a socio-cultural milieu of oppressive sexism and racism since the nineteenth centuries. *Hair Story* also recalled the 1960s moment when the Afro became the aesthetic of choice for the Black Power movement, which re-signified black hair to stand as a symbol of collective black pride. In the historical study *Hair Raising: Beauty, Culture, and African American Women* (1996), Noliwe Rooks located discourses about black women and hair in the history of black beauty entrepreneurship as well as in beauty advertisements and newspaper discourse. "Whereas in the dominant press, companies advertised... different lotions and ointments aimed at making skin look softer and more youthful," in the black press, she writes, "African American women were bombarded solely with products that promised to lighten the skin and straighten the hair."[81] While Rooks's primary focus was on the nineteenth and early twentieth centuries, she made some con-nections to contemporary hair politics, explaining how meanings and the cultural significance of black hair changed over time. Ingrid Banks's *Hair Matters: Beauty, Power, and Black Women's Consciousness* (2000) was largely a response to Rooks's quest to make connections between the representa-tion of black women's hair and black women's thoughts about their hair. In her ethnographic study of why hair matters among black women, Banks focused on how hair shapes ideas about everything from racial identity to constructions of femininity, while also explaining why, amid a media cul-ture saturated with negative messages about black hair and beauty, black women find ways to embrace and celebrate their hair. Her focus was on the importance of understanding the historical and complicated relationship between hair, power, and choice.

Other scholars such as Susannah Walker, Tiffany Melissa Gill, Julia Blackwelder, and Lanita Jacobs-Huey have expanded the scholarship on the business of black beauty. Such works have probed the "golden age of black business" (1900 to 1930), and the entrepreneurship of what Gill calls "beauty culturists" (1930 to 1960);[82] others have examined the role black beauty schools played during the Jim Crow era throughout the South and North.[83] By analyzing women's everyday conversations about their hair care, Jacob-Huey's anthropological ethnographic study sought to delin-eate the dynamics of women's beauty, that is, "how their socialization with new roles and sensibilities is negotiated in actual dialogues and hair-care practices."[84] Her work was one of the first to consider women's language, embodiment, and beauty by exploring how black women interact in beauty parlours, Internet discussions, comedy clubs, and other contexts that shape and frame how and what black women think and say about their hair today. Black feminists have also contributed to the discourse on black beauty by pointing to the wider socio-cultural milieu, where black women's bodily choices and identities are imbricated in complex relations that intersect racial, gendered, and class lines.

Scholars such as Patricia Hill Collins, bell hooks, Kimberlé Crenshaw, and Moya Bailey have all recognized, in their own unique ways, that racialized and gendered representations of black women have played a fundamental role in delineating the boundaries of what it means to be both black *and* a woman. As Collins once observed, "externally defined standards of beauty long applied to African-American women claim that no matter how intelligent, educated, or 'beautiful' a Black woman may be, those Black women whose features and skin color are most African must 'git back.' Blue-eyed, blonde, thin white women could not be considered beautiful without the Other—Black women with classical African features of dark skin, broad noses, full lips, and kinky hair."[85] Similarly, hooks has continually pointed to representations of black female bodies in contemporary popular culture as rarely subverting or critiquing images of black female sexuality that were part of the cultural apparatus of nineteenth-century racism and which still shape perceptions today.[86] In the contemporary media landscape, with the advent of social media, Bailey has taken black feminist media studies a step further by considering the fact that, as more people have access to new media tools, they are more able to create and share representations of themselves. This process of redefining representation has allowed black women to challenge the normative standards of bodily representation in popular culture.[87]

Beauty in a Box explores the same terrain as the above scholars, but its focus is on Canada, which is too often ignored in discussions of black beauty culture, among other topics. Importantly, however, this is not the first Canadian beauty culture book. Althea Prince's *The Politics of Black Women's Hair* (2009) was one of the first books by a black Canadian author to address the topic of black hair. However, Prince mostly focused on personal hair stories of black women to explore the topic. Using interviews, memoirs, and personal essays of black women from Canada, the United States, Britain, and the Caribbean, the book charted perceptions of black women's hair and how it is judged and graded in comparison to the dominant standard of beauty. *The Politics of Black Women's Hair* did not pay much attention to the symbiotic relationship between black beauty culture in Canada and the United States in terms of media, advertising, promotion, and consumerism.

Michele Tapp Roseman's *Hairlooms: The Untangled Truth about Loving Your Natural Hair and Beauty* (2017) was also driven by personal stories from African American women. Featuring thirty-two stories from such people as the late Dr. Maya Angelou, Lisa Price (founder of the natural product line, Carol's Daughter), and A'Lelia Bundles, the great-great-granddaughter of Madam C. J. Walker, *Hairlooms* also explored the emotional journey women have with their hair and the challenges some encounter when they try to "go natural" after years of chemically straightening and/or wearing a hair weave. While Roseman probed why it is still difficult for black women to embrace their natural hair, she did not examine the historical role media has played, in conjunction with retailers, in the segmentation of beauty culture, a development that made products and promotions geared toward celebrating black women's natural hair virtually non-existent until recent years when, in large part because of the Internet and black women hair bloggers, natural hair has become more celebrated.

In her ethnographic study of black British women of Caribbean descent in relation to a broader discussion of the Black Atlantic, Shirley Tate admits that she had to evolve from an earlier focus solely on the United Kingdom and United States to "thinking the Black Atlantic as a transnational structure of feeling which links diverse populations in a network of Black beauty ideology and practices... [which includes] also looking at the Caribbean and Latin America."[88] *Beauty in a Box* similarly acknowledges the transnational links between diverse populations in a network of black beauty ideology and practices while also pinpointing the ideologies and practices of the dominant beauty culture that has helped to create the hegemonic knowledge that has politicized black beauty in the first place. Tate writes that her reframing "acknowledges that Black beauty has raised the possibility for political contestations and has subverted the hegemonic knowledge as it has reaffirmed new strategies of identification."[89]

When I started my archival fieldwork for this book in 2010, I realized right away that I would need to rely on the beauty scholarship of African Americans. I also recognized shortly thereafter that there was a treasure trove of Canadian artifacts, both visual and material, that have scarcely been touched and that these materials would allow me to articulate a history of black beauty culture as existing before and after the 1960s. The lack of Canadian archival memory about black culture meant that I had to travel to the United States for most of my archival research. Over the course of four years, I travelled to Yale University's Beinecke Rare Book and Manuscript Library to review the *Ebony* magazine collection; I went to the Schomburg Center for Research in Black Culture in New York to study their manuscripts and archives collection; I also reviewed numerous African American periodicals on microfilm at the Historical Society of Pennsylvania in Philadelphia. These collections gave me a solid grounding in African American beauty culture history. Since there are no comparable research centres for black culture in Canada, I searched for materials related to African Canadian history, black women, and/or beauty culture at various sites throughout Ontario, Quebec, and Nova Scotia and relied upon virtual databases, where applicable, to piece together a national narrative. My Canadian fieldwork included trips to the Multicultural History Society of Ontario's ethnic newspaper collection, the Toronto Metropolitan Reference Library's newspaper collection, the Notman Photographic Archive at the McCord Museum, the African Canadian history collection at the Buxton National Historic Site and Museum, the University of Western Ontario's J. J. Talman Black History collection, the London Public Library's Genealogy records, and the Alvin McCurdy collection at the Archives of Ontario. I also made use of online databases at the Beaton Institute at Cape Breton University, and the Nova Scotia Archives.

At each archive, no archivists or librarians specializing in black history and/or black Canadian studies and/or beauty culture could assist me. In many instances, I also handled scarcely viewed materials, and when I asked staff about the contents of some of these collections I was often greeted with a blank stare and the statement, "I don't know, have a look and see if you find anything useful." Whenever I contacted an archivist about my research interest in black beauty, I was often told that I probably would not find much or that there was no dedicated collection related to my project. *Beauty in a Box* ultimately reflects my unrelenting refusal to take no for an answer or to be discouraged from navigating the archival record. Instead, I used my secondary knowledge of nineteenth- and twentieth-century African American history to speculate responsibly about black Canadian history in the absence of visual or textual records. If, for example, African Americans were reframing and reimagining their identities through images, consumerism, and media in the early twentieth century, it was a logical step to assume that black Canadians were doing the same thing at the same time, albeit on a much smaller scale.

Chapter 1 begins in the early twentieth century with an examination of the New Negro Woman who, like the New Woman, appeared at the turn of the twentieth century, becoming at once as synonymous with consumerism as she did with beauty, public visibility, and modernity. I explore how the New Negro Woman garnered a public visibility through cultural movements like the Harlem Renaissance and photography but also locate aspects of the New Negro Woman that can be said to have been born through editorials in black Canadian newspapers such as the *Canadian Observer* and the *Dawn of Tomorrow*. In the United States, African American beauty historians have observed that the New Negro Woman in America was "urged both to consume and to teach the ethos of consumption to their husbands and children."[90] How did the ethos of consumption affect how the New Negro Woman was "seen," but also how she "appeared" in black Canadian newspapers? This chapter provides some of the earliest evidences of a localized, diasporic black beauty culture, primarily in Toronto, in the first decades of the twentieth century. I outline the ways that African Americans and Afro-Caribbeans immigrated to cities (and provinces), establishing businesses and newspapers that reported on community news. This chapter also explores the question of how black Canadians used media, consumerism, and beauty culture to uplift the race amid a socio-cultural milieu that debased and, in some cases, blatantly restricted black progress.

Chapter 2 explains how John H. Johnson's *Ebony* magazine, when it arrived in 1945 (in Canada in 1946), presented an image of black beauty that celebrated straightened hair and lightened skin and was, for many critics, an approximation of white, middle-class values. I analyze the role that black media played in popularizing skin lightening and hair straightening products and practices in the postwar 1940s and 1950s. I also explain how African American entrepreneurs such as George E. Johnson, who in the late 1950s created Ultra Wave, the first chemical relaxer product that could be applied at home, helped to perpetuate and affirm the black beauty standard of chemically straightened hair and lighter skin. This chapter examines the life of Viola Desmond and the politics of respectability that helped to catapult her into the spotlight when, in 1946, she was arrested, jailed, convicted, and fined for sitting in the "whites only" section of the Roseland Theatre. Desmond's entrepreneurial skills, which she honed by studying in the United States under African American women and which have largely been overlooked, also helped her grow her beauty culture business in the 1940s. I consider why Desmond's beauty business efforts mark a turning point in Canada regarding the sale and manufacture of products and services. This chapter also juxtaposes, on the one hand, white-owned beauty product companies such as Max Factor, Elizabeth Arden, Avon, and Estée Lauder, which made concerted efforts to expand into Canada in the postwar 1940s and 1950s by advertising their products in the pages of *Chatelaine* magazine, and, on the other hand, local black newspapers such as *The Clarion* (1945–56), founded in New Glasgow, Nova Scotia. *The Clarion*'s editor, Carrie M. Best, believed that her publication, which first launched as a church bulletin, could address the question of racial segregation in public facilities in Nova Scotia, and she used her publication in "the interests of colored Nova Scotians" (as the paper's motto read).[91] *The Clarion* also promoted a localized black beauty culture not found in the pages of the dominant media during the period.

The rise of the Afro and the "Black Is Beautiful" aesthetic in the late 1960s signalled a major shift in the parameters of black beauty culture, not only in the pages of African American and black Canadian media, but also in the eyes of white-owned companies. Suddenly, images of black women with dark skin and Afros replaced those of black women with light skin and straightened hair. Seemingly overnight, an aesthetic that had been abhorred (i.e., tightly coiled black hair) was "in." Chapter 2 also gives an account of how this collective black aesthetic coincided with changes in Canada's immigration policies and anti-discrimination laws in the postwar era as unprecedented numbers of black people from the Caribbean (and continental Africa) emigrated to Canada. This demographic shift would be instrumental in giving birth to West Indian–run newspapers such as the short-lived *West Indian News Observer* (1967–69), which was reborn as *Contrast* (1969–91), a Toronto-based black newspaper founded by West Indian immigrants Olivia Grange-Walker and Alfred W. Hamilton, and *Share* magazine, founded in 1978 by Trinidadian-born Arnold A. Auguste, which is still in circulation today. These newspapers gave white-owned and African American–owned beauty firms an outlet to expand their operations and to promote their products in the largest market for black culture in the country. The advertisements as well as the editorials in their pages stand as roadmaps, so to speak, for how black beauty culture entered the dominant retail sector.

In chapter 3, I give detailed, year-by-year accounts of the ways in which African American–owned and white-owned American companies entered Canada's mainstream retail sector in the 1970s and 1980s. This chapter explains why (and how) *Contrast* and *Share* became the media outlets not only where companies advertised the arrival of new black beauty products but where black readers learned about the sale of products at department stores, the dates and locations of in-store demonstrations, and the goings-on at local hair shows. Today, black women can walk into most major drugstores and find the black beauty products they're looking for, from chemical hair straighteners ("relaxers") to hair oils and, in some locations, synthetic hair weaves. Prior to the late 1970s, this was not the case. This chapter explains how, when, and why this shift occurred. I also highlight the life of Beverly Mascoll, one of Canada's first black beauty product distributors, who advertised regularly in the pages of *Contrast* and *Share* for over twenty years. Mascoll's rags-to-riches tale, which saw her go from selling products out of her home to becoming the number one distributor of Johnson's Products in the country at one point in the 1970s, speaks to the cultural sentiment of opportunity that swept across Canada during the decade. For the first time in the 1980s, black beauty products also lined the shelves of retail chains in cities and town across Canada. Chapter 3 explains the strategies used by American companies to expand their black beauty operations into these spaces and places.

As Afros gave way to chemical relaxers in the late 1970s and early 1980s, local black media was there to capture it all. Chapter 3 also probes how, at the same time that black products entered the dominant consumer marketplace, multiculturalism as a policy was introduced and then promoted to black communities through advertising campaigns in *Share*. This is the moment when historically black communities, such as African Nova Scotians, were erased from the national imagination. Newly arrived black immigrants (especially those from the Caribbean) *became* Canada's black community because their arrival spoke to the new national narrative and identity centred on "cultural diversity"; as a result, new immigrant experiences were increasingly interpolated into the visual landscape of the dominant culture. This discussion helps to frame the cultural context of the 1990s, when multiculturalism morphed into a brand used by white-owned beauty companies to appear more culturally inclusive. As demographics in North America shifted, white-owned firms looked for new strategies to woo black women consumers, and many did so with "ethnic" product labelling and the expansion of existing brands.

Chapter 4 argues that ownership changes in the black beauty culture industry since the 1990s have done more than just increase the availability of products at the retail level. A "multicultural" notion of beauty has been constructed, one which has complicated the historical criticisms levied against the beauty culture industry's lack of diversity. I posit that, since the late 1990s, white-owned conglomerates have used multiculturalism and appeals for ethnic and racial diversity as a marketing tool to appear more inclusive than they have been in the past. These companies continue to perpetuate the ideal of lighter skin and/or straighter hair as more beautiful than darker skin and/or natural hair. This chapter explains how and why contemporary advertising contains similar racial biases as those found in decades past. Inclusion, I assert, has only made hypervisible the lack of commitment on the part of global beauty firms to disrupt the centuries-long beauty ideal. If the beauty culture industry has now incorporated black women into its ranks, why are issues of race, gender, hair, and skin still as politicized today as they were a century ago? Chapter 4 also provides a detailed account of the mergers and acquisitions frenzy in the 1990s and early 2000s that witnessed the takeover of the black beauty culture industry by white-owned conglomerates such as L'Oréal, Procter & Gamble, and Unilever. In this chapter, I also question how ownership shifts in the beauty culture industry have shifted the representation of black beauty in the contemporary.

Chapter 5 moves the contemporary critique a step further by examining the larger issue of racial bias that continues to permeate Western culture, primarily the politics of black hair—its texture, styling, length, and colour—and the rise in popularity of hair weaves and wigs over the last twenty years, forming part of what is known as the "global hair trade." Using examples drawn from African American films such as *Good Hair* (2009), I probe the political economy of the global hair trade, where hair is sourced in Asian and South Asian countries and shipped to wholesalers in Europe and North America, which sell the hair to beauty supply shops, beauty parlours, and hair retailers at a local level. In the 1980s, black women learned how to wear synthetic hair, and when the industry moved to "real human hair" by the 1990s and 2000s, *Contrast* and *Share* were still outlets for women to learn the latest techniques, while there was (and remains) little said about the detrimental health effects of wearing weaves. Over the last thirty years, Korean immigrants in Canada and the United States have also gained significant control of the black beauty retail end-point, a fact that has added new layers to the politics of black beauty regarding ownership and control. In this chapter, I raise further questions about why black women's hair choices still result in firing and/or reprimand at places of employment and school, over thirty years since *Rogers v. American Airlines*, discussed in chapter 3.

Beauty in a Box ultimately affirms that beauty is not just about "putting on a face" or "tightening a hair weave." Beauty is a historical, racialized, gendered construct that has played and continues to play a role in how black women think and feel about ourselves in addition to shaping how and what we consume. This book is one of the first attempts to articulate the interpolation of black Canadian women into the regime of beauty. It explains the web of social relations, institutions, advertisers, media, and consumers that gave birth to black beauty culture, while also contending with the larger question of how and why many of the politics, privileges, and contestations of early beauty culture still reverberate throughout the global marketplace today, including Canada. I firmly believe that when you know your history, you gain insight into the way things are, but you also acquire the tools to recognize and change generational patterns and pathologies. The chapters that follow will not only help black Canadian women acquire the tools to accomplish these goals but will also widen the scope of knowledge about blackness in Canada, and its linkages with transnational sites across the black Atlantic.

CHAPTER ONE

AFRICAN CANADIAN NEWSPAPERS AND EARLY BLACK BEAUTY CULTURE, 1914–1945

In December 1914 the *Canadian Observer*, a nationally distributed black-focused newspaper edited by Canadian-born Joseph R. B. Whitney and published out of Toronto, appeared. This black Canadian "war-baby" was created specifically in response to black men being barred from joining the Canadian Expeditionary Forces (CEF) during World War I.[1] In April 1915 in Halifax, Nova Scotia, the *Atlantic Advocate*, a monthly journal "devoted to the interests of colored people in the Dominion" but especially those in the Maritimes, appeared. The journal's first editor, Mowbray Fitzgerald Jemmott, was born in Bridgetown, Barbados, while the newspaper's assistant editor, Wilfred Alleyne DeCosta, was a Jamaican-born gardener and collection agent who had immigrated to Nova Scotia around 1908–9; DeCosta's wife, Miriam, served as secretary.[2] Like the *Canadian Observer*, the *Atlantic Advocate* spent several months recruiting African Canadians to join the No. 2 Construction Battalion, the segregated, all-black regiment that served for Canada during the war. These two newspapers spoke out against racial discrimination and pervasive anti-black sentiment. From today's vantage point, they provide some of the first (and only existing) material evidence of a new black identity that emerged during the first decades of the twentieth century across North America. Between 1900 and 1930, black people across the continent began to venture into new spaces and places.

In the United States during this time, millions of African Americans moved out of the rural south to the urban neighbourhoods of the north in what became known as the "Great Migration"; roughly two million black people took part in this interregional migration.³ Cities such as New York, Chicago, Pittsburgh, Detroit, and Philadelphia grew exponentially during this period; the percentage of African Americans in urban locations doubled between the years 1916 and 1940.⁴ Between 1897 and 1912, in the largest immigration Canada has ever experienced, 2.3 million Europeans and (white) Americans came to Canada, while fewer than one thousand blacks were officially admitted into the country; in the period between 1916 and 1928, official immigration figures indicate that 1,519 blacks immigrated to Canada.⁵ Importantly, it is quite possible that the actual numbers were higher, given that immigration officers often registered people by their place of birth rather than by racial criteria, which misrepresented hundreds of immigrating blacks, not to mention the fact that "official records" also did not consider illegal immigration.⁶ Given the size of Canada's black population, most scholarly inquiries into the early twentieth century with respect to shifting black identifications have predominantly focused on the African American experience, especially in cities in the north like Harlem, which became the largest epicentre for this new African American public culture.

As a large, predominantly black neighborhood in the northern section of New York City, Harlem was home to artists, educators, and writers such as Langston Hughes, Zora Neale Hurston, Josephine Baker, and Claude McKay. The neighbourhood, which stretched for many city blocks, also housed some of America's most successful black-owned barbershops, hair salons, photographic studios, restaurants, and night clubs. At the same time, as Hazel Carby notes, those blacks who remained in the southern states were "at a vast physical and metaphorical distance from those intellectuals who represented the interests of the race. After the war, black intellectuals had to confront the black masses on the streets of their cities and responded in a variety of ways."⁷ One of the responses was a new sense of collective pride that, in the new century, was urban, cultured, and would become known as the Harlem Renaissance. The New Negro and the New Negro Woman, who *appeared* and were *seen* in the public spaces of the cityscape, were born of this socio-cultural shift. This chapter is concerned with the period between the First and Second World Wars when black communities across North America went from being defined by and through the dominant cultural lens—an envisioning of black bodies as subservient and docile, and often as hoary stereotypes like Mammy, the faithful slave woman embodied in the advertising trademark Aunt Jemima—to acquiring unprecedented levels of agency via self-representation in pictures, newspapers, and magazines. As Daphne Brooks has argued, African American migration and urbanization led to a heightened rhetoric of "newness" that held a particular resonance for artists, journalists, and political leaders intent on displacing the distorted, minstrel-inspired images of African Americans that persisted in mainstream popular culture.[8] Similarly, I argue that African Canadian migration—intraregional and interregional—also led to a heightened rhetoric of "newness," albeit on a smaller scale.

The consumption of products for and in the home became a way of obtaining citizenship rights and societal acceptance within the dominant culture at large; accordingly, consumerism was viewed as tangible evidence of the efficacy of the New Negro image.[9] By the 1920s and 1930s, advertisements for black women's cosmetics and hair products began to fill the pages of African American weekly newspapers such as the *Pittsburgh Courier*, the *Chicago Defender*, and the *New York Amsterdam News*, all of which were created by newly urban, educated, and intellectual African Americans.[10] During this period, as Shane White and Graham White observe, "the swelling black populations of northern cities had created an urban African American consumer market of some significance, and commercial beauty products—at first hair oils and later creams for the face—quickly became a regular item in the expenditure of many blacks, even those who were hardly well-off," including some men.[11] For instance, in 1911, the *New York Age*, a black newspaper produced from 1887 to 1953, wryly drew attention to what it called the "latest fad," asking, "Have you had your hair straightened yet?" "Up and around 135th Street and Lenox Avenue," the story continued, "colored men can be seen in large numbers who are wont to take off their hats repeatedly…and stroke their glossy hair with their hand in an affectionate manner."[12] Elizabeth M. Sheehan opines further that the associations among femininity, visuality, and materiality intersected with debates about the political import of representing the self and the race. Thus, while black men might have been active participants in the new spaces of black consumption, "black women faced a particular burden of appearing—that is, of deploying their own status as spectacular objects and as types or representations of a collectivity."[13] Stated otherwise, black women had to both embody a "newness" and adhere to notions of femininity and respectability that pointed to uplifting the race; in this sense, they held a double burden of both race and gender.

Importantly, the appearance of—and beauty culture geared toward— the New Negro and New Negro Woman in Canada has received little scholarly attention. In their seminal text on African American photography, for instance, Deborah Willis and Carla Williams assert that the New Negro period in the United States was so defined by African American professor and philosopher Alain Locke in 1925 that it "marked the first time that black artists, particularly photographers, working in both rural and urban communities took control of their self-representation."[14] While Canada did not have stretches of city blocks catering to African Canadians or a robust visual culture, through immigration and African Canadian newspapers, the ideology and aesthetics of the New Negro and New Negro Woman became part of the cultural fabric of cities across the province of Ontario, primarily from Windsor to Toronto, and in Halifax and Montreal. Importantly, I am not arguing that there was a distinctly Canadian New Negro wholly separate from the American New Negro. Rather, I am suggesting that, in part, the images, ideologies, and aesthetic practices of the American New Negro were imported into Canada in the first decades of the twentieth century, and, in part, Canadian New Negro images, ideologies, and aesthetic practices unfolded north of the border on their own. Like the great migration of African Americans, migration and urbanization in cities such as Toronto and Montreal (and to a lesser extent Halifax) were key factors that led to a heightened rhetoric of "newness" that challenged stereotypes such as the mammy. As Sarah-Jane Mathieu observed in her examination of Canada's railway porters, "By the 1920s, the African Canadian New Negro was an informed voter, a capable citizen, an artist, a Christian, a Mason....For their part, black women exercised their citizenship by being dedicated union wives, educators, consumer advocates, shrewd voters, caregivers to the sick, and the guardians of their communities' histories."[15]

By the early twentieth century, black people, especially those who had migrated to Canada from the United States and the Caribbean, shared a collective desire to *act* rather than be acted upon, to be the *subject* rather than the object of the gaze in terms of their visual representation and their intellectual discourse. Jared Toney argues that in 1920s Toronto, for instance, West Indian immigrants forged connections with Afro-Canadians, Afro-Americans, and others of Caribbean descent in the making of a black diaspora. For West Indians in the city, Toney asserts, "businesses and churches provided some of the most prominent community leaders.... A professional class including lawyers and doctors, many of whom received formal training in the Caribbean, were also empowered as community leaders."[16] Not only did these newly arrived Afro-Caribbean people function as social ambassadors and socializing organs through which people came together and built communities, they also opened businesses and churches. At the same time, "African Canadians" in the 1910s through the 1940s were not a monolith.

West Indian immigrants during this period tended to view themselves as British subjects and were therefore more inclined to assimilate, but African American immigrants to Canada brought some of the New Negro's politics to cities such as London, Toronto, and Montreal and were thus more likely to become social activists. For example, in 1926 an editorial in the "Women's Daily Interest" section of the *Toronto Daily Star* announced the wedding of Rachel Adina Stephenson to Mr. J. R. Williams, both originally from Jamaica, at the British Methodist Episcopal (BME) Church.[17] In 1914, a church bulletin in the *Canadian Observer* listed the BME Church at 94 Chestnut Street as one of three black churches in the city—the other two were Grant African Methodist Episcopal Church (originally on Elm Street, relocating to 23 Soho Street in 1929) and University Avenue Baptist Church (at Edward Street).[18] The appearance of this editorial speaks to a kinship between the BME congregation and the newspaper's mostly British readership. "To the strains of Mendelssohn's wedding march the bridal party entered the church and took their place under the floral arch, the Union Jack and the Jamaican flag, intertwined with the roses," the *Daily Star* reported. Conversely, James F. Jenkins, an African American who moved to London, Ontario, in the early twentieth century, founded the weekly black-focused newspaper the *Dawn of Tomorrow*, and in 1924, along with J. W. Montgomery of Toronto, he formed the Canadian League for the Advancement of Colored People (CLACP).

Formally chartered in 1925 as the Canadian equivalent to the National Association for the Advancement of Colored People (NAACP) founded in New York in 1909, the CLACP differed from its American counterpart in that it never achieved national status. But as a black newspaper and a voice for New Negro politics, the *Dawn* and the CLACP shared a motto— "Devoted to the Interests of the Darker Races"—that was almost identical to the motto of the NAACP's magazine, *The Crisis*: "A Record of the Darker Races." Thus, even though Canada did not witness a "great" interregional black migration, there was a "newness" to black culture in its cities, in large part because of interregional migration from other sites of diaspora, like the United States. As Toney observes further, "There were multiple diasporas at work among West Indians in Toronto, linking them to other British nationals, Caribbeans, and peoples of African descent in North America and around the world."[19]

Importantly, one of the reasons why the black population in Canada remained relatively stagnant before the 1960s is that Canada's immigration policies in the early twentieth century directly restricted the growth of the black population. From 1896 to 1911, the Canadian homestead policy, implemented by the Liberal government of Wilfrid Laurier, together with Canada's open immigration policies, helped to attract nearly two million white immigrants to predominantly rural regions of Canada.[20] Frank Oliver's Immigration Act of 1906 introduced several new principles to Canadian immigration law, including mandatory medical and character examinations and race-based exclusion clauses.[21] Although Canada's immigration policies favoured whites, the homestead policy attracted a significant number of black immigrants, especially from states such as Oklahoma, Arkansas, and Texas, who migrated west to Alberta, Saskatchewan, and British Columbia as white settlers were encouraged to do.[22] However, news reports often contained falsified accounts and dramatic headlines such as "Black Settlers Invade the West," "Invasion of Negroes," "Negro Settlers Troop into the West," and "Negroes Ousting Whites in Canada."[23] Many of Canada's leading newspapers, including the (Toronto) *Globe*, the *Ottawa Free Press*, and the *Montreal Gazette*, also openly stated their objections to uncontrolled black immigration and supported white westerners' call for further Canadian immigration restrictions, making clear the fact that anti-black sentiment was shared nationwide.[24] On August 12, 1911, an Order in Council sought to ban "any immigrants belonging to the Negro race, which is deemed unsuitable to the climate and requirements of Canada."[25] While the ban was never written into the Immigration Act, in addition to the lack of interest in black immigration, turn-of-the-century newspaper and government discourse reveals that the theory of eugenics had deeply infected Canadian culture, as it had other Western cultures.

Since the nineteenth century, Francis Galton, Charles Darwin's cousin, had proposed that Anglo-Saxons were the pinnacle "race," coining the term *eugenics* (derived from the Greek word meaning "well-born") in 1883 to define "the study of agencies under social control that may improve or impair the racial qualities of future generations, either physically or mentally."[26] Eugenics, as a supposed science of selective breeding for the health of the "race" was one of the founding ideologies of Nazism.[27] Following Galton's lead, eugenicists argued that measures such as involuntary sterilization, marriage laws, immigration restriction, and the segregation of the mentally disabled were necessary to prevent white Anglo-Saxons from inheriting the supposed pathological traits of the "other."[28] Galton, along with Darwin's theories of "survival of the fittest," had infected the Western world with beliefs that a number of groups—notably black people, poor people, and to some extent, women—were intellectually inferior and congenitally defective. And yet, despite the Canadian government's more rigorous 1906 immigration provisions, black people still managed to circumvent these policies and enter Canada. In 1911, the Canadian population was just over seven million and the black population was seventeen thousand; by 1941, however, when Canada's population had grown to 11.5 million, the black population had still increased, though marginally, to just over twenty-two thousand.[29]

This discussion of Canada's black population and anti-black sentiment in the early twentieth century is important because it helps to explain why black Canadians have been left out of not only the history of the New Negro but Canadian history in general. In "'I'se in Town, Honey': Reading Aunt Jemima Advertising in Canadian Print Media," I examined the presence of Aunt Jemima, the prototypical Mammy plucked from the plantation South who appeared in Canadian newspaper and magazine advertising between the years 1919 and 1962. Using library catalogues and online archive holdings of newspaper and magazine advertisements and editorials, I examined over a hundred advertisements and editorials in the *Toronto Daily Star* and twenty-six advertisements in *Chatelaine* magazine; a few additional examples were drawn from *The Globe and Mail* and *The Hamilton Spectator*. Ultimately, I concluded that the idea of a selfless, sexless black woman who eagerly awaited on white families in their homes retained a persistent hold on the Canadian imagination because it helped to appease widely held beliefs that black women and men were different from white Canadians, their value assessed only by the extent of their willingness to serve and please whites, not by their acquisition of full citizenship rights.

Where African Americans were, similar to black Canadians, a small minority of the population in northern cities, "the very openness and exuberance of their public behavior attracted a disproportionate amount of attention from whites," such as racist ridicule and violence, but, given that they were "free," many African Americans seized opportunities to at least "play an active role in determining their fate, and in that lay their hope for the future."[30] Comparatively, the prevalence of racism in social practice denied black Canadians their rights as British subjects and Canadian citizens.[31] Black Canadians understood that they were not a priority as far as the Canadian state was concerned, but the real crux of the problem rested on how invested white Canadians were in defining their racial identity privileges by their ability to exclude black Canadians through anti-black racism.[32] Where, in the United States by the 1920s, "as mass consumer culture gained prominence in American life, African American marketing professionals worked to promote black consumers to national-brand name advertisers,"[33] a quick glance at the emergence of women's magazines in Canada illustrates a comparable lack of interest on the part of national-brand name advertisers to similarly promote to black consumers. Most notably *Chatelaine* magazine, one of the longest in circulation women's magazines in Canada (first appearing in March 1928), ignored black women (as readers of the magazine) throughout the 1930s and 1940s.

   Chatelaine got its name in a national contest, which offered a thousand-dollar prize and drew over seventy-five thousand entries.[34] Hilda Paine, a rancher's wife from Eburne, British Columbia, was first to suggest *The Chatelaine* (the "The" was dropped in 1930), a name that recalled the ring of keys worn by housewives in centuries past—keys to every part of the house, from the linen closet to the wine cellar.[35] The success of the magazine hinged on the fact that by the 1920s, magazines had taken on a primary role in guiding children and immigrants in the values of the dominant culture, which was unequivocally white, Anglo-Saxon Protestant, and English speaking. When *Chatelaine* appeared, it modelled itself after *Ladies' Home Journal* and *Better Homes and Gardens*, which both aimed primarily at a middle-class white female reading public.[36] Since, as Emily Spencer writes, "*Chatelaine* was unquestionably a mass circulation magazine that targeted white, Anglo-Saxon, middle-class Canadian women for its readership,"[37] when black women appeared in the pages of the magazine between the 1930s and 1940s, they did not appear as "modern" women but were depicted through the lens of a racialized, gendered Other. For example, in the December 1936 issue of *Chatelaine*, a "Mammy [Memo] Pad," was presented as "a useful and amusing novelty for the kitchen," and "Pickaninnies at Play" was described as "a very cute little pair of cross-stitch pictures for a child's room." The pickaninny, like the Mammy and the Jezebel, was a stereotype. Print advertisements urged consumers to consume racial stereotypes for their kitchen and their children, including rag dolls, cookie jars, cream-and-sugar dish sets, spice containers, cornmeal, pancake mix, cigarette lighters, Halloween masks, recipe cards, cookbooks, and syrup pitchers. These items were so beloved that, even decades later, many fondly remembered the products as part of their childhood. For example, on February 2, 1986, the *Sunday Star* printed a letter to Percy Ross's "Thanks a Million" column from a Toronto reader who had a request: "I'm hoping you can help me find an Aunt Jemima cookie jar. When I was a child it always delighted me to see these cookie jars. Nearly every home we visited had one."[38] The presence of such letters reveals how racial stereotypes were consumed by (white) families for generations.

Ultimately, the "modern appearing woman" in women's magazines, the cinema, and commodity culture did not step into modernity's symbolic systems, but, as Liz Conor asserts, "[she] was textually inscribed within its panorama. The picture formed part of her and she formed part of the picture as she became emblematic of the pictorial life of the modern scene."[39] Of the many and diverse meanings that were ascribed to feminine visibility—including artificiality, heterosexual appeal, celebrity, commodity display, metropolitan presence, fashion, whiteness, youth, and scandal— the one of overriding significance was the modern.[40] White womanhood, then, became the emblem of a modern visibility, while black women (and all other non-white women) were removed from the visual gaze of modernity. In women's magazines, by the 1930s, advertising campaigns approached the role of housewife by glorifying housework; the invention of ready-mix convenience foods—and Aunt Jemima pancake mix was one of the first—helped to "emancipate" modern white housewives while displacing the promise of racial emancipation for black women, as they were always depicted in the kitchen doing the same work that would have been expected of plantation mammies.[41] As Lola Young aptly notes, "Images are ideological, a discursive practice: in racist societies, no image is neutral or innocent of the past whether or not that past is acknowledged."[42] The images of black women—however few—in *Chatelaine* and in the catalogue pages of Eaton's, Simpson's, and the Hudson's Bay Company (the largest department stores in Canada for most of the twentieth century) are important windows into the ideological and discursive role images have played in the visioning of modern Canadian womanhood as *white* while excluding others, namely, black women, from its ranks.

As previously noted, black culture in America during the period between 1900 and 1930 was widely visible, as there existed over a hundred beauty parlours and nine toiletries companies that served black consumers in Chicago, and beauty parlours in Harlem were reportedly three times more numerous than elsewhere in New York.[43] By comparison, after arriving in Toronto from Jamaica in 1920, one black woman recalled her impression that "coloured people . . . [were] a novelty."[44] As Dorothy Williams observes, Montreal's black community was smaller than the Ontario and Maritime communities, and the small number of blacks who entered

Montreal during the last years of the nineteenth century and the early years of the twentieth did not create the same intense backlash in Montreal that occurred in these other regions.[45] I explore some of the racial tensions that existed in Ontario and the Maritimes later in this chapter.

Meanwhile, in the Maritimes, there was a continuous flow of immigrants from the Caribbean (Barbados and Jamaica primarily) who, between 1900 and 1916, arrived by ship to cities across Nova Scotia, such as Sydney, Glace Bay, Cape Breton, and Halifax. Generally speaking, however, the vast majority of black residents across the Maritime provinces were (and remain) descendants of black Loyalists and black refugees who arrived in the province following the American Revolutionary War in the 1770s and in the aftermath of the War of 1812, respectively. In many ways, African Nova Scotians share much in common with black communities in rural Ontario, places such as Buxton, Chatham, and Dresden, where large concentrations of black populations settled from the 1820s through the American Civil War in the 1860s, and where there exist black populations that have remained autonomous and separated from the white population. This chapter ultimately echoes Dorothy Williams's observation that "[black] history then is of a people whose history has been ignored, deliberately omitted, or distorted.... The writing of Afro-Canadian history re-aligns Canadian history by re-establishing continuity with the past."[46] Black communities across the country have their own unique stories, tensions, and histories and so, too, do they have a unique black beauty history that has virtually been ignored up until now. Black Canadians may not have had hundreds of barbershops and beauty parlours as African Americans did, but there is a long history of barbering and hair care in Canada, which points to the fact that, as in America's black communities, hair care and beauty have formed part of the black Canadian experience.

As early as the 1860s, almost every African Canadian community from Ontario to Quebec to the Maritimes had a barbershop. For black men who did not want subsistence employment, barbering gave them the opportunity to do something specialized that many white men often could not do themselves. Barbering in the United States also developed under similar circumstances. According to Douglas Walter Bristol, Jr., black barbers came to occupy a unique place in American society: "Even though other skilled trades excluded black men during the antebellum period," he writes, "black barbers competed against white barbers for white customers, and they won, dominating the upscale tonsorial market serving affluent white men."[47] Prior to the American Civil War, a number of black men and women in the north and south, some enslaved and some free, owned small business ventures; they were jewellers, merchants, steamboat owners, restaurateurs, grocers, real estate speculators, and, most significantly, barbers and hairdressers.[48]

In the 1861 census for Windsor, Ontario, abolitionist Henry Bibb is listed as a barber.[49] In London, Ontario, at that time, the vast majority of barbers were black, and there were several barbers in that city who appear to have been very successful, employing many other black men in their businesses.[50] In his analysis of three Ontario censuses from 1871, 1881, and 1901, historian Colin McFarquhar found that many black men were barbers, and some black women were also hairdressers: "More than one-half of the barbers and hairdressers in Essex county in 1881 were black, while such was the case for more than one-third in Hamilton, and almost one-quarter in Toronto."[51] Some men in Hamilton even reported income as a hairdresser.[52] In Montreal, barbering was among the lowest occupational jobs black men could hold, a list that included shoeshine boy and water boy.[53] In Saint John, New Brunswick, some black men established businesses and, for a time, there were barbershops in addition to restaurants, tailor shops, cartage firms, an ice business, and a dying firm owned by black people.[54]

By the 1930s, nearly all black commercial districts in the United States, even in smaller towns, hosted at least one beauty shop.[55] Black beauty shops—those catering to hair dressing and/or washing—likely were established wherever there were black women and where the vast majority of the black population lived, and, while comparable numbers are not available, it is unlikely that the number of hair salons and barbershops in Canadian cities like Toronto reached more than a dozen. Many of these early businesses were operated as storefronts or in people's homes, but there are public records of several incorporated establishments. In a rare photograph taken around 1895, Charles Duval and Fred Bolin appear in their Toronto barbershop. It stands as one of the first visual records of black men with the financial wherewithal to establish a business that catered not only to a black clientele but also to whites. Given the socio-cultural milieu of early-twentieth-century Canada, African Canadians had to rely on small but close-knit networks within black communities to learn about, consume, and promote beauty culture, for which community newspapers played a pivotal role. When advertisements for black beauty products and services first appeared in the pages of African Canadian newspapers in the first decades of the twentieth century, the socio-cultural import of the New

Negro coupled with the black diasporic presence in Toronto contributed to a thriving, albeit small, black community.

In 1911, for instance, most black community members in Toronto were multi-generational African Canadian, meaning that they could trace their ancestry back to the mid-nineteenth-century sojourn of African Americans who headed north following the Civil War and who remained. By 1919, however, there was an unmistakable Caribbean presence in the city.[56] Toronto's Caribbean community was noticeably more race-conscious and critical of what they considered the more conservative native attitudes among Canadian-born blacks toward social and race-related issues.[57] This Caribbean diaspora would play a significant role in disseminating the New Negro ideology in Toronto but also in Montreal, where African American migrants, many of whom were railway porters, established a semi-permanent community in the Little Burgundy area in the city's southwest borough. By the 1920s, the New Negro in Canada was multi-generational Canadian, Afro-Caribbean, or African American immigrant—as well as an informed voter, a capable citizen, an artist, a Christian, a Mason, and a member of the United Negro Improvement Association (UNIA).[58] While the exact numbers are not known, historians have estimated that by 1920, Montreal's black neighbourhood, "le Quartier St. Antoine," had a "solidly packed population of some two thousand blacks," of whom "at least ninety-five percent" were West Indians.[59] In large part, Montreal's black community formed through the movement of black men working on the railway as sleeping car porters. By crossing the border, not only did African American railwaymen affirm that African Canadians were included in their vision of a Great Migration, but, as Mathieu observes, African American magazines such as the NAACP's *The Crisis* and *The Messenger* (published by labour activist A. Philip Randolph and economist Chandler Owen in 1917) circulated in Canada "thanks in large part to sleeping car porters who brought them back from runs to Boston, New York, Detroit, Chicago, and Minneapolis."[60] Thus, as black men were recruited from the United States, Toronto, Montreal, and Halifax to work on the railways, these same cities became important hubs of the national rail network that linked black Canada with black America. It is this transnational, diasporic network that helped to spread the UNIA, under the leadership of Jamaican-born Marcus Garvey.

The ideology and politics of what became known as Garveyism, a Black Nationalist philosophy, along with the New Negro, spread across black communities on both sides of the border. Garvey's UNIA began in Jamaica in 1914, and by 1919, he had established chapters across the United States and Canada. The UNIA's Canadian chapters owed much of their success to the organizing efforts of Afro-Caribbean—and to a lesser degree African American—immigrants.[61] The UNIA advocated self-government and self-determination for black people in the Americas, but it also advocated race pride, building a black nation through the acquisition of capital, and repatriation to and reclamation of Africa as the true homeland for black people. Dionne Brand asserts that "Garvey fired the imagination of many Black Torontonians in the 1920s and 1930s, pointing to how Black people could actively organise against the racist social and economic conditions."[62] In addition to holding formal associational meetings and events, the UNIA in Toronto housed the United Negro Credit Union as well as the Toronto United Negro Association, both of which "sought to ameliorate the effects of discrimination and provide opportunities for black success and achievement in the city."[63] In 1925, the UNIA in Toronto had an estimated membership of seven hundred, and it was able to purchase a permanent hall at 355 College Street, while in Montreal a division opened in 1919 in Liberty Hall, housed in the Canadian Pacific Railway Building on St. Antoine Street, and there, during its first year, the UNIA successfully recruited four hundred members.[64] Meanwhile there were an estimated six hundred West Indians living in industrial Cape Breton, and there were active UNIA divisions in the industrial towns of Glace Bay, New Waterford, and Sydney, which had the largest UNIA division in eastern Canada with an active membership of approximately 250.[65] Toronto's UNIA headquarters, like the branches in Montreal and Nova Scotia, was much more than a meeting place. It was there that black culture and politics fused, and young and old met to discuss the issues of the day and to celebrate black talent.[66] In her examination of the Diamond Jubilee of Confederation celebrations in 1927, Jane Nicholas found that within the decade's cultural tides, "degeneration, decay, and effeminacy were linked to American popular cultural imports such as movies, the flapper, and jazz music, all of which were criticized for lowering the moral tone and leading to debauched incidents."[67] After World War I, many white Canadian judges, journalists, and juries concurred that jazz, drugs, and alcohol, presumably peddled by black railway porters and entertainers, many of whom were African American, jeopardized white Canadians' morality and white womanhood in particular.[68] And yet, not only did UNIA chapters flourish from coast to coast, black Canadians also created newspapers that helped to promote Garveyism, black beauty culture, and community news.

These newspapers are the starting point for locating an early African Canadian beauty culture. Their pages help to explain how the New Negro Woman in Canada *appeared* and how she was *seen*, not only within the pages of these newspapers but in women's public lives as black women. The New Negro was a shift in consciousness, but it also entailed a deliberate and prideful display of black bodies, particularly those of women, in a manner that transcended stereotypes. The clearest evidence of this shift within African American beauty comes in the form of two institutions that rose to prominence in the 1920s: the black beauty contest and the black fashion parade; the earliest evidence of this shift in Canada comes in the form of African Canadian newspapers' advertising and editorial content in the 1920s.

In 1899, there were three Negro daily newspapers and 136 Negro weeklies in the United States; these newspapers played a critical role in shaping and mobilizing black public opinion, and each also had a wide geographic reach circulating throughout the South, North, Midwest, and Southwest as "national" black newspapers.[69] Between 1891 and 1950, there were eight African American women's magazines published for a variety of audiences and purposes: *Ringwood's Afro-American Journal of Fashion* (1891–94), *Women's Era* (1894–97), *The Sepia Socialite* (1936–38), *Half-Century Magazine for the Colored Home and Homemaker* (1916–25), *Woman's Voice* (1912–27), the Home Magazine in *Tan Confessions* (1950–52), *Our Women and Children* (1888–91), and *Aframerican Woman's Journal* (1935–54). Noliwe Rooks found that each of these magazines "attempted to speak to specific political, domestic, or religious aspirations on the part of an African American female readership."[70] In the pages of these magazines, Rooks asserts further, the editors helped to create the impression that middle-class African American women were as concerned with "appearing" modern and embodying modernity's visions of women as white middle-class American women had become. The perception of oneself as "modern" was not singularly about vision; it was also an embodied experience made possible because of twentieth-century industrialized image production.[71] Those African Americans who advertised beauty products in the early twentieth century were attempting to "provide a beauty regime for African American women that would allow them to fashion and meet their own ideals as well as create career opportunities for themselves,"[72] all while asserting themselves as "modern" women akin to their white counterparts.

In addition to the lack of a national Negro press in Canada, it is also difficult to speak of an African Canadian "middle class" in the early twentieth century comparable to that in the United States. Some Caribbean immigrants living in Toronto, for example, opened businesses and churches, or became lawyers and doctors (many of them having received formal training in the Caribbean), but this group was more of a "professional class"[73] than a "middle class." As Patricia Hill Collins noted, "Being middle class requires black professionals and managers to enter into specific social relations with owners of capital and with workers. In particular, the middle class dominates labor and is itself subordinate to capital. It is this simultaneous dominance and subordination that puts it in the 'middle.'"[74] When the New York stock market crashed in 1929, for example, in the southern states, where most black Americans still lived, cotton prices fell by two-thirds; these blacks flocked north where there were no jobs and less tolerance, and by 1932, the black unemployment rate in most American cities hovered around 50 percent.[75] Despite this, African Americans were able to establish businesses and become intellectuals, and, to borrow from Pierre Bourdieu, many created "cultural capital" to symbolically and materially establish their place within America's "middle class." If cultural capital is "the set of skills that allows someone either to produce a work of art or to unpack artistic or aesthetic codes,"[76] African Americans carved out distinct spaces and opportunities to produce a visual culture equipped with their own aesthetic codes that was geared toward their own cultural reinvention.

Between 1900 and 1940, African American photographers flourished in large northern cities, and many became ambassadors for African American communities; within newspapers, magazines, and books, they published their photographic images directly to black audiences.[77] The consumption of products for and in the home also came to be viewed as a way to obtain citizenship rights and societal acceptance within America's middle class; accordingly, consumerism became tangible evidence of the efficacy of an African American New Negro in addition to the creative endeavours that gave national prominence to artists, educators, historians, and philosophers.[78] African Canadians might have lacked cultural capital comparable to that of African Americans, but there were African Canadian newspapers in the early twentieth century that provide us with tangible evidence of aspects of the New Negro identity that were born on distinctly Canadian soil. These newspapers provide some of the only existing material and visual evidence of black communities—not only in cities such as Toronto and Montreal, but also in smaller cities and towns in between—and the attempts of educated blacks to create an image of "middle-classness" in early-twentieth-century Canada that would speak to the efficacy of the New Negro ideology.

Neith, published out of Saint John, New Brunswick, by lawyer Abraham B. Walker, is the first known African Canadian newspaper, but it did not last very long.[79] Robin Winks argued that if Walker had established *Neith,* which appeared in 1903, in Ontario where there was a larger and somewhat more prosperous black audience, it might have succeeded.[80] *The Atlantic Advocate,* first published by Mowbray Fitzgerald Jemmott out of his residence at 58 Gottingen Street in Halifax, later moved to the house of Wilfred and Miriam DeCosta (the newspaper's assistant editor and secretary, respectively), then to the Keith building (now the Green Lantern Building) on Barrington Street, and finally to Dr. Clement Courtenay Ligoure's house at 166 North Street.[81] While the first issue appeared in April 1915 and the last around May or June 1917 due to the high cost of printing and materials during wartime (as well as the absence of staff, who were overseas contributing to the war effort), the *Advocate* covered a wide range of topics—historical, religious, economic, political, military, literary (fiction, poetry, songs), social, and local. Community notes were also received from across Nova Scotia—including Amherst, Digby, Halifax, Hammonds Plains, Liverpool, Shelburne, Westville, Weymouth, and Wolfville—as well as cities in other provinces, including Montreal, Saint John (New Brunswick), and Chatham and Windsor (Ontario).[82] Newspapers such as this one mirrored the Negro press in the United States as it related to morality, respectability, religiosity, and the uplift and advancement of black people. For example, the paper's editorial purpose in the first issue, published in April 1915 was stated as follows:

> We earnestly hope that all our friends will give the *Atlantic Advocate* the favorable consideration which it deserves; and the publishers in their turn shall do their utmost to place in the columns of their periodical just such news as they desire.... The *Atlantic Advocate* aims to show our people the need of unity, the desire to stand always for the right, to keep before them the dignity of true and honest toil; to teach them to keep themselves sober, temperate and honest; to encourage them to march steadily on with a true determination to work, save and endure; always keeping their mind's eye on the great goal of progress.[83]

Just as Garveyism offered a new ideology, the black press provided alternative depictions of black people and women within their communities that could contradict the negative stereotypes that were ubiquitous in the Canadian public sphere.

The *Canadian Observer*, published from December 12, 1914, to June 14, 1919, provides the most conspicuous evidence of an early black beauty culture in Canada. As previously noted, the main impetus for the newspaper was to act as a voice for black Canadians who were dissatisfied with racially biased injustices that denied them the full benefits of their rights and responsibilities as British subjects and loyal Canadians to enlist and fight "for king and country" during World War I. The newspaper helped to pressure the Canadian government to establish the No. 2 Construction Battalion that was formed during the "Great War," and even though the *Canadian Observer*'s editorial focus was to provide the black community with war news, enlistment updates, and race consciousness, Canadian New Negro Women *appeared* and were *seen* in its pages. Just as in the United States, beauty culture also formed part of the newspaper's advertising copy. While advertisements in African American newspapers promoted products and services, African Canadian advertisements in the pages of the *Canadian Observer* can best be described as localized, diasporic beauty culture that encompassed the promotion of local beauty businesses (operated by both women and men) as well as, through mail order and Canadian-based agents, the advertisement of American beauty products aimed at black Canadian women.

In January 1915, proprietor J. L. Moore posted an advertisement on page 3 of the *Canadian Observer* for his "High Class Pocket Billiards and Barber Shop" located on Toronto's York Street near University Avenue. Moore's establishment was very close to the neighbourhood known as St. John's Ward or "The Ward."[84] As John Lorinc writes, "Long before St. John's Ward came to be branded, in the early twentieth century, as Toronto's most impoverished—and most notorious—'slum,' the working-class enclave bounded by Queen, College, Yonge and University had a distinctive, diverse character that set it apart from the surrounding city."[85] In the first decades of the twentieth century, black barbershops and beauty parlours were located in one of two places in Toronto: in the Ward, or further west near the intersection of Queen Street and Spadina Avenue, where a number of Caribbean immigrants to Toronto in the 1920s had opened up barbershops.[86] In June 1915, Madame E. Young, who operated a "Hair Dressing Parlor" at Queen Street and University Avenue, posted an advertisement that read, "Special attention given. The scalp cleaned before shampooing. All combs and brushes used are thoroughly sterilised after each customer."[87] Two weeks later, Madame N. Byles posted an advertisement for her business on Nelson Street, just south of the Ward. Styling herself as a "Scalp Specialist," her ad read, "Cleans the scalp thoroughly before shampooing and pressing. Stops the hair from failing out."[88] These two examples point to a common reality for black women across the diaspora in the early twentieth century. First, contrary to popular belief, hair entrepreneurship was not primarily a male-centred business; black women also entered the black hair business. Second, the problem of scalp care and hair loss, one of the main motivators for African American beauty entrepreneurs, was also a core impetus for early African Canadian beauty entrepreneurship. Importantly, women beauty entrepreneurs were often called "beauty culturists," a term that has its origins in the nineteenth-century hair salon.

Martha Matilda Harper, born in Oakville, Ontario, is often credited as being the first beauty culturist. After moving to New York in the 1880s, she began opening hair salons, licensing her "Harper Method" in Rochester in 1890. By the 1930s, there were five hundred Harper salons.[89] Beauty culturists developed "systems" and "methods," signature programs for skin and hair care, and defined distribution networks.[90] These women (and some men) created specialized, coordinated products and step-by-step techniques that replaced the miscellaneous creams and lotions of prior decades. Where, as Peiss writes, white beauty culturists could slough off their origins to perform the American myth of self-making and individual mobility, "black entrepreneurs tended to embed their biographies within the story of African American women's collective advancement."[91] White beauty culturists may have "invented" modern beauty culture, but black beauty culturists created a new image for a new century that aligned with the New Negro Woman. To grasp the transnational collective pride of the New Negro Woman, and the development and redefinition of black beauty during what Tiffany Gill has called "the golden age of black business (1900 to 1930),"[92] the biographies of black beauty culturists are, as noted, fundamental to one's understanding of black beauty culture in Canada. The African American women (and men) who revolutionized black hair care in the early twentieth century would become the inspiration for African Canadian beauty culturists in the post–World War II era.

Anthony Overton, born of enslaved parents in Louisiana in 1864, was the first African American beauty culturist. After earning a law degree and working as a municipal judge, Overton established the Hygienic Manufacturing Company in Kansas City in 1898. Overton's fortunes blossomed after he introduced High-Brown Face Powder, which targeted African

American beauty tastes. In 1911, out of his Chicago manufacturing plant, Overton created a distribution and transportation network and hired travelling salesmen, and before long the High-Brown line was available for purchase at variety stores and neighbourhood drugstores.[93] When Overton began making High-Brown, it was designed "to harmonize with the color and skin texture of the women of our race."[94] Thus, the product was another element to the aesthetic (embodied) transformation of the New Negro Woman. Overton's success was spurred in large part by advertisements in *Half-Century Magazine for the Colored Home and Homemaker*, of which he was an editor. According to Rooks, *Half-Century Magazine* "sought to weave its story from a different, more 'modern' fiber that emphasized the cultural product of uplift in relation to fashion, race, and adornment in the context of African American migration out of the South."[95] Overton also advertised a skin-bleaching product known as Ro-Zol bleach in *Half-Century Magazine*. Even though the product was originally developed as a solution to remove various skin defects and discolorations, by the 1920s it was marketed more as a whitening agent.[96] Advertisements in promotion of hair straightening and skin lightening had long been debated within African American communities, but by the first decades of the twentieth century, even the most ardent of critics began to embrace the reality that these products were desired by black women, and that straightened hair and a "lighter" complexion had also begun to form part of modernity's vision of the New Negro Woman. Light-skinned black women with straightened hair embodied the New Negro Woman identity because black women who became highly visible in the modern panoramic cityscape were primarily light-skinned with straightened hair. Conversely, dark-skinned women, especially those with coarse-textured hair, began to symbolize the opposite of modern; they embodied a past life of enslavement and debased black bodies—engendered by the continued presence of Mammy (Aunt Jemima) in popular culture on both sides of the border.

In the Harlem jazz nightclubs of the 1920s, for example, "light-skinned" beauties such as Josephine Baker came to embody this modern New Negro Woman. Baker, in particular, is remembered as the most famous of the light-skinned beauties, but it is interesting to note that when she auditioned for Eubie Blake and Nobel Sissle's *Shuffle Along* (1921), the first all-black musical to appear on Broadway, she was not offered the job because her skin was considered "too dark" for the part.[97] When one of the regular chorus girls did not show up, Baker convinced the director to let her go on instead, and she eventually became a permanent cast member of *Shuffle Along*, which also toured Toronto in 1923 and 1924.[98] White Canadian audiences, then, would also have seen light-skinned, straight-haired black women as emblems of the New Negro Woman. Significantly, however, "lighter" skin was not only a black woman's preoccupation in the 1920s; beyond the mere use of powders for a clearer complexion, bleaching creams and/or whitening agents and ointments were also used by the New Woman, who was white, middle class, and increasingly, a beauty consumer.

Incorporating whitening creams or concoctions into one's skin care regimen enhanced the Victorian ideal of being a "natural"-faced, genteel woman, and in the twentieth century advertisers relied on traditional appeals to gentility, social climbing, and Anglo-Saxon superiority to market these products. For example, Dorothy Dignam's advertisements for Nadinola skin bleach and Nadine face powder, which appeared in mass-circulation women's magazines, resurrected the Old South with an appeal to the "gentility" of whiteness.[99] The whiter the skin, the more likely a white woman could climb the social ladder, and a return to the Old South was a strategy to bring back a time when whiteness was believed to be "pure." While there is no such thing as a "pure" race, especially given the ubiquity of miscegenation (interracial sexual relations) in antebellum America, beauty companies actively sought to market this idea of purity in the context of black migration from the south to the industrial cities of the north. But if women's magazines encouraged the New Woman to use skin-bleaching products and whiteness was associated with "purity," how did advertisers target the New Negro Woman? What did skin bleaching and hair straightening mean to black women in the 1920s?

In his 1922 study, *The Negro Press in the United States*, Frederick G. Detweiler noted that "the persons and firms who do hairdressing or sell skin bleaches and hair straighteners are legion."[100] In every sense, from the late nineteenth century onward, black women were bombarded with messages to alter their hair texture and skin colour. Even the *Christian Recorder*, one of the oldest existing black periodicals (first published on July 1, 1852), was riddled with advertisements for skin-bleaching and hair-straightening products. In one representative advertisement for a product called Scott's White Lily Toilet Wash, appearing in September 1886, potential buyers were told: "NO LADY is Really BEAUTIFUL without a CLEAR, White COMPLEXION."[101] The product was not overtly marketed as a skin lightener, but the ad did make it clear that attaining white skin was the optimal outcome. The woman featured in the advertisement had European features, and a portion of the advertising copy read, "a valuable discovery that causes the cheek to glow with health and rival the lily in whiteness." Robert E. Weems, Jr., asserts that "advertisers, consciously or unconsciously, deemed the natural physical attributes of black women 'ugly.' Consequently, black women...were urged to buy a myriad of concoctions to straighten their hair, whiten their teeth, and thin their lips."[102] In the late nineteenth century, most of the advertisers argued for the desirability of changing the physical characteristics of an African body (especially dark skin and coarse-textured hair) by juxtaposing the characteristics of a light-skinned, straight-haired woman with a dark-skinned, "kinky-haired" woman. Some of the earliest examples of this racialized juxtaposition were produced by the Chicago-based, white-owned, Ozonized Ox Marrow Company.

Between 1866 and 1905 Ozonized Ox Marrow regularly advertised in black newspapers, making frequent use of "before and after" images. In February 1901, for example, the company placed an advertisement in the *Christian Recorder* that featured a black woman with dark skin in before-and-after shots. The woman's "before" hair was dishevelled while her "after" hair was coifed and straightened. Late-nineteenth- and early-twentieth-century beauty companies depended on the commonly held belief of a racial hierarchy and maintained it in their advertisements. Skin lighteners and hair straighteners marketed by white companies suggested to black people not only that they needed to change their physical features but that class mobility within their communities and social acceptance by the dominant culture depended on it. Except for wig manufacturers, no other companies advertised products aimed at enhancing black beauty.[103] Packaged in attractive boxes with fancy names, most of these early products contained nothing more than chalk and grease; later, formulas did lighten the colour of the skin, but they were equally as harsh as homemade concoctions and usually damaged the skin.[104]

Within black communities, skin bleaching came to be viewed as a "cure" to remove a disabling African heritage, dark skin. To "fix" this problem, some black women (and men) would rub sodium hydroxide, also known as caustic soda or lye, directly onto their skin. Others applied harsh acidic products made for removing dirt and grime from floors and walls, while still others prepared homemade concoctions of lemon juice, bleach, or urine to smear on the skin—all designed to "get the dark out."[105] These methods usually left women with blemishes, burns, and uneven skin. While white-owned companies might have promoted the idea that black women had to alter their appearance to achieve beauty, African American newspapers also valorized lighter skin and straighter hair as the epitome of black feminine beauty. In 1923, for instance, an advertisement from the Beautiwhite Company appeared in the *Chicago Defender* using before-and-after head shots of a black woman who had purportedly used the product to lighten her skin. The advertising copy explained that, at a church dance the week prior, Helen Powell of Brooklyn, New York, surprised her friends, both men and women, when, after using the Beautiwhite product, she showed up at the dance with "a clean, light, radiant complexion that attracted all the men."[106] "You too can lighten and beautify your skin and improve your looks over one hundred per cent," the advertisement stated, adding, "Beautiwhite lightens your skin quickly. It cleans, dark, muddy skins and gives you that delicate light appearance which so attracts." Considering that by 1915 the *Chicago Defender* reached its peak circulation of about 230,000, and through the actions of railway porters it circulated nationally, as well as transnationally to Canada, Gerald Horne estimates that its actual readership may have surpassed one million.[107] Thus, advertisements for skin lighteners in its pages would definitely have reached African Canadian women.

With respect to hair straighteners, an advertisement for No-Mor-Kink, produced by the Hawaiian Beauty Products Company, appeared in the *Chicago Defender* in 1929, declaring it to be "Hollywood's gift to all who desire beautiful, straight, lustrous hair."[108] The company, playing off the "flapper" image, used a facial profile of a woman whose hair mirrored the short, lacquered style of Josephine Baker. The advertisement also pointed to the collective reality that many of the techniques for hair straightening could potentially cause hair loss or damage to the scalp. "Without the least injury to the scalp or hair," the advertisement read, "you can now have that smart, fascinating appearance which comes only with long, soft, beautiful STRAIGHT hair."

When the *Dawn of Tomorrow* appeared on July 14, 1923, it became the third nationally distributed African Canadian newspaper of record. While the *Nova Scotia Gleaner*, founded by British West Indies–born Frederick Allan Hamilton, circulated in 1929 as a monthly publication with offices in Sydney, it did not last long.[109] The *Dawn of Tomorrow* provided opportunities for the transnational promotion of black beauty products and opportunities for local black beauty culturists to promote their products and services—and, it promoted images of New Negro Canadian Women. As previously noted, the *Dawn* was founded in London, Ontario, by James F. Jenkins, an African American who had moved to the city from Georgia and who also created the CLACP in 1924 along with J. W. Montgomery of

Toronto. London was an ideal place to launch a newspaper because it was a chief metropolitan centre for blacks between Toronto and Windsor, and many African Americans had also been present there since the nineteenth century. Although the *Dawn* relied heavily upon the Chicago-based *Associated Negro Press* for a lot of its editorial news, the majority of its pages were dedicated to black Canadian developments. Between 1923 and 1927, for example, it covered the establishment of a black community centre in Montreal; the activities of the British Methodist Episcopal Church, including meetings that were held in London, Chatham, and North Buxton and an international conference held at Owen Sound in 1927; and reports on UNIA events, such as an annual convention that was held in Montreal in 1923.[110] By 1925, the paper had reduced its publishing frequency to twice a month; when Jenkins died suddenly in 1931, his widow, Christina Elizabeth, continued the publication on a monthly basis until her death in 1967.[111]

At its height, the *Dawn* reportedly had a readership of five thousand and a circulation that included countries in Africa as well as England, Brazil, the West Indies, Bermuda, and New York.[112] In addition to its editorials, the *Dawn* modelled itself after its African American counterparts in its promotion of skin-bleaching and hair-straightening products. While the newspaper never explicitly defended its promotion of these products, in its pages we find a sample of advertisements comparable to the African American Negro press at the time. The *Dawn* also shared with its African American counterparts a preference for featuring black women who were generally light-skinned, straight-haired, and middle class in appearance. These images ran in editorial pages as the pride of the New Negro Woman. For example, the *Pittsburgh Courier* typically placed a photograph of an African American beauty in the upper-left corner of the front page in the 1920s, a prominent location bespeaking the image's importance.[113] The *Dawn* followed a similar style. On July 28, 1923, a photograph of Miss Ethel Shreve, a light-skinned, straight-haired teacher of shorthand and typewriting at the Wilberforce Institute in Chatham appeared on the newspaper's page 2.[114] A month later, a photograph of Madame Berry-Hunter, a graduate of the State Normal Teachers Institute of Frankfort, Kentucky, also appeared on the cover page.[115] Her hair is straightened, and the photograph is so large that it takes up almost the entire top half of the front page. These two examples confirm that the *Dawn*'s layout and editorial content mirrored that of the Negro Press in the United States.

In April and November 1924, an advertisement for a hair-straightening product from the white-owned Ozonized Ox Marrow Company with the

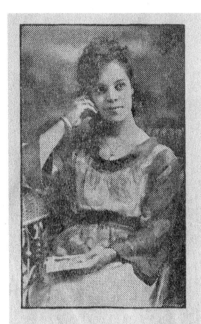

MISS ETHEL SHREVE, teacher of shorthand and typewriting in the Wilberforce Institute, Chatham, Ont. She is a graduate of the Chatham Business College.

Figure 2. Miss Ethel Shreve, 28 July 1923, *Dawn of Tomorrow*, p. 2. Archives and Special Collections, Western Libraries, Western University, London, Canada.

tagline "Have better hair...Everybody likes to look their best," appeared in the pages of *The Dawn*.[116] "By using Ford's Hair Pomade and Ford's Hair Straightening and Shampoo Combs, stubborn, harsh, snarly and unruly hair becomes softer, straighter, more pliable, and easier to dress and put up in any style," the advertisement proclaimed. The Ozonized Ox Marrow Company is an enduring example of how white-owned companies preyed on the insecurities of black women on both sides of the border by promising a "cure" for the curse of "kinky hair"; it also speaks to an image of black womanhood that could be circulated across time and space. From today's vantage point, these advertisements read more like demeaning insults than encouragements, but in context, they reveal plenty about the ways in which black newspapers were active participants in shaping what its readers consumed and purchased in terms of beauty.

When African Canadian beauty culturists began to advertise hair products in the *Dawn*, they did so on the heels of several African American

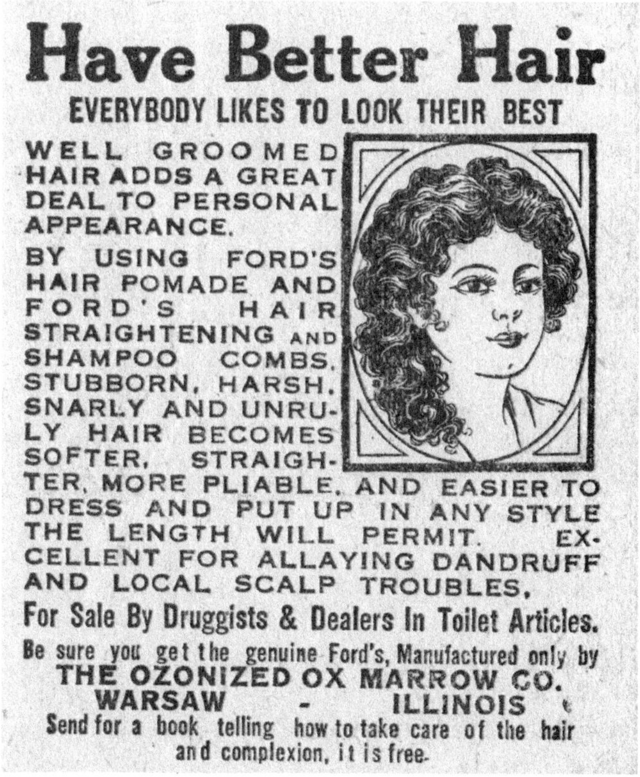

Have Better Hair
EVERYBODY LIKES TO LOOK THEIR BEST

WELL GROOMED HAIR ADDS A GREAT DEAL TO PERSONAL APPEARANCE.

BY USING FORD'S HAIR POMADE AND FORD'S HAIR STRAIGHTENING AND SHAMPOO COMBS, STUBBORN, HARSH, SNARLY AND UNRULY HAIR BECOMES SOFTER, STRAIGHTER, MORE PLIABLE, AND EASIER TO DRESS AND PUT UP IN ANY STYLE THE LENGTH WILL PERMIT.   EXCELLENT FOR ALLAYING DANDRUFF AND LOCAL SCALP TROUBLES,

For Sale By Druggists & Dealers In Toilet Articles.

Be sure you get the genuine Ford's, Manufactured only by

THE OZONIZED OX MARROW CO.

WARSAW   -   ILLINOIS

Send for a book telling how to take care of the hair and complexion, it is free.

Figure 3. Ozonized Ox Marrow advertisement, 12 April 1924, *Dawn of Tomorrow*, p. 6. Archives and Special Collections, Western Libraries, Western University, London, Canada.

women who were first to market hair-straightening products as agents of collective pride rather than as a sign of disavowing oneself, as white-owned companies had done. Annie Turnbo Malone was the first African American woman to do this. Born in 1869 in Metropolis, Illinois, Malone was orphaned as a child, but by the 1890s, she had managed to become an ardent entrepreneur by experimenting with preparations to help black women, like herself, care for their hair and scalp. Many black women needed remedies for common problems at the time, such as hair loss, breakage, and tetter (a skin ailment), and they also considered lush, well-groomed hair a sign of beauty.[117] When Malone relocated to the predominantly African American town of Lovejoy, Illinois, she began to manufacture Wonderful Hair Grower and went door to door to sell it. While her hair products contained common substances such as sage and egg rinses, by canvassing among other black women, she became living proof of the financial benefits of hair care. In 1906, as competitors began to imitate her product, Malone registered the trade name "Poro," a Mende (West African) term for a devotional society, and by 1914 Malone's Poro was a thriving enterprise.[118] With little apparent awareness of the social and psychological aspects of hair straightening, particularly among black women, Horne observes that the *Associated Negro Press* lavished positive press coverage on entrepreneurs like Annie Malone, and later, on one of her former employees, Madam C. J. Walker, who witnessed Malone's success and was inspired to start her own hair care business.[119]

Born Sarah Breedlove in 1867 in Delta, Louisiana, Madam C. J. Walker had worked in the cotton fields alongside her parents and siblings as a child, though she was the first member of her family to be born free. In 1910, she married C. J. Walker, and although they would divorce a few years later, she continued to use his name. Walker was a true anomaly. She was a poor, dark-skinned, large-framed woman who had worked as a laundress; the odds that she would eventually become the world's first woman millionaire had to have been a billion to one. By 1912, Walker claimed to have trained a thousand women at the Walker College of Hair Culture, and when she died in 1919, newspaper articles stated that she had employed more than ten thousand women at the Madame C. J. Walker Manufacturing Company, headquartered in Indianapolis, Indiana.[120] Like that of Malone before her, Walker's product line included a hair grower, "Glossine" (pomade), a vegetable shampoo, "Tetter Salve" (an anti-dandruff treatment), and "Temple Grower." Often referred to as the "Walker system," the product line was unique because it had to be used in conjunction with a shampoo-press-and-curl method of straightening hair. The shampoo-press-and-curl method involved the use of light oil and a wide-toothed steel comb heated on a stove. Although many African American historians often credit Walker for inventing this "hot comb," French hairdresser Marcel Grateau first invented heated metal hair implements as early as 1872, and straightening combs were also available in Sears and Bloomingdale's catalogues in the 1890s.[121] Walker diverged from Malone's method of hair straightening, but both women used a door-to-door and pyramid-type selling strategy, methods they undoubtedly borrowed from the California Perfume Company (later known as Avon), founded in 1886 by David H. McConnell. What Malone and Walker also did was modify existing formulas and improve hot combs that were already on the market, adjusting them for the condition and texture of black women's hair.

Significantly, in the 1880s Malone developed another system known as "pullers," which flattened the hair by pulling it, but upon Walker's invention of the shampoo-press-and-curl method in 1905, Walker immediately warned against working two combs at once (a common practice that often led to burns to the hair) and discouraged the use of hair pullers, which stretched and straightened the hair by aggressively pulling it, because it damaged and ultimately thinned the hair.[122] Many women were dissatisfied with the slick, flattened appearance the pullers created and found Walker's hot comb a huge improvement in hair straightening. Ultimately, Walker (and Malone) promoted the idea that *all* women had the potential for beauty, no matter their hair texture or skin colour, and by the 1920s, the Walker system became the industry standard for black hair care.[123] Following their lead, Sara Spencer Washington achieved large-scale success as a beauty culturist in the early twentieth century.

Born in 1889 in Berkley, Virginia, Washington opened her first beauty shop in 1918 in Atlantic City, New Jersey, and soon thereafter she began to market her own line of products. Following the death of Walker in 1919 and the decline of Malone's business following a divorce from her husband and a fight over control of her business, Washington's Apex Hair and News Company became one of the largest black-owned businesses in the 1920s and 1930s.[124] Like Walker, who grew her business through a chain of beauty schools, Washington added several beauty schools to her operations before the beginning of World War II. While Washington is often overshadowed by Walker and Malone, she was instrumental in the expansion of black beauty schools across the south and north. And even though Washington's Apex Beauty System was introduced roughly a decade after Malone and Walker had built sizable manufacturing plants, unlike them, she added wigs and other hairpieces to the general line of hair products that they had marketed.[125] In chapter 2, I explain how Halifax-born Viola Desmond, who trained at Washington's beauty school, learned not only the business of hair care but also how to produce and market hairpieces and hair products across the Maritimes. To date, I have not located any examples of advertisements placed by Malone, Walker, or Washington in black Canadian newspapers; however, there is material evidence that, as early as 1922, Malone's Poro College boasted of "enthusiastic agents in every state in the United States and in Africa, Cuba, the Bahamas, Central America, Nova Scotia and Canada."[126] By the first decade of the twentieth century, African Canadians began to post advertisements for hair care products as well as for hair care services. In many cases, these advertisements referred to black women as "Canadian Agents" for American companies. This suggests that a transnational black beauty culture existed not only in Toronto and Halifax, but in other black communities across the country.

In September 1916, for example, Mrs. George Green, the Windsor agent for a hair grower firm based in Denver, Colorado, posted an advertisement in the *Canadian Observer* with a headline reading, "A Marvelous Discovery that Will Positively Grow Hair on BALD HEADS."[127] The advertisement continued, "An excellent Hair Dressing, producing a healthy lustrous growth of hair. Stops failing hair, positively eradicates dandruff and gives that brilliant, natural color to gray or faded hair. Real Hair Grower should be used twice a week, rubbing it well into the scalp. If hair is dry and harsh, use often as described." In 1917, in one of the last available editions of the *Canadian Observer*, an advertisement promoting "real, handmade human hair" and an "electric straightening comb" by mail order appeared.[128] This advertisement points to two shifts in black hair care during the first decades of the twentieth century. First, in addition to straightening the hair, black women bought hair to add length and/or texture to an existing style or to hide baldness and/or hair loss caused by harsh hair care methods, such as pullers. Second, by the end of the 1910s, "straightening combs" had become standard equipment in the maintenance and care of black women's hair. In 1924, for example, Mesdames Wells and Hunter, a London, Ontario–based duo advertised a hair straightener and hair grower product in the *Dawn* as follows: "It makes your hair soft and silky, gives life to stubborn hair. Why not have a beautiful and luxuriant head of hair?"[129] A month prior, the paper had printed a photograph of Madame Lillian D. Wells on its front page, proclaiming that Mesdames Wells and Hunter "conduct one of the finest hair dressing parlors in the Dominion."[130] As previously noted, Madame Hunter's photograph also appeared in the *Dawn* in 1923. These women were black, and while there is little known of their biographies, they were beauty culturists, operating a beauty parlour in addition to selling their own products. Importantly, there are numerous examples in the *Dawn* of local black hair care operations in Toronto, Montreal, and London throughout the 1920s.

In March 1924, J. M. Jefferson Hair Dressing and Shaving Parlor in Montreal (Verdun) posted an advertisement for its "hair dressing and shaving" services,[131] and in November 1927, beauty salons like the Yale Tonsorial and Beauty Parlors in Toronto's Queen West offered a range of hairstyles from the "Marcel wave" to curls.[132] Grateau might have created the heated comb, but François Marcel Woelfflé, who later changed his name to François Marcel, obtained US patents for the curling iron in 1905, and by the 1920s electric curling irons were used not only in white-owned salons but also in barbershops and black hair salons. Black women occasionally requested hairstyles such as the "finger wave," a styling technique in which the hair is wetted with a setting lotion before waves or curls are arranged by crimping hair between the index fingers of the hands or curling the hair around the finger, but white salon clients more frequently requested Marcel waves.

The fact that black barbers in Toronto were, by 1927, well versed in the hairstyling techniques of the dominant culture illustrates the extent to which black people in Canada were attuned to the beauty trends of the time. The appearance of an advertisement in 1925 for the sale of a three-chair barber business in London with "fifty years practice in the same building" also points to a long history of barbering in that city, and another advertisement two years later for the Wolverine Barber Shop on Toronto's Queen Street West with the tagline, "ladies hair cutting, my speciality" suggests that male barbers might have outnumbered female beauty stylists, which is why some barbers also specialized in cutting women's hair.[133] When William L. Berry, a London-based product distributor, advertised his Wavine Hair Preparations and Beauty Treatment in the *Dawn* in June 1930, it stands as one of the first examples of a product advertisement from a Canadian company offering not just shampoos and soaps but also skin-bleaching creams, "hot-comb" pressing oils and hair dressing oils.[134] Importantly, wig advertising was also a prominent feature in the *Dawn* as the 1920s progressed. Throughout 1924 and 1925, New York City's Alex Marks posted advertisements in the newspaper for her mail order catalogue which consisted of "wigs of natural human hair made to your measure."[135] The appearance of human wigs from an African American firm suggests that Canada still lacked an infrastructure for the sale and advertisement of wigs geared toward black women at both the retail and door-to-door levels. It is difficult to make claims about African Canadian women's desires for wigs in the early twentieth century, as compared to African American women, but the appearance of these advertisements signal that there was a market for these products north of the border, however small it might have been.

While the *Dawn* was an African Canadian newspaper, by the 1930s and early 1940s, white-owned beauty companies began to advertise in its pages. In May 1937, an advertisement for Harriet Hubbard Ayer's "Beautifying

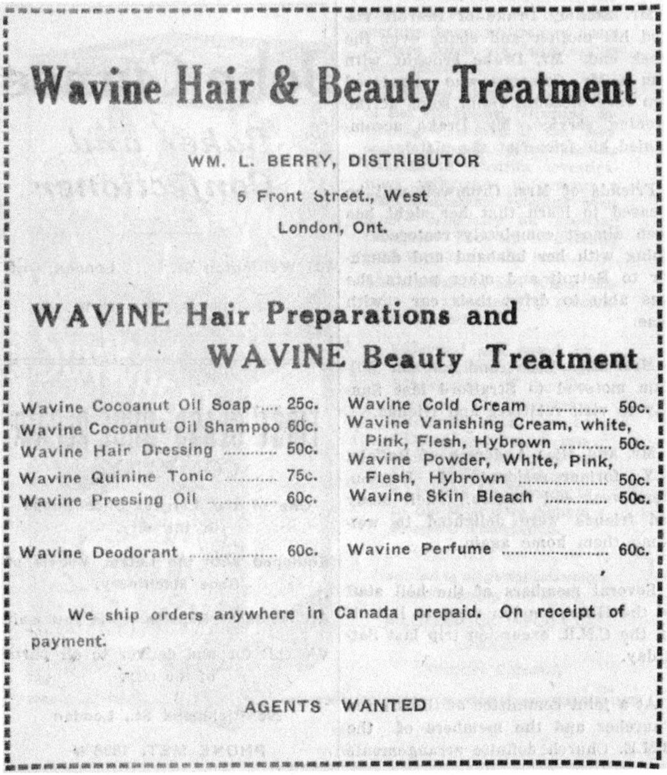

Figure 4. Wavine Hair & Beauty Treatment advertisement, *Dawn of Tomorrow*, 20 June 1930, p. 6. Archives and Special Collections, Western Libraries, Western University, London, Canada.

Face Cream" appeared in the newspaper.[136] Ayer, who had established her business in 1874, is often credited with launching the first cosmetic firm in the United States. The company's products were typically geared toward the higher-end beauty market; as such, the presence of an advertisement from Ayer in an African Canadian newspaper is significant. Another popular cosmetics firm geared toward white women was Du Barry Beauty Preparations. Established in 1874, the company created advertisements that highlighted the idea of a glamorous romantic beauty. In a representative Du Barry advertisement for "weathered skins" appearing in the *Dawn* in April 1942, the firm proclaimed, "Soft, glamorous beauty—one must possess it to look right in the new clothes."[137] Du Barry's products were offered for sale at Strong's Drug Store in London, Ontario. Where African American newspapers and magazines saw little advertising revenue from national brand companies in the 1920s and 1930s, apart from black women's cosmetics and hair product advertising,[138] throughout the 1920s and 1930s the *Dawn* was riddled with non-beauty-related ads from local Canadian companies and national firms.

McClary's, a London-based household products store with locations in Toronto, Montreal, Winnipeg, Vancouver, Saint John, Hamilton, Calgary, Saskatoon, and Edmonton, regularly advertised in the newspaper. Advertisements from smaller companies, such as cash-and-carry stores, funeral and undertaking businesses, furniture stores, florists, and retailers based in London, St. Catharines, and Toronto also appeared. In 1932 Zeller's, the discount retailer founded in 1931 by Walter P. Zeller, also placed ads in the *Dawn*. In August 1946, Eaton's even promoted its Fall and Winter Catalogue for 1946–1947 in the newspaper.[139] This support for the *Dawn* among white businesses that would accept black patronage points to a desire to cultivate African Canadian consumers, even as black women continued to be ignored in the catalogue pages of retailers like Eaton's and the editorial pages of *Chatelaine*.

In September 1946 the *Dawn* announced the arrival of *Ebony* magazine in Canada.[140] Dubbing itself a magazine in promotion of "National Negro Life," *Ebony* modelled itself after *Life* magazine, and in its first few years it contained frequent references to blacks in Canada.[141] The first issue of *Ebony* appeared in November 1945, and although no advertisements were included in the first issues, advertisements from major white-owned companies began appearing in 1946 after publishing magnate John H. Johnson persuaded white advertising and corporate executives to give *Ebony* the same consideration extended to *Look* and *Life* magazines.[142] Almost immediately after its arrival, the magazine took it upon itself to be the "voice of black America." Numerous other mass-market black magazines also appeared in the 1940s and 1950s. As well as *Ebony*, Johnson's publications included *Negro Digest* (1942–76), *Jet* (1951–2014), *Hue* (1953–59), *Tan* (1952–71); additionally, there was John P. Davis's *Our World* (1946–57) and George Levitan's *Sepia* (1947–83). All of these were photograph-filled publications aimed at black readers. By the late 1940s *Ebony* had become the most read of all the publications founded by Johnson. As *the* voice for black America at a time when most of the images of black people in the dominant culture remained negative stereotypes, it helped to usher in a new image for a new time. Black beauty culture from the postwar years onward became embodied through the photographic images of black woman in the pages of glossy magazines, and the display of black "middle-classness" helped to reposition lighter skin and straightened hair as emblems of black American "progress." Given that *Ebony* was also in Canada, it played a role in shaping African Canadian middle-class tastes as well. According to Laila Haidarali, to overturn the racist stereotyping of black women as dark-skinned, unattractive mammies, maids, and laundresses, magazines like *Ebony* endowed black women with attributes historically denied African American women—beauty, poise, and success. Black woman, she writes further, "began to visualize a different public racial reality, with the 'Brownskin' woman—the polished 'Brown' diamond—at its center."[143] This image also coincided with black respectability politics.

Historically, respectability politics have been viewed through the prism of racial uplift, but they also acquiesced to the dominant beauty ideal. As Evelyn Brooks Higginbotham observes, "By claiming respectability through their manners and morals...black women boldly asserted the will and agency to define themselves outside the parameters of prevailing racist discourses,"[144] but, she writes further, "the politics of respectability constituted a deliberately, highly self-conscious concession to hegemonic values."[145] The "Brownskin," as a gendered and commodified representation, emerged from the need of advertisers to "attract a newly important demographic: the African American consumer"[146] who, in the post–World War II era, no longer desired to be viewed through the derogatory image of the mammy. Marketers warned white advertisers about the use of skin tone in their advertisements, and they were told to use "brown-skinned girls for illustrations" because the image of the dark-skinned, fat woman too closely resembled the desexualized Mammy image.[147] During the war years, the "Negro Market" emerged in business periodicals and marketing magazines as a consumer demographic; in a 1943 article in an issue of *Sales Management*, for example, readers were cautioned, "Don't Do This—If You Want to Sell Your Products to Negroes!"[148]

The "Brownskin" woman ultimately struck a happy medium—she was black but removed from the image of the dark-skinned black servant. Throughout the 1940s, the "Brownskin" beauty in the pages of *Ebony* helped to valorize straightened hair and lighter skin and in tandem forged a new form of black consumer capitalism that encouraged black women to buy products from both white-owned and black-owned firms alike. Because Canada lacked a distribution network and there was no interest on the part of Canadian drugstores, grocery chains, and department stores throughout the 1940s and 1950s to sell products geared toward black women, *Ebony* made it possible for African Canadians to aspire to a new standard of black beauty that the magazine helped to create. In 1946, when Viola Desmond was arrested, jailed, sentenced, and fined for sitting in the "whites only" section of a theatre in New Glasgow, Nova Scotia, her story shed light on the tension between respectability politics and African Canadian communities, as well as on the opportunities, however limited they were, for beauty culturists to succeed in postwar Canada. Glossy magazines, the expansion of beauty product distribution, respectability politics, and chemical advances in hair straightening would, from the late 1940s to the late 1960s, fundamentally transform the scope and scale of black beauty culture in North America.

CHAPTER TWO

FROM *EBONY'S* "BROWNSKIN" TO "BLACK IS BEAUTIFUL" IN THE *NEWS OBSERVER*, 1946–1969

In March 2017, *Canada: The Story of Us* premiered on CBC Television. The ten-part historical drama aimed to "tell the extraordinary tale of some of the people, places and events that shaped Canada—stories of change makers and rule breakers, dreamers and visionaries, scientists and entrepreneurs who forged a nation in a vast and harsh land."[1] The show featured two black Canadians. In episode 5, "Expansion (1858–1899)," John Ware appeared. Ware, an African American, born into slavery, who became one of the best horsemen in the American West, settled in Alberta's Amber Valley in the 1870s. Episode 9, "A New Identity (1946–1970)," highlighted the life of Viola Desmond, who, after refusing to give up her seat in the "whites only" section of the Roseland, a segregated theatre in New Glasgow, Nova Scotia, was arrested, jailed, convicted, and fined. Canadian media sojourns into the past through images, stories, and legends are not so much lies as expressed truths aimed at idealizing certain aspects of our collective identity while demonizing others. We select events and institutions that seem to embody important cultural values and elevate them to the status of legend; and we vilify, or at least marginalize, anyone who seems to be frustrating the main cultural project.[2] Chapter 1 established an early history of African Canadian newspapers and beauty culture. This chapter elucidates the extent to which beauty practices in Canada became interconnected with the United States due in large part to rapid expansion and growth in the black beauty culture industry in the postwar years.

My arguments borrow from Inderpal Grewal's work on late capitalist consumer culture in India, where she suggests that "Americanness was produced transnationally by cultural, political, and economic practices, so that becoming American did not always or necessarily connote full participation or belonging to a nation-state."[3] Consumption practices, she writes further, "which were part of the imaginary community formed by 'American' nationalism through discourses of the 'American way of life,' were conveyed through transnational media advertising as a dominant white lifestyle of power and plenty as well as a multicultural and 'global' one."[4] While Grewal's focus was on the question of identity and citizenship in a liberalized India/America in the 1990s, I argue that a liberalized Canada/America in the post–World War II years similarly denoted a space where African Americanness was produced transnationally by cultural, political, and economic practices, so that becoming *black* did not always or necessarily connote full participation or adoption of a national identity, in this case, African Americanness, but engendered a form of transnational, global *black* identification. I explore how consumer markets geared toward black women produced a multiplicity of identities that proliferated in black media on both sides of the border such that by the 1960s, these identities were created and co-created through socio-cultural struggles around subjectivities, civil rights, and black nationalist discourses. This chapter ultimately argues that consumer culture, in the two decades following World War II, provided the modalities through which national and transnational forms of blackness were imagined, reimagined, and then produced and disseminated via black media.

By 1940, manufactured beauty formed a major sector of the United States economy and informed the everyday practices of women; in the decades that followed, mass media tied cosmetics ever more closely to notions of feminine identity and self-fulfillment, proliferating images of flawless female beauty as youthful, white, and increasingly sexualized.[5] In response to this ubiquitous image of beauty, African American magazines created the "Brownskin" ideal—a heterosexual and feminine woman who was visibly black and whose stylized display of respectable, feminized heterosexuality embodied the crowning glory of an attendant African American middle class.[6] As Laila Haidarali argues further, "ubiquitous in early postwar popular magazines, the gendered image of the 'Brownskin' became a signifier of democratic promise by representing economic and social triumph in a period when these goals remained unfulfilled for many African Americans."[7] Two of the most prominent representatives of the

"Brownskin" beauty in the 1940s and 1950s were Lena Horne and Dorothy Dandridge, both of whom appeared in adoring publicity stories in African American media. These women achieved commercial success at least in part because they fit a beauty ideal perpetuated in the mainstream and African American media, that of light skin and straightened hair.

Importantly, the roots of the light-skinned, straight-haired black ideal can be traced back to the black church, and the sentiment of racial uplift, as discussed in chapter 1, that circulated at the turn of the twentieth century, when many light-skinned blacks who had built America's black churches and schools also began to live together in segregated communities.[8] These "mulatto elites," as they were called, could be found in virtually every major urban centre across America where predominantly light-skinned blacks resided. In Philadelphia, communities predominantly inhabited by light-skinned blacks were unofficially called "lighty brighty" and "banana block"; in Chicago, this group could be found in Chatham and East Hyde Park, and in New York, certain sections of Harlem were reserved for light-skinned elites.[9] Black churches played a key role in framing the respectability politics of middle-class African Americans, especially as it related to who could and could not gain entry into the light-skinned elite class.

The earliest church in America established exclusively for blacks was the African Methodist Episcopal Church (AME) founded in Philadelphia in 1793. By 1870, colour increasingly divided America's AME worshippers, as lighter-skinned members split off to form their own denomination, the Colored Methodist Episcopal (CME; in 1954 the "C" was changed to stand for Christian).[10] The black church is central to the politics of respectability that would come to define the photographic and advertising imagery of African American magazines by midcentury. It was the place where, as Evelyn Brooks Higginbotham explains, a mythos of religiosity was tied to an ethos of respectability, which "held an identifiable and central place in the philosophy of racial self-help. It entrusted to blacks themselves responsibility for constructing the 'Public Negro Self' (to borrow from Henry Louis Gates, Jr.), a self presented to the world as worthy of respect."[11] In 1914, for example, the Woman's Convention, an Auxiliary to the National Baptist Convention, established Negro Doll Clubs. These clubs were "an attempt to instill in young black girls pride in their skin color.... The dolls were advertised as exhibiting the grace and beauty of a 'refined American Negro woman.'"[12] The dolls also attempted to refute unflattering images of black women, along with the idea that beauty was "flaxen-haired, blue-eyed, rosy-cheeked."[13] As Robin Bernstein points out, "African American adults championed beautiful black dolls as a direct cause of racial uplift."[14] As noted in chapter 1, these dolls stood in direct opposition to pickaninny dolls, which depicted a debased black child. At the same time, the notion of respectability engendered an in-group form of prejudice that created a double bind on black women and the pursuit of "feminine" beauty. On the one hand, a "feminine" sensibility enabled black women to cultivate a gendered space in a patriarchal society where they could establish a modicum of sisterhood with white women; on the other hand, the boundaries of femininity carried the cultural baggage of middle-class respectability and Christian virtue.[15] The link between black "feminine" beauty and Christian morality, for instance, was made when black families wishing to join colour-conscious congregations often had to pass skin colour and/ or hair texture tests known as "the paper-bag, the door, or the comb test." Accordingly, the paper-bag test involved placing a prospective member's arm inside a brown paper bag, and only if the person's skin was lighter than the colour of the bag would they be invited to attend church services. The comb test involved hanging a fine-toothed comb on a rope near the front entrance of the church, and if one's hair was too coarse and snagged the comb, one's entry to attend service was denied. The door test, conducted at some churches, involved painting the doors a light shade of brown, and anyone whose skin was darker than the door was politely invited to seek religious services elsewhere. Some historically black colleges and universities (HBCUs) also discriminated against dark-skinned blacks, denying them admission regardless of their academic qualifications if their skin was "too" dark.[16] Christian religiosity and church codes of conduct as they related to beauty played a significant role in the business lives of hairdressers; united by a broadly shared body of religious values, beauticians regularly turned to African American Christian principles.[17]

The history of racial uplift, respectability politics, and the business lives of African Canadian beauty culturists in the postwar years has largely been ignored in the literature on black Canada. What did the politics of respectability mean to African Canadian women in the postwar 1940s and 1950s? What role did the black church play in regulating black women's beauty choices in postwar Canada? Noliwe Rooks found that "from the late 1940s, with the rise of the liberal consensus in America and hegemonic integrationist legal and political efforts in African American culture, a notable ideological difference can be seen in ads promoting products manufactured by white-owned as opposed to African American–owned companies."[18] Drawing on comparative examples from the United States during the period from the late 1940s through to the late 1960s, this chapter uses a discursive, historical lens to explore the rise of liberal consensus in Canada and the hegemonic legal and political efforts that led to shifts in the public discourse on race and anti-black racism. While some of these developments parallel those in the United States, some of them were unique to the Canadian context. For instance, the American civil rights movement has been publicized, mediatized, and politicized, but the Canadian civil rights movement has been mostly ignored, undervalued, and depoliticized in the historical record. Between 1944 and 1967, the passage of anti-discrimination laws and race-neutral immigration policies helped to increase the visibility of black people in Canada's public sphere. These legislative and demographic changes transformed the segregated Canada of the 1940s into the increasingly diverse Canada of the 1960s, but they also proved to be ineffective when it came to eliminating anti-black sentiment and, in some cases, acts of violence in black communities.

The first civil rights shift occurred in 1944 with the passage of the Racial Discrimination Act in Ontario, which prohibited the public display in any form of signage that showed discrimination based on race, ethnic origin, or religion. The Racial Discrimination Act led to a wave of civil rights legislation across the country. In 1945, the province passed the Fair Employment Practices Act, followed by the Fair Accommodation Practices Act in 1954. In 1953, Nova Scotia passed the Fair Employment Act, followed by the Equal Pay Act in 1956 and the Fair Accommodations Act in 1959. Ontario and Nova Scotia might have been the first provinces to legislate (in the absence of civil protest) anti-discrimination laws designed to prevent racism and other forms of discrimination against non-whites, but in the 1940s, 1950s, and 1960s, several incidents involving African Canadians in small cities and towns turned a spotlight on the practice of de facto segregation, proving that top-down legislation could not eradicate deep-seated prejudices. Desmond's 1946 case has been highly publicized. In December 2016, in a public ceremony in Gatineau, Quebec, Finance Minister Bill Morneau accompanied Wanda Robson, Desmond's younger sister, on stage to announce that Desmond would appear on the new ten-dollar bill in 2018, becoming the first Canadian woman to appear on a regular-circulation banknote. Back in 2010, Mayann Francis, Lieutenant Governor of Nova Scotia (2006–12), the first black person to hold that position, granted an official apology and posthumous pardon to Desmond, also in a public ceremony. In 2018, Toronto City Councillor Neethan Shan introduced a motion to initiate the process of renaming Hupfield Park in Scarborough (a suburb east of the downtown core) after a celebrated individual in Canadian history who had demonstrated values of diversity and equity through their work. The motion passed unanimously at Toronto City Council, and the new name, Viola Desmond Park, was formally approved unanimously by Council in June of that year. While this recognition is important, less attention has been paid to remembering other black Canadians who endured racial prejudice in 1940s Canada.

In Toronto, for example, a 1947 editorial in *The Globe and Mail* asked, "Have We a Color Line?"[19] The editorial, written by Ross Perry, focused on Marguerite Bradley, a black woman who wanted to be a hairdresser, and who, after graduating from Malvern Collegiate, sent an application to the Marvel Hairdressing School. While Bradley initially received a letter back accepting her application with a request for a twenty-five-dollar advance payment for the course, which she sent by return mail, "when she reported to the school and they saw her for the first time she was told that because she was colored the school could not accept her and her $25 was returned," Perry reported, noting that the school accepted Chinese and Japanese students. While Bradley was later accepted by another school, after graduating, she tried to get a job in twenty-five beauty parlours across the city and no one would take her. This discrimination occurred despite the presence of a Fair Employment Practices Act passed just two years earlier. Bradley ultimately found work as a sewing machine operator in a tailor shop, but Perry concluded that her case was typical of black women and men in 1940s Toronto.

In her writing about black women in Canada who worked outside the home between the world wars, Dionne Brand interviewed Addie Aylestock (1909–98), a minister of the British Methodist Episcopal Church, and the first black woman to be ordained in Canada. Aylestock, who also helped organize BME congregations in several communities in Ontario, as well as in Montreal, Africville, and Halifax, recalled that, when she first came to Toronto in the 1930s, "there weren't many opportunities for black girls."[20] Violet Blackman, the only woman of Caribbean descent in Brand's oral histories, who came to Toronto in 1920, also observed that "you couldn't get any position, regardless who you were and how educated you were, other than housework because even if the employer would employ you, those that you had to work with would not work with you."[21] Yet there is little collective memory about the pervasiveness of anti-black racism at schools and places of employment, except for the Desmond case in recent years. As Graham Reynolds writes, the study of black people in Canada, "has not been a part of the mainstream of Canadian history, and it remains a marginalized subject, largely overshadowed by the study of other racial-ethnic groups. For this reason, the history of racial segregation and the experience of blacks in Canada are not well understood, and what Canadians do know is often the American example or merely a fragment of the larger narrative."[22] Another example of Canadian historical amnesia with regard to white racism and black Canada can be found in the story of Dresden, the southwestern Ontario town where two restaurants refused to serve a black couple from Toronto in 1954, despite the Fair Accommodation Practices Act.

After taking their plight to the media, the couple in the Dresden case proved that anti-discrimination policy was not being enforced on the ground. The National Film Board of Canada film *Dresden Story* (1954) by director Julian Biggs revealed that although black residents made up 12 percent of the town's population, since the 1840s, they had not attended white churches, white-owned barbershops, or any other establishments with "whites only" policies. Local black residents did not go to the poolrooms, service clubs, or beauty parlours. In 1949, journalist Sidney Katz visited the town, and in an exposé for *Maclean's* titled "Jim Crow Lives in Dresden," he noted, "Although Dresden citizens do not like to talk about it, Negroes cannot eat at the town's three restaurants serving regular meals."[23] Just as in Desmond's case, Jim Crow segregation was alive and well in Ontario in the 1940s and 1950s. By the 1960s, led by the establishment of Ontario's Human Rights Code (1962) and the Nova Scotia Human Rights Act (1963), other comprehensive human rights legislation passed across the country—in Alberta (1966), New Brunswick (1967), Prince Edward Island (1968), British Columbia (1969), Newfoundland (1969), Manitoba (1970), and Quebec (1975). These policy changes were important steps forward but they, too, did little to shift anti-black sentiment.

In 1971, historian Robin Winks published *The Blacks in Canada: A History*. It represents the first attempt at a comprehensive chronicle of the black experience in Canada; however, he has been (rightfully) criticized for relegating the voices of black people to the capacity of passive recipients. Specifically, Owen Thomas observed that while Winks's writings reflect the real racial hurdles that people of colour had to endure, "he largely ignores the importance of historical continuity within the African Canadian community."[24] In October 1968, Winks published an article in *The Journal of Negro History* titled "The Canadian Negro: A Historical Assessment" that affirms Thomas's concerns about his writings.

This two-part examination of "the Negro in the Canadian-American relationship" pointed to a uniquely Canadian contradiction. On the one hand, Winks observed that "as in the United States, the Negro was a convenient figure around which to shape a moral and sexual mythology. Countless lavatory graffiti testified to the greater attractiveness of what with surpassing vulgarity was called 'black meat'; Negro chorus lines were reportedly the most risqué of all in Montreal, and a West Indian nightclub singer in Winnipeg was barred before he could perform on the well known principle that Calypso songs are objectionable."[25] On the other hand, he argued that most white Canadians interacted with, and in some cases had knowledge of, black people only through an "American lens refracted by Canadian institutions" such as television and newspaper reports on the black American experience. "*Life, Newsweek, Time*, and *Look* have effectively championed Negro rights, and readers of these magazines in Canada have learned much of the subject as it relates to the United States," wrote Winks, adding "Canadian magazines, too, especially *Maclean's, Saturday Night*, and *Canadian Forum*, have kept their readership well informed of developments with respect to race relations."[26] For his part, Winks failed to consider the media that black Canadians interacted with, and the extent to which race relations in black Canada were being shaped by developments in black America. While Canadian media actively reported on racial incidents in the United States, for the most part, the same acts of racial violence and discrimination in the Canadian context were often minimized as "isolated" or being the actions of a few, not reflective of long-standing, community-wide anti-black racism.

In Nova Scotia, black communities in small rural areas such as Truro had become known as "Little Mississippi," in large part because white and black people rarely interacted in the province, with black people living in segregated and often poorly serviced communities such as North Preston and Africville, a black community on the outskirts of Halifax that was frequently referred to as "Nigger Town" by many white Haligonians through the 1960s.[27] Africville was founded by black Loyalists and black refugees in the 1840s but in the 1960s, it was bulldozed by the city of Halifax to make way for private housing, ramps for the A. Murray MacKay Bridge, the Fairview Container Terminal, and a dog park called Seaview Park. In February 2010, Halifax Mayor Peter Kelly apologized for the razing of Africville, and a settlement with the residents and descendants of Africville was made that included the apology, a hectare of land on the former site to rebuild the community church, and $3 million towards the building's cost. In 2016, up to three hundred former Africville residents and descendants attempted to join a class-action lawsuit against the City of Halifax over the loss of their land in the 1960s. In 2018, however, a Nova Scotia Supreme Court judge denied the proposed class-action lawsuit on the grounds that those who were seeking compensation through the class action brought by Nelson Carvery, a former resident, had failed to meet the requirements of the Class Proceedings Act; specifically, Carvery, as plaintiff, had not demonstrated that there was a second member of the class and that there was a common issue among possible class members. Africville still remains largely removed from the national Canadian historical memory. Similarly, anti-black sentiment in Quebec and Ontario has largely been forgotten, even though it was equally as rampant, although black populations did not necessarily live in communities segregated from white populations, as in Nova Scotia.

In the early 1940s, most hotels in Montreal refused to serve black customers,[28] and a Quebec cemetery where black slaves are believed to be buried about eighty-three kilometres south of Montreal was called "Nigger Rock" up until 2015 when the Quebec Toponymy Commission ordered name changes for it and ten other provincial sites whose names contained the word "Nigger." In August 1965, a month and year most remembered for the Watts riots in Los Angeles and riots in other cities across America, there were five intense days of racial incidents in the southwestern Ontario town of Amherstburg. At the time, there were three hundred black residents in Amherstburg who lived alongside four hundred white residents.[29] Amherstburg was also a historically black town, as it had been a stop along the Underground Railroad by which enslaved African Americans had travelled to freedom in the nineteenth century. A Baptist church was built there in 1849, and, in Harriet Beecher Stowe's novel *Uncle Tom's Cabin* (1852), it was the meeting point where Eliza Harris, who flees with her young son over ice floes on the Ohio River, is reunited with her husband, George.

Over a period of five days in 1965, a cross was burned in the town centre, threatening phone calls were made to black residents, the black Baptist church was defaced, and the sign welcoming visitors to the town was spray-painted "Amherstburg Home of the KKK [Ku Klux Klan]."[30] While the American Klan was created in December 1865 in Pulaski, Tennessee, the Canadian Klan has been active since the 1920s. In October 1921, a headline in the *Montreal Daily Star* read, "Ku Klux Klan being organized in city; trouble expected."[31] In 1923, Klansmen toured the country vowing that the hooded empire would "soon be operating over all the Dominion."[32]

A photograph on the front page of the *Hamilton Herald* on March 20, 1925, also captured members of the Grand Executive of the Women's Canadian Ku Klux Klan in full white robe and hood regalia.[33] By 1930, branches of the Klan had opened in Montreal and Vancouver and across Ontario, New Brunswick, and Nova Scotia, and Klan activity was recorded in Saskatchewan, Alberta, Manitoba, and throughout Ontario.[34] For example, one night in February 1930, seventy-five Klansmen appeared in Oakville, a city between Toronto and Hamilton, marching through "the principal streets clad in their white gowns and black hoods."[35] By the 1960s, the Klan was not something imported from the United States into Canada; it was a homegrown institution that was active in cities and towns across the country.

In the United States, the Klan steadily declined during the Reconstruction era (1865–77) in the period following the Civil War, but after D. W. Griffith's *The Birth of a Nation* (1915) became a smash hit, the Klan found a resurgence. The film told the story of the Old South, the Civil War, the Reconstruction era, and the emergence of the Ku Klux Klan. It depicted old faithful black servants on the one hand and uneducated boors or half-crazed savages on the other, incapable of common courtesy let alone self-government.[36] As the first full-length feature film, *The Birth of a Nation* justified the need for Jim Crow segregation to be maintained, inciting white fear of black (male) violence, whether directed toward poverty or toward white women, and affirming beliefs in the inherent danger posed by black sexuality.[37] The Canadian expansion of the Klan, on the other hand, was buoyed by interwar anti-immigrant sentiment, which had deep roots since Confederation, and concerns over "vice"—in the form of alcohol, drugs, and homosexuality—that was often prejudicially associated with ethnic minorities.[38] At the same time the Canadian Klan might have formed under different cultural circumstances, as Sarah-Jane Mathieu observes: "Canadians opposed to black migration persistently conjured up images of the black rapist, made popular in D. W. Griffith's internationally celebrated film *The Birth of a Nation*, when making the case for blocking passage of blacks in Canada."[39] The black population in Canada may have been significantly lower than the white population, but they were certainly not shy about voicing their opinions about anti-black propaganda, which *The Birth of a Nation* unequivocally was. According to the *Winnipeg Free Press*, *The Birth of a Nation*'s initial release in 1915 had sparked public outcry "by delegations of colored citizens" denouncing its racist content.[40] On December 4, 1915, the African Canadian newspaper the *Canadian Observer* also reported that Windsor's black residents had succeeded in suspending a planned theatrical production of *The Birth of a Nation* in the city.[41] These examples reveal that, despite the lack of political capital, African Canadians were not afraid to use their voices to speak out against prejudice.

In response to Amherstburg, Daniel G. Hill, an African American who moved to Toronto in the 1950s and who became the first director of the Ontario Human Rights Commission (OHRC), the agency responsible for enforcing Ontario's Human Rights Code (1962), spearheaded an investigation that eventually led to increased integration in the town. In the end, however, no arrests were made. What is significant about Amherstburg is the tone and focus of the reporting in Canadian media at the time. Most notably, on August 12, 1965, a *Globe and Mail* editorial on Amherstburg, titled "Burning Cross Hoodlum's Work, OPP Says," quoted Deputy Attorney General A. Rendall Dick, who dismissed the five-day affair, stating that "if any crimes were involved in these incidents they were of the petty types" and that overall, "there was no organized racial disturbance."[42] Thus, by the 1960s, it was very clear from coast to coast that there was widely held anti-black sentiment, and even with anti-discrimination legislation, public officials often minimized and hyper-localized overt racist acts of violence, like those at Amherstburg. Where legislation would not eradicate racial prejudice, governments continued to turn to policy to shift the Canadian cultural climate. Anti-discrimination legislation also corresponded to changes in immigration policy.

With the passage of the Immigration Act in 1952, and its implementation in 1953, long-standing patterns of racial discrimination that had contributed to the stagnant growth in the black population prior to the 1950s were removed as de facto practice. Back in 1947, Liberal Prime Minister William Lyon Mackenzie King had stated in the House of Commons that "Canada is perfectly within her rights in selecting the persons whom we regard as desirable future citizens. It is not a 'fundamental human right' of any alien to enter Canada. It is a privilege."[43] Quite clearly, these comments would have been deemed highly offensive to West Indians who were regularly barred and deterred from emigrating to Canada. Thus, changes to immigration policy in the postwar years explicitly prohibited the exclusion of immigrants for reasons of nationality, citizenship, ethnic group, and geographical area of origin. In 1952, the Immigration Act set up the basic framework for an immigration system based on merit. As Joseph Mensah notes, Canada formally revoked the preferential treatment given to white immigrants, and for the first time in Canadian immigration history, emphasis was placed on education and professional skills and not on race or ethnicity. "Applicants from all countries were (purportedly) treated equally," Mensah notes, "and skilled and professional blacks from the Caribbean and Africa were able to come to Canada on their own merits."[44] Canadian immigration policies fundamentally changed in 1967 with revisions to the Immigration Act that became known as the "points system," which stipulated that all immigrants, irrespective of their country of origin and racial and ethnic background, were to be assessed on nine factors. These factors included education and training, knowledge of English and French, personal assessment by an immigration officer, occupational demands, occupational skills, arranged employment (or designated occupation), a relative in Canada, employment opportunities in the destination point, and adaptability.

With an emphasis on education and professional skills and not race or ethnicity, by the late 1960s, Caribbean and continental Africans began to immigrate to Canada in unprecedented numbers. The West Indian immigrant population gradually increased annually after 1962, more than doubled between 1966 and 1967, and tripled again by the mid-1970s; by the time of the 1971 census, there were 68,000 West Indian-born residents in Canada, and the decade of the 1970s saw the arrival of nearly 140,000 more.[45] The opening of Canadian immigration offices in Jamaica and Trinidad and Tobago in 1967 and later in Haiti, Barbados, Kenya, and Côte d'Ivoire was another significant factor in the immigration wave of blacks to Canada in the 1960s and 1970s.[46] This second wave of Caribbean immigration (the first wave occurred in the 1920s) not only changed the demographics of Canadian society, it also helped to create a critical mass in cities like Toronto and Montreal. Because many of the newly arrived West Indian immigrants spoke English, it was much easier for them to settle in Toronto than, for instance, in Montreal. By the 1970s, these immigrants would help to foster a homegrown black beauty culture.

In the late 1960s, black newspapers in Toronto would for the first time become instrumental in contributing to a growing black diaspora that was no longer on the fringes as it had been in the early decades of the century but was now increasingly becoming an important part of the city's cultural fabric. These newspapers also played new roles in the promotion and sale of black beauty products in the postwar years. Importantly, these newly formed black newspapers in the 1950s also played a vital human rights role in eradicating anti-black racism from public schools, another aspect of Canadian society prior to the 1970s that has received little attention. Since the late nineteenth century, dehumanized depictions of black children as pickannnies, black women as servile mammies, and black men as Sambos—an all-purpose nickname to denote any smiling, servile black male, from railway porters to hotel bellhops to restaurant waiters and cooks—continued to occupy more than their share of space in the cultural imagination. For example, in 1884 the N. K. Fairbank Company introduced the cartoon images of two "pickaninnies," the Gold Dust Twins (Goldy and Dusty), to promote its brand of soap. The company even hired black children to hand out product samples and pamphlets at the 1904 St. Louis World's Fair.[47] In 1897, an advertisement for Gold Dust Washing Powder appeared in Toronto's the *Daily Mail and Empire*.[48] The first protest against the children's book *Little Black Sambo*, written and illustrated by Helen Bannerman in 1899, took place in 1954 when Daniel Braithwaite, who was born in Sydney, Nova Scotia, launched a campaign in Toronto to ban the book from Ontario's public schools because of its derogatory depiction of black children. Braithwaite mobilized support from the railway employee unions and community service organizations and gathered letters from black community newspapers like the *Canadian Negro* (1953–56). His efforts, along with those of Daniel Hill, led to the banning of both the book and the film from Ontario schools in 1956.[49]

The *Canadian Negro*, launched by the Canadian Negro Publishing Association, and edited by Roy Greenidge and Donald Carty, emphasized "social and church news, sporting events, and hortatory articles dealing with racial history."[50] Like J. R. Whitney's *Canadian Observer* and James F. Jenkins's *Dawn of Tomorrow*, the newspaper was a voice for and of black community at a time when there was no visible black presence in Canada's dominant media and when cases of discrimination were framed as isolated, such as in 1950s Dresden. While black-themed stories did make their way into the pages of daily newspapers, black community newspapers, especially in the postwar years, took on new importance as black people sought to acquire higher levels of social and political capital. Whereas, by comparison, there were 255 African American periodicals as of 1945—110 general newspapers; 45 religious, college, advertising, fraternal, and other miscellaneous papers; and 100 magazines and bulletins[51]—Canada lacked (and continues to lack) the infrastructure for dozens, let alone hundreds, of African Canadian newspapers. The lack of a national black press and the inadequate nature of the reporting on black communities across the country points to a form of black regionalism that is unique to Canada. By the mid-twentieth century, black communities were separate from one another—those living in Halifax's black communities in the 1960s, for example, were removed from those living in communities in southwestern Ontario—despite clear parallels and shared experiences of discrimination and anti-black racism. Black immigrants to Toronto and Montreal during the same period remained connected to other sites of blackness such as the United States and Caribbean while paradoxically disconnected from black communities across Canada. Thus, black Canada in the postwar years can only be described as a disjointed community connected through similar entanglements with the dominant culture but disconnected—geographically, spatially, and politically—from one another.

This chapter ultimately tackles the question of how black beauty culture developed in postwar Canada despite the lack of a highly defined national infrastructure akin to that which formed in postwar America. It also provides one of the first accounts of the strategies used by African American and white-owned beauty firms to advertise and promote black beauty products in Canada prior to the 1970s. The two questions underpinning this chapter are as follows: If *Ebony* magazine, the first magazine geared toward a specifically African American audience, "popularized a new visual discourse on middle-class life with the 'Brownskin' woman at its center,"[52] how did African Canadian-run newspapers in Halifax and West Indian-operated newspapers in Toronto do the same thing? Second, how did the "Brownskin" ideal, popularized in African American glossy magazines, appear in Canada's community newspapers? The biography of Viola Desmond provides us with a window to gain a deeper understanding of black beauty culture and black Canada in the 1940s. As in Ontario, newspapers in Nova Scotia would prove to be more than just newspapers; they became a voice and platform for African Canadian civil rights, and most notably, they helped to catapult Desmond into the public sphere not just as a "victim" of racism but as an example of African Canadian respectability.

Viola Desmond was born Viola Irene Davis in Halifax in 1914. She grew up in a prominent, middle-class, self-identified "coloured" (the term used to refer to blacks until the 1950s) family. Her father, James Albert Davis, was black, and her mother, Gwendolin Irene Davis, was white.[53] Desmond was destined to be an entrepreneur: her paternal grandfather was a self-employed barber who established the Davis Barber Shop in Halifax's north end, and her father briefly worked there until he established a career for himself managing real estate and operating a car dealership.[54] For a brief period, Desmond was a teacher at racially segregated schools in Preston and Hammond Plains; as Robson writes, "In the early '30s, Halifax schools did not hire black teachers . . . [so] if you were black and going into Grade 12 and wanted to be a teacher, you could take a test to attain a special certificate which allowed you to teach in the black schools—a kind of dispensation. Viola attained one of these certificates."[55]

Institutional racism across the province meant that self-employment was one of the few options available to African Canadians, allowing them to accrue not just status in their communities but also the ability to construct a dignified "public self." Accordingly, Higginbotham argues that one of the tenets of respectability politics is the demand that "every individual in the black community assume responsibility for behavioral self-regulation and self-improvement along moral, educational, and economic lines. The goal was to distance oneself as far as possible from images perpetuated by racist stereotypes" because individual behaviour, black Baptist women contended, ultimately determined the collective fate of black people.[56] For Desmond, owning a beauty business was her ticket to achieving this. In this regard, the opportunities that hair care afforded black women in Canada paralleled those of African Americans, especially in the early twentieth century when beauty schools, hair salons, and beauty culturists became ubiquitous fixtures in black communities. Black women entrepreneurs such as Annie Turnbo Malone, Sarah Spencer Washington, and Sarah Breedlove (Madam C. J. Walker) amassed fortunes and created jobs for African American women in cosmetology, hair care, and product distribution. These African American beauty culturists were so influential in shaping African Canadian women's business choices that in her book about Desmond, *Sister to Courage*, Robson recalls:

> Viola read about Madam Walker. And she was inspired. This woman's success is what got Viola going. She studied how Madam Walker started her own business. . . . Now, Viola wanted to study at [Madam Walker's beauty school], in New York, and that's where she eventually went. . . . She also earned a diploma from Madam Sara Spencer Washington's Apex College of Beauty Culture and Hairdressing in Atlantic City in 1940, and then a certificate from the Advanced Hairstyling Studio in New York in 1941.[57]

Whereas Canada's beauty culture was still segregated into the 1940s—specifically, "all of the facilities available to train beauticians in Halifax restricted black women from admission,"[58]—in the United States, things had begun to change.

Malia McAndrew observes that in the postwar economic boom of the late 1940s, 1950s, and 1960s, "African American hair care professionals had a new opportunity to expand their business interests in the United States and abroad."[59] Historically, the black hair care industry had depended upon segregated markets for its success, but as large white-owned firms began to move into the black hair care industry in the 1950s and 1960s, African American entrepreneurs had to reconceptualize the scope of their business practices.[60] In Canada, white-owned firms and the dominant beauty industry continued to ignore black women in the 1940s, 1950s, and 1960s. For example, in 1950, *Chatelaine* had an annual circulation of 378,866; over the next decade, its circulation almost doubled, reaching 745,589 by 1960, and, according to a *Chatelaine* advertisement, "by 1959 one of every three English-speaking women in Canada, or a total of 1,650,000, read each issue of Chatelaine."[61] And yet, black-focused topics were virtually excluded from its pages until 1959, when the magazine made two controversial topics—interracial dating and immigration—its focus.

In a May 1959 editorial written by Rita Cummings and titled "My Daughter Married a Negro," the personal story began, "I was convinced I was free of race prejudice and proudly raised my children to believe in the equality of all men. Now I was being called on to test the depth and sincerity of my own words."[62] The story outlined how Cummings, who lived in Winnipeg, was having a difficult time adjusting to the idea of her daughter being in a relationship with a black man. "You'll be asking for nothing but trouble if you go into a life like that," Cummings recalled advising her daughter, adding, "I don't think mixed marriages bring happiness to anybody."[63] In September of that year, another first-person narrative graced the magazine's editorial pages; this time it was the personal narrative of Yvonne Bobb, a West Indian immigrant to Canada, as told to *Chatelaine* staff writer Jeannine Locke. Titled "Are Canadians Really Tolerant?" the piece recounted Bobb's experiences—her inability to meet other Canadians, the subtle yet systematic racism she encountered, her difficulty in finding an apartment, and her simmering resentment—without any sugar-coating for the magazine's primary audience, middle-class white women.[64] Bobb, like thousands of other West Indian women, had come to Canada via the West Indian Domestic Scheme initiated in 1955. To be eligible for the scheme, an applicant had to be a single woman between the ages of 18 and 35, in good health, and with a minimum Grade 8 education. At first, the scheme was limited to a hundred women annually from Jamaica and Barbados, but it expanded both in numbers and in the sites of recruitment. Gradually, the government increased the annual quota for the scheme to 280 people drawn from a wider range of Caribbean nations, including Trinidad and Tobago, Antigua, British Guyana, St. Vincent, Dominica, Grenada, Montserrat, St. Lucia, and St. Kitts, with the largest numbers still from Jamaica and Barbados.[65] While most of the women worked in Toronto and Montreal, some black women also went to Ottawa and Vancouver. By 1965, it is estimated that 2,690 West Indian women had been admitted under the scheme, more than all the West Indian immigrants who had come to Canada before 1945.[66]

Under the Canadian government classification, black domestic immigrants were under contract for a predetermined period; although the contract conditions were difficult, many of these immigrants wanted employment, so Canada was able to capitalize on the strong demand, particularly from middle-class black women immigrating directly from the West Indies who wanted to escape the depressed economies of the region.[67] Many of the women who came to Canada as domestics did so not just because of the lack of employment opportunities in the Caribbean, but as a means to escape boredom, and to travel. For a minimum of one year, these women were essentially indentured servants for well-to-do white Canadians, and while technically the women were "free" to remain in Canada to pursue other careers or to continue their education and training after one year, after their first year few had the opportunity or the time.[68] As Mensah observes, "Most of the women who came under the...scheme had not been domestic servants at the time of their application. Nurses, secretaries, clerks, and teachers took advantage of the scheme to establish a foothold in Canada, as that was virtually the only means by which they, as black women, could enter Canada at the time."[69] While the Domestic Scheme was cancelled in 1967 following the introduction of the points system, it had a lasting impact on black community. As Dorothy Williams observes, "Men in particular, looked down on the domestics, regardless of their background. Domestic service in West Indian culture was perceived as a sign of low class standing. There is little wonder that many black women domestics felt no sense of belonging or acceptance. They were invisible in their own community, and...the very nature of their work—with its long hours—made it impossible for them to participate in community events."[70] Thus, when Bobb spoke of her experiences, she was speaking on behalf of black women who, like her, had come to Canada under the scheme, and who were also finding it difficult to assimilate into Canadian society.

The opening teaser in the 1959 exposé drew a symbolic line between Bobb and *Chatelaine*'s (white women) readers: "We smugly boast that we have no racial barriers, but, says this young West Indian, in practice we're as prejudiced as any nation. We just dodge the issue by keeping the colored people out."[71] If we put this editorial in context, it speaks to how black women were excluded from Canada's mainstream beauty culture through the 1950s. Rather than appear in a beauty editorial and/or advertisement, when the magazine was at its height in the 1950s and 1960s, black women appeared in *Chatelaine* only under the purview of "diversifying" the breadth of the magazine's social awareness, not with regard to its beauty imagery—that remained an exclusively white woman's domain until the 1970s. In her examination of department stores, Belisle also found that these spaces of consumption helped to build and represent a vision of Canada that was exclusionary and based on class and race privileges rooted in the social relations of empire and bourgeois class formation.[72]

In 1937, when Desmond returned to Halifax from her beauty schooling in the United States, she immediately opened Vi's Studio of Beauty Culture on Gottingen Street in the north end of Halifax's downtown, a predominantly African Canadian community that was segregated from the parts of the city inhabited by whites. Her salon sat alongside the barbershop of her husband, Gordon (Jack) Desmond, whom she had married in 1936. Robson explains further that "[Viola] put her name on the windows, and she would later put her name on her products—just like Madam C. J. Walker.... And the business grew."[73] Specializing in shampoos, press-and-curl, hair straightening, chignons, and hairpieces and wigs, as Desmond's business expanded, she eventually branched out into chemistry, learning how to manufacture specialized beauty powders and creams, which she marketed under the label "Vi's Beauty Products."[74] Desmond's beauty salon, products, and the Desmond School of Beauty Culture, which she opened after a few years, drew black women from across Nova Scotia, New Brunswick, and Quebec. Her business was undoubtedly modelled after the African American women who had trained her. Black beauty schools, primarily in the eastern, southern, and midwestern United States were experts on teaching black hair care methods. As Bonnie Claudia Harrison asserts, women who attended these schools "learned technologies to straighten, and therefore lengthen, the diversity of curl in the hair of African descended customers. In this era...it was particularly critical for striving black women to achieve a well-groomed appearance that was complimentary and socially presentable."[75]

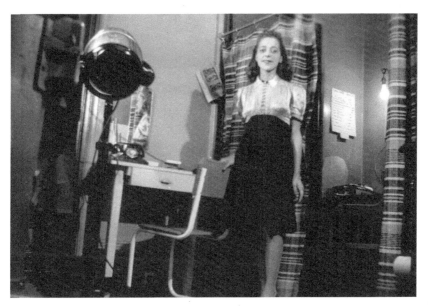

Figure 5. Viola Desmond in her studio, ca. 1938. Wanda and Joe Robson Collection, MG 21.14, 16-87-30227. Beaton Institute, Cape Breton University.

Desmond's "well-groomed appearance" is partly what catapulted her into the spotlight following the Roseland Theatre incident, as members of black community wondered how a "respectable" black woman could be treated like a lesser citizen in the country of her birth. As in most segregated places, middle-class respectability politics imposed upon black women an imperative to appear well groomed in public, especially with respect to their hair, to avoid negative attention from whites. From the public spaces of buses and streets to the private spaces of their individual homes, the behaviour of blacks was perceived as ever visible to the white gaze.[76] Desmond embodied the "Brownskin" ideal of middle-class femininity espoused by magazines like *Ebony* and upheld in black communities across North America during the period. As Backhouse explains, Desmond was "described as both 'elegantly coiffed and fashionably dressed,' a 'fine-featured woman with an eye for style.' Her contemporaries recall that she was always beautifully attired, her nails, make-up, and hair done with great care.... Desmond was a well-mannered, refined, demonstrably *feminine* woman."[77] When her ordeal was brought to the attention of prominent members of Halifax's black community such as Pearleen Oliver, the first black graduate of New Glasgow High School, and her husband, the Reverend William Pearly Oliver, it became

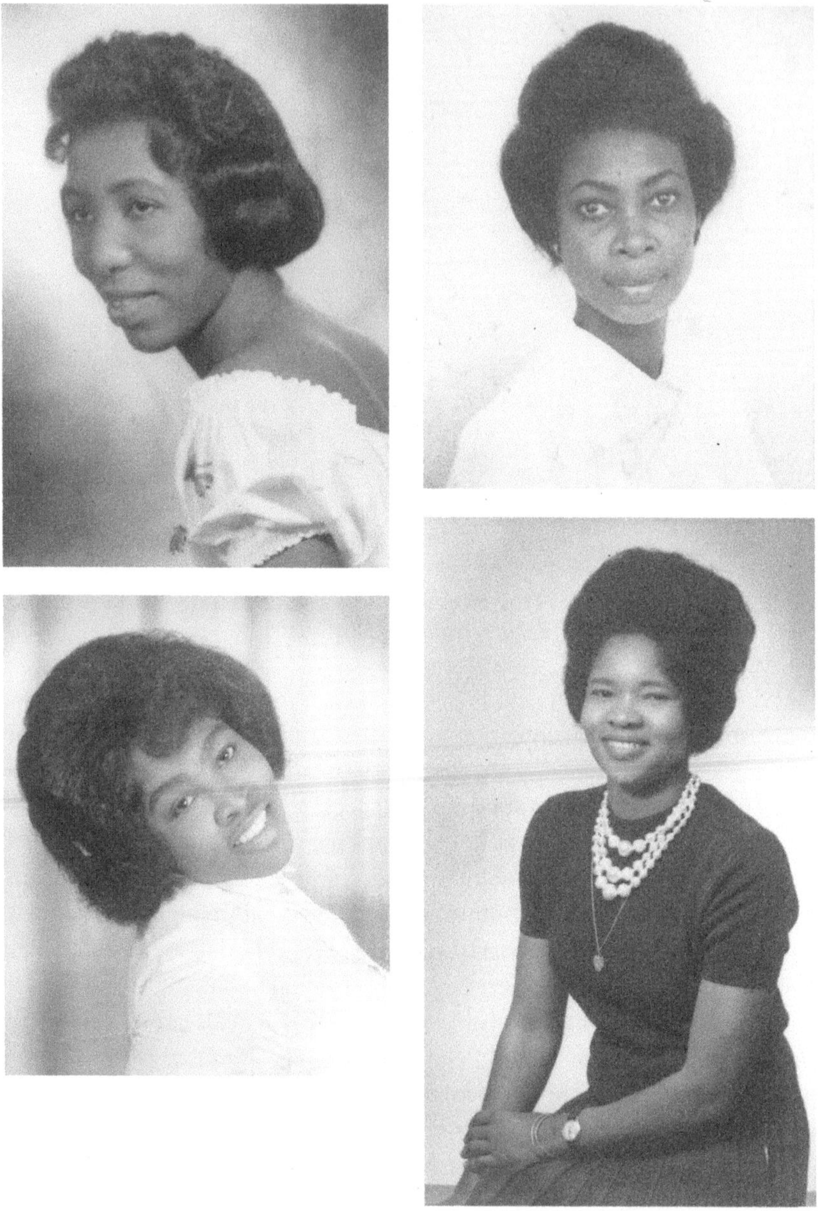

Figure 6. Black women with well-groomed appearance, family photographs, late 1950s/early 1960s.

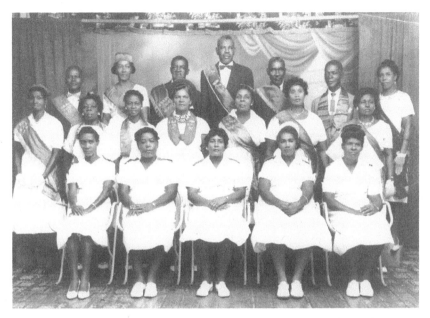

Figure 7. My grandmother, Lena Wilson (1912–2003), middle row, fourth from the left, Baptist church group, Kingston, Jamaica, ca. 1950s.

more than just another racist incident: Desmond became the face of de facto segregation in Maritime Canada.

The Olivers presided over an almost exclusively black congregation at Cornwallis Street Baptist Church, centrally located in downtown Halifax.[78] In 2017, in response to protests to remove a public statue of Edward Cornwallis, founder of Halifax and an oppressor of First Nations people, Cornwallis Street Baptist Church's current pastor Rhonda Britton said publicly that the church—named after the street it sits on, not Cornwallis the person—would undergo a name change to reflect the church's solidarity with the oppressed. This move speaks to a mythos among black Baptist women who, historically, have embraced the philosophy of racial self-help as they infused concepts such as equality, self-respect, professionalism, and nationalist identity with their own intentions and interpretations.[79] For instance, my grandmother, Lena Wilson, was a Baptist woman her entire life until she passed away in 2003 at the age of ninety-one. She ardently followed the ethos of Baptism, which was to espouse the importance of "manners and morals." For her, and other Baptist women like her, the concept of respectability signified self-esteem, racial pride, and something more—it signified the search for common ground on which to live as citizens with citizens of other racial and ethnic backgrounds.[80]

When Desmond sought the assistance of the Olivers, she was not just doing so because of the visible bruises and humiliation she had suffered at the hands of the Roseland Theatre staff and the New Glasgow police; it was also about her public image and the Baptist belief in cultivating a public self based on respectability. As Higginbotham writes further, "The Baptist women's adherence to temperance, cleanliness of person and property, thrift, polite manners, and sexual purity served to refute the logic behind their social subordination. The politics of respectability, as conceived by the black Baptist women, formed an integral part of the larger resistance that would eventually nullify unjust laws."[81] Pearleen Oliver had long believed in fighting to overturn unjust segregation practices in Nova Scotia. In 1944, she spearheaded a campaign of the Halifax Coloured Citizens Improvement League to remove from the province's public schools racially objectionable reading material such as *Little Black Sambo*, and she campaigned to eliminate racial barriers from the nursing profession.[82] It was Oliver, at Desmond's request, who sought public support from the Nova Scotia Association for the Advancement of Colored People (NSAACP), which led to Desmond's story being featured on the front page of the *Clarion*, a newspaper launched by Carrie Best, a black woman who also fought to end racial discrimination in Nova Scotia.

In 1941, Best had challenged long-standing racially segregated seating at the Roseland Theatre in New Glasgow, her hometown.[83] *The Clarion*, like other African Canadian newspapers before it, became an outlet for her to fight for racial equality. First published in 1945 as a single sheet, the newspaper later expanded into a church bulletin in 1946, and in 1947, it was incorporated as the Clarion Publishing Company Ltd.[84] The image used for Desmond's 2012 commemorative Canada Post stamp—her hair in a pageboy style, where the hair is straightened then curled under at the ends, with bangs—is taken from the December 31, 1946, issue of *The Clarion*. This hairstyle had become quite popular among middle-class African American women during the 1940s and 1950s. Variations on the pageboy hairstyle included "cluster curls," which was a modified pageboy: instead of bangs, the hair was curled in the front. "Chignons" and "feather curls," finely textured, layered hairstyles, were also deemed acceptable because they met the standards of the "Brownskin" ideal and were also deemed "most attractive" to men. In a November 1956 editorial in *Ebony*, for example, titled "Women's Hair Styles That Men Prefer," an unattrib-

THE CLARION

49 Connsval...

Published in the Interest of Colored Nova Scotians

VOL. 1., NO. 1.   NEW GLASGOW, N. S.   1946   DECEMBE..

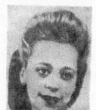

MRS. VIOLA DESMOND

Locals

The Season's Greetings to

All Our Readers

M.. and Mrs. James MacPhee have moved into their new home on South Albert Street.

Calbert Best, student at King's College, Halifax, will spend the Christmas recess with his parents, Mr. and Mrs. A. T. Best.

Congratulations are being extended to Rev. and Mrs. Thomas for their Christmas Calendar. It is a lovely job!

Miss Evelyn Williams, daughter of Mr. Norman Williams, stenographer with the Pay Roll Department at Ottawa, will be home on Dec. 20th to spend the Christmas holidays with her family.

Friends will be interested to know that Miss Thelma Parris, formerly of this town, has become an American citizen. She is making her home in Cambridge, where her mother, Mrs. Douglas Gordon, resides.

The Ladies' Auxiliary of Second Baptist Church held a successful sale and tea in the Church Hall on Dec. 10th. A lovely display of fancy work was noted.

Mr. and Mrs. Lemuel Mills left Saturday, Dec. 14, for Boston, where they will spend Christmas with their daughters, Mrs. Thornton Harper and Mrs. Bennie Shepherd.

Johnnie Mills met a deer—DEER, that is, recently, while driving his mother to Halifax. The deer darted out on the highway near Elmsdale and hit the side of the car. Not seriously injured, the deer soon scampered off, none the worse of the impact.

Word has been received that Miss Irma Halfkenney will be a participant in the St. John Music Festival in May. A student at Mount Allison School of Music, Miss Halfkenney is a soprano of promise, and that she will make a creditable showing goes without saying.

The Senior B. Y. P. U. of Second Baptist Church chartered a bus and motored to Riverton where they held a service for the inmates of the Pictou County Home. Among those who took part were Rev. H. D. Thomas, Howard Lawrence, Miss Althea Lawrence and Mrs. Gordon Clark. About twenty-five persons made the trip.

The Ladies' Auxiliary of the Second Baptist Church had a surprise party early in December for Rev. and Mrs. Thomas, at the Parsonage, Washington St. The gifts included china, linen, etc., and each gift was accompanied by an original verse. Typical of the verses was the one accompanying the crocheted doily gift of President Mrs. L. Mills:

"I may be small, but my mission is great, I'm here to decorate your cake plate. Your cakes I have are a treat to eat, So use me when next your guests you treat."

Takes Action

Mrs. Viola Desmond, 32-year-old Negro beautician, arrested and fined $20 and costs by Magistrate Rod G. MacKay, of this town, for sitting downstairs in the Roseland Theatre while holding an upstairs ticket.

Mrs. Desmond was fined for defrauding the Federal Government of one cent, the difference in the Amusement tax on an upstairs ticket of two cents and a downstairs ticket of three cents.

Counsel for Mrs. Desmond, F. W. Bisset of Halifax, has served a writ against Henry MacNeil, manager of the theatre, charging false arrest, false imprisonment, assault and malicious persecution.

E. M. Macdonald, K.C., of New Glasgow, is acting for Mr. MacNeil.

Mrs. Desmond, the former Viola Davis, daughter of Mr. and Mrs. James Davis, of Halifax, is well known throughout the Province. She is a graduate of the Halifax High School, and is also a graduate in Beauty Culture from a leading Beauty College in New York. She is a niece of John Davis, Civil Service employee (Post Office Division), Halifax.

Viola Desmond's Appeal

Just as we go to press we are in receipt of a letter from Mrs. Bernice Williams, Sec'y N. S. A. A. C. P., informing us that an appeal trial of the Viola Desmond case will be held in Halifax on Dec. 27th, also a Viola Desmond Court Fund has been established by the Association soliciting contributions. A public meeting will be held by the Association on Dec. 22nd in Halifax asking everyone to attend and give their donation.

The N. S. A. A. C. P. is the Ladder to Advancement. STEP ON IT! JOIN TODAY!

Did You Know?

(a) That Adult education in rural communities is being sponsored by the N. S. A. A. C. P.

(b) That the Educational Department of the Province of Nova Scotia is supporting the movement.

(c) That a class has already started in Hammonds Plains and is progressing favourably.

(d) That the C.G. I. T. group of Cornwallis Street Baptist Church, Halifax, raised the sum of $35.00 at their Christmas Sale. Mrs. Oliver is leader and all girls are under 16 years.

(e) That the money will be used for the work of the Summer Camp at Fall River.

(f) That Mr. Horborn, of Fall River, gave the use of an island near the Cornwallis Street Church camp site for the promotion of the Young People's work of that Church.

(g) That two Colored girls are enrolled as student nurses in two Halifax hospitals. They are Miss Gwendolyn Barton of Halifax and Miss Ruth Bailley of Toronto.

(h) That J. Calbert Best of King's College, Halifax, will write for the Afro-American, one of the largest weekly Negro newspapers in the U. S. A. Mr. Best has been asked to prepare a 700-word article on Canada. The weekly circulation of the Afro is 200,000.

The N. S. A. A. C. P.

The Nova Scotia Association for the Advancement of the Colored People was organized in 1945:

(a) To improve and further the interest of the Colored people of the Province.

(b) To provide an organization to encourage and promote a spirit of fraternity among its members.

(c) To co-operate with Governmental and private agencies for the promotion of the interest and the welfare of the Province or any community therein, wherein Colored People are resident, and particularly in reference to said Colored people.

(d) To improve the educational opportunities of Colored youth and to raise the standard of the Colored people of the Province or any community therein.

The following people comprise the charter members of the Association:

Arnold P. Smith, Richard Symonds, William Carter, Bernice A. Williams, Carl W. Oliver, Walter Johnson, Pearleen Oliver, William P. Oliver and Ernest Grosse.

Join the N. S. A. A. C. P.

Write BERNICE A. WILLIAMS, Sec'y

186 Maynard Street.

Halifax, N. S.

Figure 8. Viola Desmond on the front page of *The Clarion*, December 1946. Nova Scotia Archives, Microfilm 4350.

uted writer told readers that men preferred women who looked "feminine," which meant longer hair, not "mannish" cuts.[85] The assumption was not only that all black women wanted shiny, wavy hair and would not hesitate to straighten and style their hair to achieve this look, but that long straightened hair (coupled with light skin) was the only measure of black beauty.

In the 1950s, white women popularized short hairdos, especially the pixie. Most notably, Leslie Caron and Audrey Hepburn introduced the style in the films *An American in Paris* (1951) and *Roman Holiday* (1953), respectively. As Grant McCracken observes, "They gave the look new credentials. They made it a refuge for women who wished to escape the big hair enthusiasms of 1950s America and embrace something more continental, artistic, sophisticated and even slight *demi-monde*. The pixie was a way out of the '50s construction of self."[86] In the pages of *Ebony*, however, black women were told to avoid short hair in favour of more "feminine" hairstyles like the pageboy. Throughout the 1940s and 1950s, *Ebony* positioned the "Brownskin" as the embodiment of black progress, but this depiction was not without criticism. In her study of letters to the editor in *Ebony* and *Negro Digest*, Joanne Meyerowitz found that reactions to the "Brownskin" model's display of femininity, beauty, and middle-class respectability ranged from disgust at the "immoral" displays of sexualized femininity to appreciation of the "racial advancement" of beauty as inclusive of African American women.[87] The portrayal of happy marriages, successful careers, dutiful motherhood, and efforts to stay physically fit all while "having fun" rendered the "Brownskin" model in *Ebony* not merely commercial models, but "also as models for African American womanhood. Presented to the average woman was the ultimate ideal of African American middle-class womanhood—balancing glamourous work with home and husband and attaching greater status to the husband's job."[88] Middle-class black women of the 1940s and 1950s typically wore their hair in one of four pageboy styles. Some continued to wear their hair short in a pixie or bob either because they liked the style or because their hair had never grown to the lengths that other looks demanded, but most black magazines frowned upon either hairstyle. Importantly, the "feminine" hairstyles projected onto middle-class black women required false hair attachments for length and texture. The market for "falsies," as they were called, also boomed in the postwar era.

According to a June 1947 *Ebony* feature, four million African American women used an average of two cranial falsies each year to achieve the above hairstyles. The feature, titled "Hair Attachments," explained that before World War II, China had been a huge exporter of hair to the United States, but it shut its doors after the United States entered the war in 1941. "During the war years, no hair imports were coming through save from India but today the market is flooded and a genuine boom in freshly-styled wigs and pompadours is in full swing," *Ebony* noted.[89] Two of the biggest hair attachment firms at the time were the Howard Wig Company and Bell and Hudgins Company, both located in Harlem. In comparing a sample of hair from 1919 with some 1947 samples, the article continued, "both leading hair attachment firms see emerging a new type of Negro hair, 'less kinky, more wavy, finer-textured.'"[90] In addition to China, other countries, such as Italy, Czechoslovakia, Sweden, and Norway were also key exporters of hair. The *Ebony* article explained that the sterilization of the hair involved a twenty-two-hour boiling process during which one-sixth of the raw hair was lost. The likes of Madam C. J. Walker and Viola Desmond might have offered solutions to black women, but their products could not produce the miracle of long, flowing hair so many desired.

Significantly, by the late 1940s, *Ebony* was littered with advertisements from hair businesses in New York and Chicago selling not just hair attachments but also the image of straightened hair as the epitome of the "Brownskin" beauty ideal. As of 1946, *Ebony* was also available in Canada and "Pan-American Countries" (as they were listed on its pages) for four dollars a year, and single copies were priced at thirty cents. If the "falsies" market continued to grow throughout the decade in the United States, interest in hair attachments undoubtedly grew in Canada, as well. That same year, *Ebony* paid special attention to black Canada in a December 1946 four-page editorial titled, "Canada's Crimeless Colored Community," in which the magazine described to African Americans the complexity of black Canada's demographics. "Most of [Canada's black population] are the descendants of the more than 50,000 slaves who fled the South via the Underground Railroad to Canada. The bulk of the others are British West Indians and their offspring," *Ebony* explained.[91] At the same time, *Ebony* pointed out to readers that, in the absence of a Jim Crow policy, a de facto colour line still impacted black life north of the border. "Despite the lack of any segregation in Canada," the magazine stated, "there are several virtually all-Negro communities in the country, mainly in Ontario where most of the Fugitives from slavery ended their perilous journey to the North."[92] *Ebony* made mention of black Nova Scotia, but it mostly highlighted the southwestern Ontario town of North Buxton, a rich farming district at the time that also had a dwindling population because of a "lack of jobs for its young people, who have been going to the United States," the magazine concluded.[93] This editorial stands as a reminder that *Ebony* stood as arguably the most important transnational black media outlet in the postwar years, not only disseminating editorials on black culture, but also cultivating an image of blackness with respect to culture, appearance, and respectability.

Hair attachments were popular with black women because many continued to suffer hair loss and damage to the scalp due to insufficient hair care products and/or improper straightening techniques. Many black women continued to long for solutions to an age-old problem—hair that did not stay "straight" for extended periods. While hot combs or thermal methods of hair straightening may have "straightened" the hair, when met with humidity, rain, sweat, or physical activities such as swimming, the hair reverted back to its natural state, a process often known as "turning back." Around 1940, chemical hair straighteners—known as "perms" or "relaxers"— made with sodium hydroxide (lye) were introduced to the mass market.[94] These products offered a solution to the "turning back" problem. As noted in chapter 1, since the nineteenth century, lye had been used as a chemical to straighten black women's hair, but when formulated as a chemical treatment, it straightened the hair and prevented the treated hair from "turning back" for several weeks. Chemical hair-straightening products also provided a "safer" alternative to pure lye because it did not burn the scalp as severely, and people believed it was less damaging to the hair follicle. By the late 1940s, several men developed businesses built around chemical hair-straightening methods. While Mexican-born José Baraquiel Calva was the first of these men, he could not have promoted his products to the extent that he did if not for *Ebony* magazine.

In 1948, Calva's company, the St. Paul, Minnesota–based Lustrasilk, announced in *Ebony* that its product was "a gift to humanity from a distinguished scientist…long lasting hair beauty, your dream of dreams has come true!"[95] The company's advertisement also subtly addressed the "turning back" problem: "Swing, dance, work, play effective, safe, clean and wholesome, professional."[96] The chemical straightener, Lustrasilk Permanent, was available to licensed beauty shops as of May of that year in New York, Baltimore, Atlanta, Philadelphia, Chicago, Birmingham, St. Louis, Detroit, Memphis, Cleveland, New Orleans, and Washington, DC. Like Anthony Overton's Ro-Zol bleach product, which was not originally intended for use on black women's skin, Lustrasilk Permanent was not originally intended for hair care. In June 1948, Calva, in a feature in *Ebony* titled "New Hair Culture Discovery," explained that his venture into black hair straightening occurred while he was searching for a process to turn raw sheepskin into luxury furs.[97] Noliwe Rooks posits that Lustrasilk argued that black women's lives would be "substantially changed by the purchase of this product. If African American women want a 'different' life, complete with 'beauty, comfort and lasting peace of mind' as well as a 'smile of confidence,' they must use this product."[98] The chemical relaxer was the first advancement in black hair care since the Walker System's shampoo-press-and-curl, and even though it was not created with "racial uplift" in mind, it signalled and affirmed to black women (and some men) that straightened hair equalled beauty. By the early 1950s, several other chemical hair straighteners hit the market, such as Ultra Wave Hair Culture, Silky Strate, Perma-Strate, Hair Strate, and Sulpher-8. These products would not appear in advertisements in black Canadian newspapers until the late 1960s.

Between the 1940s and 1950s, however, only a few black Canadian newspapers were in circulation. In addition to *The Clarion*, there was *Africa Speaks* (1953), and for a few months, the *Afro-Beacon* did just as the *Canadian Observer* had done during World War I, encouraging blacks to assist with World War II efforts.[99] In 1949, when Best sought national circulation for *The Clarion* under a new name, the *Negro Citizen*, the costs of the venture proved to be disastrous; subscription rates subsequently doubled, circulation declined, and the newspaper eventually folded in 1956.[100] The newspaper was instrumental in shining a light onto Desmond's case, helping her hire a lawyer to appeal her conviction, but in the end, her case was dismissed. In 1947, Desmond graduated her first large class of students from her beauty school; many of her students subsequently found employment in various parts of Nova Scotia, New Brunswick, and Quebec, but within a few years, she ended up closing down her beauty shop, abandoning her product line, and moving to the United States.[101] Desmond had planned to establish a business in New York, but she fell ill, and on February 7, 1965, at the age of 50, she died of a gastrointestinal hemorrhage. Desmond's refusal to adhere to the Roseland Theatre's policy of segregation occurred nine years before Rosa Parks refused to give up her seat on a Montgomery bus. If racism had not stalled Viola Desmond's beauty business, instead of drawing comparisons to Rosa Parks we might be remembering her as Canada's Madam C. J. Walker. The Desmond story ultimately illustrates the fact that tolerance, as an ideological concept, does very little to shift discriminatory practices when prejudice and racism are deeply embedded within institutional structures as well as within the minds of tight-knit communities who see racial diversity as posing a threat to their "way of life."

Significantly, while *The Clarion* contained few advertisements for hair salons or barbershops (in the small and closed black communities within cities like Halifax, such advertising was scarcely needed, since an effective grapevine kept black people informed of where their patronage was

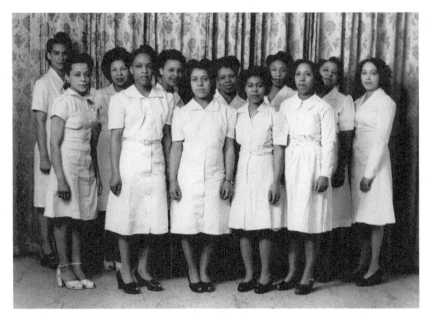

Figure 9. Viola Desmond with School of Beauty Culture graduates, ca. 1947. Wanda and Joe Robson Collection, MG 21.14, 16-87-30227. Beaton Institute, Cape Breton University.

welcomed), a rare advertisement for a line of hair products called Mirror Tone appeared in February 1949.[102] The product was offered for sale "coast to coast" and a photograph of a black woman and man with straightened hair accompanied its slogan, "Use Mirror Tone Hair Products to Beautify Your Hair." Along with pomade and glossine, pressing oils were also included in Mirror Tone's product line. The Mirror Tone advertisement contained a list of retail locations (and private homes) where patrons could buy the products: New Glasgow (McLeod's Drug Store), Glace Bay (Miss Shirley King), Truro (Mrs. Merle Chase), and Halifax (Pat's Beauty Parlor). Where by the 1880s, pharmaceutical houses, perfumers, beauty salons, drugstores, wholesale suppliers, mail order, and department stores had all provided the infrastructure for beauty culture geared toward white women,[103] there was no such infrastructure for beauty culture geared toward black women in Canada, and to a lesser extent, in the United States. Thus, local distribution networks like the above, especially in tight-knit black communities in the Maritimes, were extremely important.

As early as 1917, the United Drug Company, which distributed Rexall products, dispatched product demonstrators to small-town drugstores

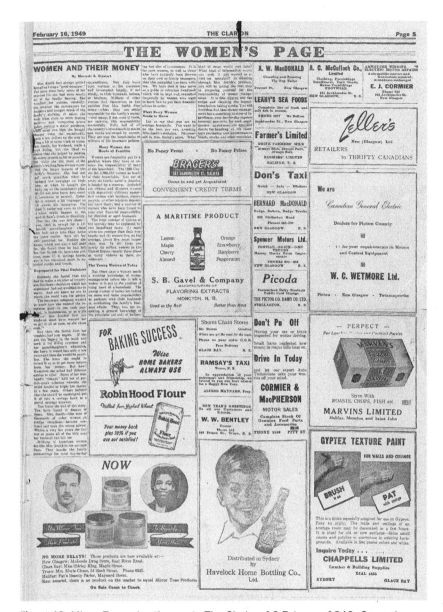

Figure 10. Mirror Tone advertisement, *The Clarion*, 16 February 1949. General Collection, Beinecke Rare Book & Manuscript Library, Yale University.

in the United States.[104] By the early 1920s, both drugstores and department stores in America were regularly sponsoring "beauty marts" and "beauty weeks" filled with lectures, makeup sessions, and free samples.[105] In Canada, when *Chatelaine* magazine launched in 1928, in addition to newsstands and bookstores, it was also available for sale at drugstores.[106] With respect to drugstores and the infrastructure for beauty culture geared toward black women, there has been little research on the role small-scale retailers played in the expansion of not just black Canadian beauty culture but Canadian beauty culture in general prior to the 1970s. It is therefore difficult to know what other products were advertised to black women consumers. *The Clarion*'s Mirror Tone advertisement ultimately holds a lot of significance because it is one of the few glimpses into African Canadian beauty culture at a time when racial segregation was rampant as well as when there was no defined distribution network for black beauty products in Canada. Through it, we gain deeper understanding of how black beauty products were distributed, albeit on a much smaller scale than in the United States, before large-scale promotional campaigns appeared in the 1970s.

Importantly, the image of middle-class femininity in *The Clarion*, as in *Ebony*, mirrored the images of white womanhood that proliferated women's magazines such as *Chatelaine* in the 1940s and 1950s. When Max Factor, Helena Rubinstein, Avon, and other cosmetics firms entered Canada in the postwar years, each geared their products and advertisements exclusively toward white, middle-class women who were homemakers and mothers. In the decades that followed the war, mass media increasingly tied cosmetics to notions of feminine identity and self-fulfillment, proliferating images of flawless female beauty—mostly youthful, white, and increasingly sexualized women. For the woman of the 1940s who had survived the Depression and a world war, cosmetics bespoke an "American way of life" and a free society worth defending; white women who wore makeup became global commodities and symbols, exported in Hollywood films and promoted by cosmetics firms.[107] When these firms advertised in *Chatelaine*, it reflected economic expansion but also signified the reification of the American pursuit of individual happiness in Canada. The first beauty mogul of the twentieth century to expand into Canada was Max Factor.

Born Maksymilian Faktorowicz in Poland in 1877, Factor brought theatrical makeup to the mass retail market. After immigrating to the United States in 1904, and after four years in St. Louis, Factor moved to Los Angeles in 1908 and quickly established a barbershop, wig business, and makeup studio.[108] In 1920, he introduced Society Makeup, a cosmetic line for everyday use, but it was not until 1927 that he achieved national distribution, and a year later, Factor's first advertisements ran in mass-circulation movie and romance magazines.[109] In August 1940, Max Factor of Hollywood announced in *Chatelaine* magazine that it had arrived in Canada "with the make-up secrets of the screen's beautiful stars."[110] Using the image of RKO radio star Irene Dunne, the advertisement was the first from a global makeup firm to appear in the Canadian women's magazine. Apart from Max Factor, the only pre–World War II makeup companies that managed to grow into global corporations were Maybelline and Revlon, founded in 1914 and 1932 respectively. Both companies began as specialty firms—Maybelline producing mascara, Revlon nail polish—but grew after the war into general cosmetics firms. Andrew Tobias found that "the year lipstick was added to Revlon's line of nail-care products, 1940, sales more than doubled over the previous year, to $2.8 million."[111] During the postwar years, Factor's biggest rivals were Helena Rubinstein and Elizabeth Arden, who also launched their businesses around the turn of the century. Unlike Factor, who singularly attached cosmetics to Hollywood and stage actors, Rubinstein and Arden each opened beauty salons that emphasized the importance of skin care and the luxuriousness of cosmetics.[112] By all accounts, the development of the modern makeup industry was in large part due to Rubinstein's and Arden's efforts.

Like Factor before her, Rubinstein was born in Poland in 1870. She arrived in the United States following the outbreak of World War I and opened her first salon in New York City in 1915. Arden, whose real name is Florence Nightingale Graham, was born in Woodbridge, Ontario, in 1884. When her elder brother moved to New York City in 1908, she followed him and eventually ended up working for a pharmaceutical company where she learned about skin care products. After changing her name to Elizabeth Arden, she opened a beauty shop and in 1918 began selling products.[113] Both women strategically placed advertisements in women's magazines such as *Town and Country* and *Vogue*, which targeted the specific consumers (upper-class white women) they both sought.[114] Their advertisements in *Chatelaine* were also geared toward a similar demographic. Rubinstein and Arden followed Factor's lead with advertisements in May 1944 and February 1945 editions of *Chatelaine*.[115] In September 1945, an advertisement in *Chatelaine* for Rubinstein's skin-toning lotion and face cream proclaimed, "Many, many ladies there are whose beauty lies a-drowsing because they've trusted to luck instead of logic, and dreams instead of creams. Here are special awakening aids by Helena Rubinstein—preparations fashioned with scientific care, and skillfully designed to arouse dormant loveliness."[116] In September 1953, Elizabeth Arden told *Chatelaine* readers: "TODAY is the time to consider the future and Start Building Beauty."[117] "Use the famous Elizabeth Arden Essentials night and morning to cleanse, refresh and smooth...be loyal to Elizabeth Arden's matchless makeup...and realize that fine preparations are an economy in the end," the ad declared. In November 1945, advertisements from Avon appeared in *Chatelaine*.[118]

Avon, with its door-to-door sales strategy, made cosmetics accessible to the middle-class homemaker on a budget. Founded in 1886 by David H. McConnell, the California Perfume Company changed its name to Avon in 1929. Significantly, the company never marketed its products under the allure of luxury; instead, it emphasized convenience and affordability. Although the company had been in Canada since the 1930s, the 1940s marked a period when it increasingly advertised in Canadian women's magazines. In June 1946 an Avon advertisement proclaimed, "Let Beauty be Brought to You!"[119] The advertisement also instructed readers on how to purchase Avon products in the "privacy of your own home through the well-informed Avon Representative who calls on you with these exquisite preparations." By 1952, Avon established its Canadian headquarters in Montreal to directly appeal to its Canadian customers' growing interest in lower-cost cosmetics.

While some of these firms had targeted the black beauty market since the early twentieth century, in the 1950s and 1960s these companies made concerted efforts to cultivate black female consumers. African American Avon representatives, for example, first appeared in black neighbourhoods in the 1940s, and Avon established ties to the black cosmetics market by placing advertisements in *Ebony* magazine as early as 1961.[120] From the 1940s onward, the beauty industry in the United States fit into three categories: dedicated cosmetics makers, large consumer-products companies, and proprietary drug producers. Canada's beauty industry, by comparison, was still largely a localized sector with boutiques, mail-order operations, and select products available for sale at small-scale drugstores—this was true for white women and black women alike. When Estée Lauder entered the beauty culture market, however, the breadth of American beauty culture expanded beyond the United States and Canada to Europe and Asia.

In 1930, Josephine Esther (Esty) Mentzer married Joseph Lauter; a few years later, she changed her married name from Lauter to Lauder, and thereafter she was known as Estée Lauder.[121] By 1946, the Lauders had founded Estée Lauder Cosmetics, targeting a small number of fine department stores such as Saks Fifth Avenue, Neiman-Marcus, Bloomingdale's, and Marshall Field's. By the 1950s, Lauder's products were competing alongside those of Factor, Rubinstein, Arden, and Revlon, expanding eventually into the fragrances market. In 1968, Estée Lauder's products were also available for purchase at Eaton's. In March of that year, the department store advertised in the *Toronto Telegram* the arrival of Estée Lauder cosmetics at its Queen Street, College Street, Don Mills, and Yorkdale locations in Toronto.[122] Yorkdale Shopping Centre had opened on February 26, 1964. It represented the growth of Toronto's northern suburb of North York and the expansion of department-store shopping—Yorkdale was the first mall in Canada to house two department stores, Eaton's and Simpson's—beyond the city's downtown core, where most of its shopping had taken place before the 1960s. By the early 1970s, firms like Revlon began to realize the untapped market potential of the black community; before then, however, the Revlons, L'Oréals, Max Factors, Estée Lauders, and Helena Rubinsteins of the beauty culture industry ignored black women altogether, and until the late 1960s, Hollywood, television, magazines, and even Miss America contests had ignored black women, as well.

Thus, the consistent deployment of the image of the "Brownskin" in black magazines in the postwar era participated in producing a new iconographic understanding of African American womanhood, redressing the denigrating and pervasive stereotypes of black women in the dominant media culture, but such imagery did little to disrupt dominant understandings of racial and gender identity.[123] Similar to the skin-bleaching advertisements in the Negro press in the 1920s, black women in the pages of *Ebony* through the 1940s and 1950s were still being told to lighten their skin in order to attract black men and achieve beauty. For editors, these products were uncontroversial—so much so that it caught them by surprise when in 1966, as Kathy Peiss notes, readers "complained about the magazine's long-time depiction of black women, which featured models and beauty queens with European features, light complexions, and straightened hair."[124]

Nadinola, the skin-bleaching cream manufactured by the J. Strickland Co., of Memphis, Tennessee, also advertised in *Ebony* on a regular basis. The white-owned company first entered the black hair care market in 1936, marketing such products as Royal Crown and Magnificent in addition to its skin-bleaching cream Nadinola. In one of the first issues of *Ebony* in 1946, however, a Nadinola advertisement featured a light-skinned woman with straightened hair and a caption that read, "There's no greater beauty price than a light, clear, smooth complexion. And there's no better way to win lovelier skin than with the help of NADINOLA Bleaching Cream."[125] By 1957, Nadinola's advertisements continued to instruct *Ebony* readers that the product provided "a complexion he'll love to remember...so clear and bright and kissable."[126] Importantly, *Ebony* also drew upon foreign examples to help in its construction of the "Brownskin" ideal. One such example appeared in the magazine's February 1956 issue in a report on Jamaica's "Ten Types, One People" beauty contest.[127]

With a headline reading "Ten Types of Colors of Beauties Emphasize Racial Harmony of West Indian Island," *Ebony*'s article featured a photograph of the contestants, with a description for each participant. There was "Miss Ebony," for black-complexioned women; "Miss Mahogany," for women of "cocoa-brown complexion"; "Miss Satinwood," for "girls of coffee-and-milk complexion"; "Miss Golden Apple," for "Jamaican women with a peaches and cream complexion"; "Miss Apple Blossom," for "a Jamaican girl of white European parentage"; "Miss Pomegranate," for "white Mediterranean women"; "Miss Sandalwood," for women of "pure Indian parentage;" "Miss Lotus," who was a "pure Chinese woman"; "Miss Jasmine," for "a Jamaican girl of part Chinese parentage"; and "Miss Allspice" for "part-Indian" women. While *Ebony* viewed "Ten Types" as proof of a racial paradise that might offer hope to blacks in America, it failed to grasp the nuances of race that had historically divided Jamaican society.[128]

Starting in the 1940s, beauty contests in Jamaica had been open exclusively to white Creole girls (i.e., whites born in the Caribbean). The first beauty pageant, the Miss Jamaica contest, was held in Kingston in a racial landscape where femininity was the guarded domain of white Jamaican females and they were put on a pedestal for what Natasha Barnes describes as "respectability and civility that was denied to black people in general and black females in particular."[129] The contest was, from the outset, a politicized event because of its white bias, which excluded the black majority of the population in addition to Chinese and East Indian Jamaicans from participation.[130] Andrea Shaw writes, "The ideological disparity between the ethnicity of the contestants and the racial composition of the Jamaican population drew varying efforts to placate an increasingly disenchanted public."[131] Thus, "Ten Types" was an attempt to universalize a feminine standard by showing that women of different racialized bodies could conform to a recognizable Western ideal, an ideal that had long established that in addition to light skin, beauty queens also had to be slim and petite in frame. The contest also affirmed that there was a universal beauty standard to which all Jamaican women had to conform to, and one that the islands' various ethnic groups needed to mimic to *become* modern women.

Another example of the African American press's lack of understanding concerning Jamaica's racial politics occurred in 1954, when the first Miss Jamaica winner, Evelyn Andrade, a woman with a Syrian-Jewish father and a "coloured" mother, appeared at the Miss Universe contest. In November of that year, *Ebony* magazine declared, "Jamaican girl is the first Negro to enter top beauty contest."[132] In his examination of slave dress in Jamaica, Steeve Buckridge found that *whites* in this context referred to people from Europe or those of unmixed European descent, including locally born whites; and whereas in the United States, as he explains, "all persons of African ancestry, of whatever degree, were categorized as Negro, or black,"[133] in Jamaica, *coloured* persons consisted of all people of African-and-another ancestry. Thus, where for *Ebony*, blackness was identified through the presence of a black progenitor, in Jamaica, the progressive whitening of the island's elite "mulatto" caste (coloureds) made individuals of Andrade's background—irrespective of black ancestry—white to most Jamaicans.[134] In the parade of feminine beauty at Jamaica's beauty pageants, the array of light-brown beauty queens may have outwardly suggested "the pre-eminence of brownness as a social category in the ascendency, worthy of broad national representation"[135] but for black Jamaicans, it symbolically represented the valorization of whiteness as the ideal beauty.

Historically, light-skinned women have been the overwhelming favourites to win the Miss Jamaica title, despite public outcry. When Lisa Mahfood, a light skinned, straight-haired Jamaican of Middle Eastern ancestry, was crowned Miss Jamaica in 1986, for example, the crowd erupted in shouts and jeers and hurled debris on the stage. Even though Miss Jamaica 2015, Sanneta Myrie, was the first contestant with dreadlocks to win the crown, she was also light-skinned. In 2017, however, Miss Jamaica broke all the rules when she appeared at the Miss Universe pageant. Davina Bennett, a twenty-three-year-old model and philanthropist who is dark-skinned, wore an Afro hairstyle during the competition. "I did not win but I got what I was seeking," she wrote on Instagram following the competition, "I stand as the first Afro queen to have made it thus far."[136] While Bennett is a welcome change to the norm, ultimately, since the 1950s there have been few exceptions to the straight-hair rule that has been the unequivocal standard of beauty for black women in the beauty pageant world.

When George E. Johnson entered the chemical relaxer business in the 1950s, his products had the biggest impact on the demand for chemical hair straighteners. Johnson is often referred to as a pioneer of the black hair care industry because he was the first African American to take his company public in 1971, when Johnson Products became the first black-owned firm to be traded on the American Stock Exchange. Born in Mississippi in 1927, Johnson began his career as a chemist for the Fuller Products Company, founded by Samuel Fuller (publisher of two African American newspapers, the *New York Age* and *Pittsburgh Courier*). In the early 1950s, Johnson collaborated with a Chicago barber, Orville Nelson, to improve a hair-straightening product that he used in his barbershop.[137] After consulting another chemist at Fuller Products, in 1954, they developed Ultra Wave Hair Culture, a chemical straightening system ("relaxer") that could be purchased at retail and applied at home.[138] Johnson perfected the formula by mixing lye with petroleum instead of potatoes. During and after slavery, lye was the most toxic chemical used to straighten black hair. Women (and men) would mix it with potatoes to decrease its caustic nature and apply it to their hair. Black women would also put butter or bacon fat on their hair, then straighten the hair with a butter knife heated in a can over a fire as a crude version of a hot comb.[139] This was an extremely painful process. Johnson's invention made hair straightening less painful, but, as I explain in chapter 3, it did not eradicate the pain entirely.

There are three reasons why Johnson, rather than José Baraquiel Calva, is credited as being the first inventor of the chemical relaxer. First, Johnson's Ultra Wave Hair Culture was the first straightening system that could be purchased at retail and applied at home; unlike Calva's Lustrasilk, it did not require a visit to a salon (in 1956, Lustrasilk offered a permanent straightener that could be applied at home). Second, by 1964 Johnson's company recorded $1 million in revenues, due in large part to the launch of the Ultra Sheen Permanent Creme Relaxer in 1958, which catapulted Johnson to the top of the black hair care industry.[140] Third, as noted above, Johnson Products became the first publicly traded African American company and black beauty firm, and as such, he was celebrated as an innovator. In January 1963, for example, Johnson's picture appeared in the *Chicago Daily Defender* in a feature titled "How the Male Entered Beauty Culture Field."[141] The article spoke of the black woman beauty culturists—Madam C. J. Walker, Annie Malone, and Sara Spencer Washington—who had created the black hair care industry, and went on to say that hair care was increasingly becoming a black man's business, in which Johnson was seen as the pre-eminent force. These factors all combined to catapult Johnson and his Ultra Sheen product line to the top of the black hair care industry by the early 1960s. It is important to note, however, that chemical relaxers are not truly "permanent." These products are called "permanents" or "relaxers" because they straighten or relax tightly coiled hair without thermal combs and because they also keep the hair straight for weeks at a time; for these same reasons, they have always been marketed as "freedom" products. In 1964, for instance, the *Chicago Daily Defender* noted that more women were becoming aware of chemical hair relaxers, showing more interest, and adopting this "modern method of hair care."[142] The article estimated that five out of every hundred women chose relaxers over other methods. "The working girl finds it brings assurance of being well-groomed without the fuss and bother of previous hair care methods. The housewife discovers daily chores can be completed leaving the hair well groomed and suitable for attending any evening affair," the editorial explained. "Professional women can enjoy an impeccable hair appearance throughout the day. Even school girls have discovered this modern type of hair technique permits them to participate in all sports and yet be presentable for other activities. The little girl can be taken out on spur-of-the-moment trips without worry about her hair."

While older women continued to use the Walker hot-comb method of hair straightening, throughout the 1950s the chemical relaxer became the most popular hair-straightening method among young black women, especially middle-class women, in large part because it minimized the "turning back" problem attached to thermal straightening. Straightened hair was more than just a preference; it also signalled one's progressive social status. Since I was a child, my mother has often shared stories of her experiences working in an office environment in Jamaica, and how, when she immigrated to Canada, she maintained a professional appearance, which included thermally straightened hair. In fact, chemical straightening was so popular in the postwar era that even African American men were encouraged to straighten their hair. Hairstyles such as "the conk," famously worn by Duke Ellington and heavyweight boxing champion Joe Lewis, had also been a popular style among black men since the 1920s. Spike Lee's 1992 film *Malcolm X*, based on Alex Haley's *The Autobiography of Malcolm X* (1965), famously captured how black men "conked" their hair. The chemical process contained harsh amounts of lye that could, if applied improperly, result in severe scalp burns. The conk had even been popular among members of the Harlem Renaissance, and when these artists immigrated to Paris in the 1920s, Petrine Archer-Straw observes, they "bleached their skins, straightened and conked their hair ... in order to

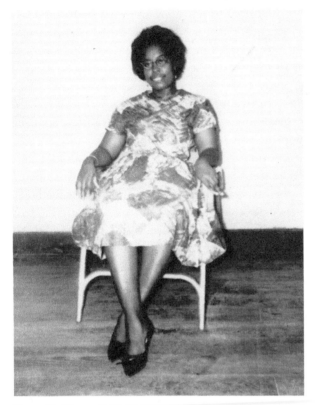

Figure 11. Thermally straightened hair: my mother, Syrilin
Thompson, Toronto, 1960s.

assimilate better."[143] Josephine Baker, for example, famously wore her hair
in a short, lacquered hairstyle. By the 1950s, Murray's Hair Pomade and
King Konk, leading producers of hair-straightening products for men, simply filled a desire among black men that had existed for decades. Between
1964 and 1966, however, "coloured people" and "Negroes" became "black"
and, with this name change, black people on a global scale began to adopt
a new, African-identified visual aesthetic, known as the Afro.

In the 1950s, the earliest female Afro wearers came from the fringes
of African American society—avant-garde artists, intellectuals, and elite
urban trendsetters[144]—and, as Robin D. G. Kelley notes, in some bourgeois high fashion circles in the late 1950s "the Afro was seen by the black
and white elite as a kind of new female exotica.... The Afro entered public
consciousness as a mod fashion statement that was not only palatable to
bourgeois whites but, in some circles, celebrated."[145] However, against the

backdrop of the assassination of two African American activists, Medgar Evers and Malcolm X, the rise of the Black Panther Party, founded by Huey Newton and Bobby Seale in 1966, and the work of other activists such as Stokely Carmichael, the movement that became known as Black Power gave new symbolic meaning to the hairstyle. In Canada, Black Power could be seen in the formation of the Black United Front of Nova Scotia (also known as BUF, this was a Black Nationalist organization founded by Burnley "Rocky" Jones in Halifax in 1965 that modelled itself after the Black Panther Party), Halifax's Kwacha House, and Toronto's West Indian Federation Club, the venue used to launch Austin Clarke's early novels. The Congress of Black Writers held at McGill University in October 1968, followed by the February 1969 protest at Sir George Williams University—in which mostly black West Indian students occupied the computer room in an act of protest against the alleged racism of a white professor—also announced that a socio-political shift was occurring within Canada's black communities.[146]

Black Power was not only about political and social change and the reclaiming of Africa as the literal and symbolic homeland for black people; it was also a celebration of the natural texture of black hair (hence the colloquial term "the natural"). The Afro, which stood as the primary hairstyle of the movement's leaders, became an aesthetic of political change and black self-love/knowledge. It was one of many cultural symbols and practices in the late 1960s that had a powerful message to convey about racial pride and solidarity. When black women and men stopped wearing wigs and stopped straightening with chemicals or conking their hair, it was initially a way to directly reject commercially promoted European standards of beauty. For the first time, Afros and other natural hairstyles such as braids and cornrows (or canerows, as they are called in the Caribbean) became the valorized signifiers of this new black beauty ideal. Importantly, black women continued to face tremendous socio-cultural pressures to straighten their hair, especially in the workplace. Susannah Walker found articles about the Afro "trend," written in the late 1960s, that mentioned that some women wore wigs over their naturals when at work in order to avoid trouble with white employers.[147] For the most part, before 1966, the Afro was hardly commercially popular, as the vast majority of black women continued to straighten their hair. Even during Black Power, black women continued to use chemical relaxers. For example, an article appearing in the *Chicago Daily Defender* in August 1966 promoted the arrival of a new relaxer, Epic Soft-Styling. The article began with a title that asked, "Why Use Chemicals for Modern Day Hair Care?" and went on to inform

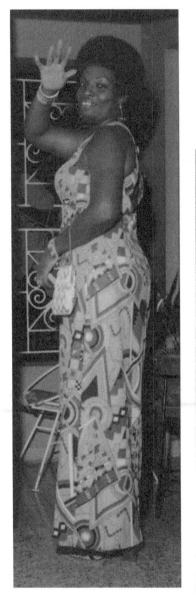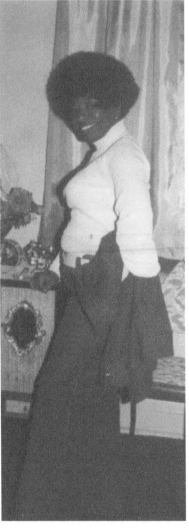

Figure 12. My cousin Dorothy Adams (left), family photograph, Yonkers, New York, 1972; and my godmother Cecilia Butler, family photograph, Toronto, Ontario, 1970s.

readers as follows: "Whether at home, work, play, school, church, or a social affair, the impeccable hair appearance throughout the day...should create greater confidence for a woman. Why? Because it makes her always ready to 'go,' rain or shine."[148] Significantly, the Afro was also complicated by skin colour.

For the first time, in the mid-1960s, dark-skinned women *became* beautiful—in some cases, more beautiful than light-skinned women. The darker one's pigment and the larger one's Afro, the more authentically "black" one was thought to be. This sentiment was also embedded within the "Black Is Beautiful" slogan, which became a badge worn by those in the movement. Even though political activist Angela Davis was (and remains) one of the symbols of Black Is Beautiful, she garnered most of her attention despite her light skin. Her famously large Afro contested the white beauty ideal, but it also gave light-skinned blacks (and some whites) permission to align themselves with the aesthetics of black liberation. For the first time, having light skin was a political liability. Some dark-skinned civil rights leaders even questioned the militancy of light-skinned blacks, believing that they had too long benefited from colour privilege to understand oppression. For most black women, however, the Afro was not just a political statement; it meant that, for the first time, when people said, "Black is beautiful," it was not in jest. In the hope of securing black business while at the same time acknowledging this socio-cultural shift, many white-owned companies were faced with increased pressures to make their products more racially inclusive. Several companies responded with strategies for market expansion and segmentation. Initially, however, many of these efforts did not include Afro styling products.

For instance, at the height of the Black Is Beautiful movement, Revlon developed a line of chemical relaxers, and Alberto-Culver and Clairol also expanded their appeals to black consumers with hair-straightening products.[149] By 1969, products from Raveen Hair Sheen to Afro Sheen to Ultra Sheen and other Afro hair care products dominated black hair care advertising. Clairol, however, which had courted black consumers since the early 1960s by placing advertisements for its hair colouring in *Ebony*, began to conduct research on potential black consumer markets for its products by sending representatives and demonstrators to black hair shows in order to sell products catering to the Afro.[150] In doing so, Clairol became the first white firm to attach itself to Black Is Beautiful. In 1968, other advertisements for Afro products, including Afro wigs, could be found in the pages of *Ebony*. A product called Raveen Au Naturelle appeared in the November

1968 issue with the caption, "easy-to-comb to condition your hair,"[151] and in December 1970, one's of Clairol's first advertisements for Afro products appeared.[152] The product, Afro hair setters, promised to "free the 'fro"; the ad stands as an example of how white-owned beauty firms began to co-opt the vernacular of Black Power and Black Is Beautiful. Clairol's use of slang vernacular not only trivialized the significance of black resistance, it diminished the political significance of the Afro itself.

Like Lustrasilk in the 1950s, Clairol failed to focus on what was naturally beautiful about black women's hair; instead, the company only pointed out what black women needed to fix. Of all the white-owned companies during this period, L'Oréal, a company founded in Paris in 1907 by French chemist Eugène Schueller and originally called the Société Française de Teintures Inoffensives pour Cheveux (the Safe Hair Dye Company of France), would become the most influential in the beauty culture industry. Initially, L'Oréal's primary product was hair dyes, and its primary market was Parisian hairdressers. By the 1950s, however, it became a competitor of the American brand Clairol in the global hair-colouring market. Clairol, launched in 1931 by Americans Lawrence M. Gelb and his wife, Joan Gelb, has been part of the personal care product division of the Procter & Gamble Company since 2001. Since 1959 Clairol has arguably been the leading American brand of hair dyes. The company's "Does she…or doesn't she?" advertising campaign, launched in 1956 helped to catapult it to top of the hair dye market, and throughout the 1960s, both Clairol and L'Oréal's advertising campaigns would help to transform blonde hair into a symbol of beauty.[153] The roots of the concept of "the blonde beauty" began in "the circum-Atlantic vortex in which whiteness covers over blackness."[154] Like the Victorian fashion of whitening one's skin, the blonde beauty was also a fabrication of British culture, and the use of blonde wigs, and the dying of one's hair, "expressed a need to artificially construct whiteness in an effort to emphasize difference—to make the whiteness of whiteness hypervisible."[155] By the early twentieth century, however, pageants and the emergent film industry had entrenched the notion of blondeness as a precursor for beauty.

In 1921, the first Miss America, Margaret Gorman, was a 15-year-old with blue eyes and blonde hair.[156] As the chemical hair-colouring process advanced through the 1920s, the first widely available commercial hair dyes became available first in Europe, and by the 1930s, the filmic heroine also had *become* blonde, blue-eyed, and white. Jean Harlow, for instance, created the iconic "platinum blonde" when she appeared in *Hell's Angels* (1930) and then *Platinum Blonde* (1931). A string of other Hollywood blonde films throughout the 1930s and 1940s, notably *Blonde Crazy* (1931), *Blonde Venus* (1932), *Blonde Fever* (1944), and *Blonde Trouble* (1944) further cemented blonde hair as a prerequisite for beauty. Even though Harlow was already blonde, when she came to Hollywood and Max Factor lightened her hair to a shade called "platinum blonde" she became a star. Harlow's look was widely replicated by other white women in Hollywood, such as Mae West, Marlene Dietrich, and Jayne Mansfield. Significantly, Harlow was one of the first blondes in Hollywood to garner the title of "blonde bombshell," but within a few years she fell ill and eventually died of kidney failure in 1937 at the age of 26.[157] In order to become platinum blonde, highly toxic substances such as peroxide, ammonia, and Clorox bleach were applied to Harlow's hair, chemicals that unequivocally contributed to her untimely death. By the 1950s, when the most famous blonde movie of all—*Gentlemen Prefer Blondes* (1953) starring Marilyn Monroe and Jane Russell—appeared, the trope of the blonde heroine as "light and fun" as opposed to dark-haired women as "knowing and dangerous"[158] had become a naturalized representation. When Clairol, which launched its hair dye campaign in 1955, conceived the idea of depicting the women in their advertisements as the girl next door, having colour-treated hair was no longer limited to actresses and high society mavens; now every woman could look like a movie star. As had been done with the use of lipstick and rouge in the late nineteenth century, dying one's hair was now represented to white women as a "natural" beautification practice.

To introduce its Miss Clairol home hair-colouring kit, the company created one of the most memorable advertising campaigns of the twentieth century with the phrase, "Does she...or doesn't she?" After the advertisement appeared in *Life* magazine in the fall of 1955, sales of the company's Hair Colour Bath soared. The women in Clairol advertisements were not glamorous models; instead, they looked like "attractive, everyday people." To attract these everyday people, the company ran advertisements featuring "mothers" with similarly blonde-haired "daughters." During this period, L'Oréal also produced a series of advertisements that claimed that its formulations were superior and more "natural" looking than those made by competitors, namely, Clairol. By the 1960s, hair dyes marked the return of a hypervisible form of whiteness: to go blonde was not singularly about changing one's hair colour, it was also about the construction of a new embodied gendered identity. In the pages of *Chatelaine* throughout the 1960s and 1970s, hair dye advertisements reflected white women's increased purchasing power while also piggybacking on the sexual revolution of the period.

In the 1960s, the inside front cover of almost every issue of *Chatelaine* was devoted to Miss Clairol products. The first of these advertisements appeared in October 1960. The full-page advertisement featured a close-up headshot of an attractive, well-coiffed brunette below the trademarked caption, "Does she . . . or doesn't she?" The model is leaning to one side while holding a child's toy. In the background, a young boy with blonde hair—presumably her son—is playing outside, perhaps at a park, and the text invites the viewer to look again and re-evaluate this image of a married woman: "Hair color so natural only her hairdresser knows for sure!" Clairol's message was clear—hair dyes were respectable, and married, middle-class women had a right to look beautiful, an image which dispelled previous notions that only women of disrepute "coloured" their hair.

Between 1960 and 1965 the women in Miss Clairol advertisements were always shown with a child, even though the image seemed at odds with the product's "Miss" name. In her biography, Shirley Polykoff, the creator of the Miss Clairol ads, confessed that she worried that the women in the ads would be interpreted as unwed mothers, so she halted production, and each model was then given a gold ring for her ring finger.[159] The Miss Clairol advertising campaign reflected the growing tension that emerged in the 1950s and 1960s between traditional and modern ideas about white womanhood. On the one hand, white women were becoming "liberated" from the domestic sphere, but on the other hand, marriage and children were still symbols of a normative, heterosexual feminine ideal. The valorization of white womanhood as the epitome of beauty had long marginalized black women. This dichotomy between the dominant beauty culture and black beauty culture was made most apparent in 1968 at the Miss America pageant. As the beauty pageant was under way on the boardwalk in Atlantic City, New Jersey, roughly a hundred (mostly white) women, who identified themselves as members of the women's liberation movement, dumped bras, girdles, makeup, curlers, hair spray, and other "beauty aids" into a trash can in protest of the contest, which they had equated with sexism and the exploitation of women. Several blocks away at the Ritz Carlton Hotel, the National Association for the Advancement of Colored People (NAACP) staged the first Miss Black America pageant as a "positive protest" against the exclusion of black women from the Miss America title. This protest sought to denounce the very idea of a beauty contest because "beauty" up until this point had been nothing more than a synonym for white womanhood. While the boardwalk protest captured the mainstream media's attention, as the image of unruly white women mocking symbols of American beauty was broadcast by the media as one of the first public displays of what become known as "second-wave feminism," the Miss Black America protest, as Maxine Leeds Craig argues, "*was* a beauty contest."[160] The 1968 Miss America protest is so set in the memory of second-wave feminists that today few even remember the Miss Black America pageant (or think of it as a protest) and others also forget that until the 1980s (Vanessa Williams in 1984) no black woman had been crowned Miss America. As Natasha Barnes notes, by contesting the racial bias of beauty pageants, "black feminists sought to challenge Eurocentric ideologies that denied their identity as women, however much this focus on 'negative imagery' may [have seemed] politically misguided to their white feminist sisters."[161]

While some black women participated in the protests and marches in support of the 1960s feminist movement, such as the Reverend Dr. Pauli Murray who, along with Betty Friedan, author of *The Feminine Mystique* (1963), had been instrumental in the founding of the National Organization for Women (NOW) in 1966, black women generally felt disconnected from women's liberation. As Lisa Farrington observes, many black women "believed themselves to be already 'liberated' because, unlike so many of the white middle-class proponents of the women's movement, their presence in the work force was strongly felt, although their jobs earned them far lower wages and inferior working conditions."[162] As a result, black women defined their own feminism, and the Afro was at the centre of this new identity.

A new group of African American artists, for example, such as Betye Saar, Freida High W. Tesfagiorgis, and Faith Ringgold, challenged commodity stereotypes, such as the Aunt Jemima trademark, making it their feminist issue by offering up reinterpretations of the trademark through the eyes of a black woman. Other artists incorporated the Afro into their art as a form of social protest, a rediscovery of the African diaspora, and a symbolic affirmation of the new politically conscious black subject. Joe Overstreet's *The New Jemima* (1964), Murry DePillars's *Aunt Jemima* (1968), and Jeff Donaldson's *Aunt Jemima (and the Pillsbury Dough Boy)* '64 (1963–64) also moved the trademark from a demeaning continuation of slave iconography to a black militant by appropriating the aesthetics of Black Power and turning the prototypical Mammy into a symbol of the necessity of physical resistance to white domination.[163] Additionally, in Barbara Jones-Hogu's silkscreen *Unite (AfriCOBRA)* (1971), the Chicago-born artist captured how the Afro, as a symbol of black protest, challenged the dominant culture and was also a nod to the defiant raised fist made infamous by Tommie Smith and John Carlos during the medal ceremony at the 1968 Summer Olympics in Mexico City. There are parallels to be drawn between women's liberation of the 1960s, women's hair colouring, and Black Is Beautiful. Most notably, each offered women some form of emancipation. Hair dyes, however, gave white women something that political movements did not—the immediate transformation of themselves as opposed to long-term socio-cultural change, which the Afro ultimately pointed to. When traditional beliefs about women's sexuality gave way to a new sense of sexual liberation, companies like Clairol positioned blonde hair dyes as the embodied expression of this cultural shift. In the pages of *Chatelaine*, the sexual revolution hit the advertising pages at the same time feminism hit the editorial pages.

In April 1966, an advertisement for Clairol's Born Blonde Lotion Toner featured a cropped image of a blonde-haired woman that revealed one eye in a seductive stare above a caption that read, "Maybe the real you is a blonde."[164] The advertising copy continued: "Every smart woman keeps searching for her identity—the inner woman she really is, and the outward expression of it. She looks for a special way to shape her mouth or tilt her chin...a new color that will light up her skin.... Often a woman who looks merely pleasant with dark hair could be a beauty as a blonde." Between 1966 and 1969, Clairol advertisements in *Chatelaine* also equated blonde hair with freedom and choice. Advertising copy read: "If you're going to be a blonde be a good one," "Blonding Simplified," "Clairol thinks if you're lucky enough to be a blonde (one way or another) you ought to make up like one," "Even the Atlantic Ocean can't wash Naturally Blonde out of your hair," and "Go blonde...what a way to go!"[165] Through the late 1960s, *Chatelaine*'s advertising pages still presented an image of white femininity as a blonde. It is interesting to note, however, that brunette hair dyes dominated the magazine's pages throughout 1970, perhaps as a response to the feminist movement. In 1973, Clairol ditched the "Does she...or doesn't she?" tagline and portrayed women as artists, doctors, and politicians alongside the feminist-slanted slogan "To know you're the best." Soon thereafter, L'Oréal also adopted the tagline "Because I'm worth it." Ultimately however, blonde hair was here to stay in the pages of women's magazines; as one representative Revlon advertisement encouraged in October 1971, "Brunettes, now you can go up to three shades blonder...with no pre-lightening."[166] When Rona Maynard became editor-in-chief of *Chatelaine* in the 1990s, she even admitted that while the magazine made attempts over the years at diversity on its covers, in its articles and advertising, "The truth is that blondes still sell more, they do. We have to remember that our job is to sell magazines, not to be politically correct."[167]

Blonde hair dyes permitted white women to change their identities, and, by extension, it gave ethnic white women an opportunity to acquire a form of whiteness that was sanctioned by the dominant beauty culture. At the same time blonde hair made the whiteness of white women hypervisible, by the late 1960s, the Afro made the blackness of black women hypervisible. The Afro stood in direct opposition to one of the "truths" that black beauty culture had, up until the late 1960s, rested upon—that long, flowing, straight hair equalled black beauty. In direct response to Black Is Beautiful, African American entrepreneurs created a market for black beauty products that did not denigrate black women but sought to give them the tools to acquire their own beauty, enhancing (not removing) the hair texture and skin colour they were born with. At the same time, African Canadians also entered the business of beauty, but unlike their African American counterparts, they found themselves faced with two realities. First, there was a lack of interest within Canada's white beauty culture to sell products geared toward black women. Second, African American beauty companies controlled the sale and advertisement of black beauty products, and a result, while a few black beauty entrepreneurs established businesses in the late 1960s, these were localized ventures that were not scaled to reach national or global markets. However, by reading the newspaper discourse of the era we can gain a sense of how black Canadians replicated the Black Is Beautiful sentiment and where they departed from black Americans in terms of how they interpreted the symbolic meaning attached to black aesthetics. While there were no known artists with a national profile commenting on Canada's cultural and political hegemonic institutions in the 1960s, by the1970s there were Afro-wearing black feminists who began to challenge the white, mostly British view of Canadian history.

In 1975, Rella Braithwaite produced one of the first books exclusively on black women's history in Canada, *The Black Woman in Canada*. In Halifax, Iona Crawley became one of the first child-care activists,[168] and in London, Ontario, Elaine Crowell was instrumental in the organization of a black Canadian cultural workshop in 1975, which was "aimed at making whites in the city more aware of black heritage and contributions to society."[169] As a black woman of Antiguan descent living in Toronto in the 1960s, Canadian scholar Althea Prince recalls how, when black American singers adopted the Afro aesthetic, it had a big impact: "In 1968, when James Brown intoned, 'Say it loud—I'm Black and I'm proud,' it became an anthem for Black people because they were ready to live it."[170] In 1969 Nina Simone belted out, "To Be Young, Gifted, and Black," and her neatly coiffed Afro coupled with her dark skin also had an impact on Black Is Beautiful. Simone's "Four Women," released on her 1966 album *Wild Is the Wind*, was a song about black women of varying skin tones and hair textures that questioned ideas of beauty and the connection between these ideas, self-acceptance, and love. Singer Abbey Lincoln also began to wear a natural, and the Jackson Five helped to popularize the Afro aesthetic among black youths.

While the Afro sparked generational conflicts between black parents, grandparents, and children who all had differences of opinion on what hair was "appropriate" for one's appearance, hair care companies soon stepped in to capitalize on the hairstyle's popularity among black women and men of all ages and every socio-economic class. Johnson Products, which continued to promote its Ultra Sheen brand of straightening products throughout the 1960s, launched an Afro Sheen line of conditioners, shampoos, and sprays, the first of which appeared in *Ebony* in November 1968. One representative advertisement proclaimed, "Natural hair hangs out. Beautiful! But Mother Nature doesn't care. She rains. She blows. She dries out hair. Afro Sheen cares. That's why we created a shampoo and a conditioner-hair dress that really takes care of the business."[171] When *Essence* magazine appeared in 1970, it also incorporated the Afro aesthetic and the politics of black liberation into its editorial content.

In May of that year, *Essence* magazine became the first African American periodical "to fill its pages with stories and photo layouts of wigs (including Afro wigs), weaves, hairpieces, and straight styles alongside styles for natural hair."[172] In December 1972, for instance, an *Essence* editorial declared, "You're Not A Black Woman. You Are Five or Six Women. All Black. All Beautiful."[173] In an advertisement published in the magazine in November 1970, Clairol also declared, "No matter what they say . . . Nature Can't Do It Alone! Nothing pretties up a face like a beautiful head of hair, but even hair that's born this beautiful needs a little help along the way."[174] This shift in tone from 1968 to 1970 reflects how, for the first time, companies like Clairol were paying attention to the needs of their black women consumers, who sought to embrace the natural texture of their hair, not to alter it. However, although salon owners and cosmetic companies began to offer black women an array of products and services to help them achieve the new, racially conscious hairstyle, a January 1969 *Ebony* article titled "The Natural Look—Is It Here to Stay?" revealed that many black hairdressers were against the new hairstyle.[175] "As recently as three years ago," the article stated, "it was almost possible to determine the degree of a woman's militance by the state of her hair," adding that "naturals were encountered almost exclusively on picket lines, at civil rights meetings and protest demonstrations."[176] By 1969, however, sentiments had changed. A "midwestern stylist" complained to *Ebony* that the Afro had negatively affected many black hair businesses: "People do all this talking about black power and going 'natural,'" the stylist lamented, "but they don't stop to think that it might all backfire.... If they go all the way with this thing, they'll just be putting people out of work."[177] Compared to chemically relaxed hair, Afros did not require frequent visits to a hair salon for maintenance, thus, many salons feared the loss of clientele. Despite such worries, the Afro became a youthful, "hip" style that beauty companies promoted in conjunction with new, gentler chemical relaxers that came onto the market in the 1960s, and with the arrival of a second wave of African Canadian newspapers launched by West Indian immigrants in cities such as Toronto, the promotion of black beauty culture dramatically changed.

When the *West Indian New Observer* (1967–69) appeared, it did not just contain advertisements for the Afro, it celebrated the hairstyle in several editorials, even though its pages were mostly filled with advertisements from local hair salons, barbershops, and mail-order businesses. In November 1968, six black women with Afros of varying shapes and sizes appeared in a *News Observer* feature titled "For Women Who Wear It Like It Is."[178] The size of each Afro, from small to large, was given a name: the "Petite," "Ebonette," "Princess," "First Lady," "Elegante," and "Afrique." The "Petite" was a small, round Afro; the "Ebonette" was slightly larger and more oval in shape; the "Princess" was a large, round Afro; the "First Lady" was a medium-sized, round Afro; the "Elegante" was a short cut Afro, and the "Afrique" was a coiffed Afro that was curved and elongated at the front. In an accompanying editorial titled "Black Is In," the newspaper proclaimed that the black woman who wears her hair natural, or Afro, with minimal makeup was "in."[179] Quoting New York wig makers, the article noted that "Afro-styles, real hair wigs, and synthetic Afro-wigs are now greatly in demand." The *News Observer* also profiled black hairstylists who, like their African American counterparts, were contesting the Afro. In December 1968 Azan's Beauty World, a beauty shop opened by Kemeel Azan in Toronto, appeared in a feature. "I do not promote the Afro-look," said the Trinidad-born hairstylist to the *News Observer*. "I do not think the black woman needs the Afro-look to identify herself.... Just being black, dignified and proud of it is all I think she needs to portray a true black identity."[180] Unlike African American hairdressers who worried over the economic impact of the natural, Azan's Beauty World points to a cultural difference between Canada and the United States. In Toronto, some stylists were not principally concerned about the potential loss of income resulting from the Afro; instead, they opposed the rhetoric that positioned the Afro as the only signifier of one's socio-political consciousness.

In January 1969, the *News Observer* ceased publication. One month later, under the editorial guidance of Jamaican-born Olivia Grange-Walker and Alfred W. Hamilton, it was reborn as *Contrast*. The newspaper was initially published biweekly, but in 1972 it increased the frequency to weekly, at which time its circulation, around ten thousand, included West Indians but also blacks across Canada.[181] Throughout the 1970s, *Contrast* became the primary outlet for white-owned and African American–owned beauty companies to advertise where black beauty products could be purchased at department stores, the date/location of in-store demonstrations at drugstores, and the goings-on at hair shows across Toronto and eventually cities in the Greater Toronto Area, Montreal, and Calgary. From the outset, *Contrast* ran editorials on the Afro, as a trend and a political statement. In an April 1969 article, "Todays Look—The Natural You," in the column Primarily For and About Women, *Contrast* declared that for some, wearing their hair in its natural state—also referred to as the "Freedom Cap" or the "Nappy Explosion"—was "a significant cultural trend" and yet to others, it was "simply a fashion."[182] Similar to the *News Observer* before it, *Contrast* supported the Afro but also promoted beauty salons that specialized in hair straightening. For instance, when the Ken and Tony of Jamaica Beauty Salon placed a large advertisement in the newspaper in April 1969 to announce their grand opening on Bathurst Street in downtown Toronto, the advertisement read, "Specialists in All Types of Hair-Dressing. Cold Wave, Hair Straightening, Colouring and Styling."[183] *Contrast* also reported on one of the first hair presentations for hair-straightening products in Toronto, which had taken place at The Four Seasons hotel earlier that month.[184] The presentation included a chemical relaxing clinic for hairdressers, who were shown how to use Johnson's Ultra Sheen and Ultra Wave (used primarily by men). "The general consensus of opinion after the show was unanimous: ULTRA SHEEN is a tremendous breakthrough in the relaxing field for the beauty industry," the article noted.

By the end of 1969, black women in Canada, like their counterparts in the United States, continued to use chemical hair relaxers, and it was just as common for women to grow their hair into an Afro as it was for some women to wear Afro wigs. For example, even though the number of advertisements in *Ebony* promoting hair-straightening and skin-lightening products declined between 1949 and 1972 (the most dramatic drop occurring between the years 1968 and 1972), the magazine continued to promote hair-straightening products.[185] With the arrival of *Contrast*, if black women in Toronto wanted to find out about new beauty products, when and where the latest hair demonstration was taking place, and which department stores and drugstores carried products specifically "for them," the newspaper was there. In May 1969 an article in *Contrast* titled "Keep Your Natural Looking Great" profiled two black women: one wore an Afro wig, the other a naturally grown Afro.[186] The article, which provided maintenance tips for both options, explained that for women who wore a "natural" Afro, they should shampoo it at least two or three times a week with a non-alkaline shampoo, but for the Afro wig wearer, it "should not be washed or become wet because most of them are made of nylon. To clean the Natural or Afro wig, use an aerosol spray cleaner [and] spray the wig completely," the article advised. By the early 1970s, the Afro (whether one's natural hair or a wig) had transformed into a freedom hairstyle for black women because it *freed* them from the constraints of hot combs and other hair straightening products as well as from the parameters of the "Brownskin" ideal. Over the course of the 1970s and 1980s, Toronto became not only an epicentre for a localized black beauty culture but also the primary location for white-owned and African American–owned beauty product companies' expansion into Canada.

CHAPTER THREE

BLACK BEAUTY CULTURE IN THE PAGES OF *CONTRAST* AND *SHARE*: LOCAL BEAUTY SALONS, DEPARTMENT STORES, AND DRUGSTORES IN THE 1970s AND 1980s

In the 1970s, Canada garnered its international reputation as a "multicultural" nation, and cultural institutions began to promote multiculturalism as our national brand. The term *multiculturalism* was first used in the 1960s to counter "biculturalism," which was an ideology popularized by the Royal Commission on Bilingualism and Biculturalism (also known as the Bi and Bi Commission) established in 1963 by the government of Prime Minister Lester Pearson. The Commission sought to formulate steps that would move Canada toward finding equal partnership between the two founding cultures, English and French, while considering the contributions made by other ethnic groups to the cultural fabric of Canada. This was the precursor to multiculturalism as not only a policy but a Canadian ethos. In 1971, when Liberal Prime Minister Pierre Trudeau declared in the House of Commons the Canadian government's commitment to the principles of multiculturalism, he paved the way for a formalized policy that would "protect" and "promote" diversity. His 1971 statement also recognized the rights of Aboriginal peoples, cultural diversity, and support for the use of Canada's two official languages. The concept of diversity, as Melissa Aronczyk notes, is a structuring aspect of the Canadian nation itself: "It is its primary source of pride, embedded at once in its policies of cultural rights and recognition, its principles of political liberalism, and its practices of civility and tolerance."[1] Trudeau's recognition of cultural diversity would help to inspire a new generation of Canadians to view the aforementioned principles as Canadian "values" to be upheld and embraced. If it is to mean anything, in the deeply personal sense, Trudeau said, national unity "must be founded on confidence in one's own individual identity; out of this can grow respect for that of others and a willingness to share ideas, attitudes, and assumptions."[2] In 1967, when Toronto's West Indian community organized a Caribbean festival called Caribana (today it is known as Peeks Toronto Caribbean Carnival) in celebration of Canada's centennial year, it was also in recognition of the country's newly embraced ethos of cultural pluralism and diversity, concepts that Canadian governments, post-1967, have consistently promoted in the public sphere.

In 1968, the *West Indian News Observer* featured three articles about Caribana. In the first, appearing in July, the newspaper explained, "Caribana started one year ago, as West Indians took the opportunity of Canada's Centennial year to give some further insight into what constitutes the West Indies, their way of life, their joys, their struggles."[3] Caribana came on the heels of Expo '67 in Montreal, which was Canada's main celebration during its centennial year. Expo '67 was the first attempt to bridge the "two solitudes"—French and English—but on another level, it was the first public display of Canadian diversity and an attempt to show the world that Canada was a united country and a place of tolerance where people from all over the world lived together in one harmonious nation. Importantly, as David Trotman observes, "by the time Caribbean immigrants started arriving in Ontario in large numbers, the historical black population was considerably reduced and resident largely in the rural provinces of southern Ontario."[4] The city of Toronto itself seemed to erase from its collective memory the existence of a prior black population, including a black Alderman and acting mayor of Toronto, William Peyton Hubbard (1842–1935), and the black population seemed to have left little traces of its existence, save a number of black churches like the African Methodist Episcopal (AME) Church founded by Reverend Richard Allen (1760–1831), who was born into slavery in Delaware and who ministered to AME congregations across Toronto until the church settled at 23 Soho Street in 1929, one block north of Queen Street West. Until recently, few had even heard of Albert Jackson, Toronto's first black letter carrier (a job he held for thirty-six years until his death in 1918), who was also born into slavery in Delaware, and who endured unimaginable racism delivering the mail in the Annex neighbourhood in nineteenth-century Toronto. Post-1967, Canada's West Indian immigrants, primarily from Jamaica, Barbados, and Trinidad and Tobago, *became* the black community, not just in terms of their presence but because of the erasure of historical black communities in Toronto, Montreal, Vancouver, Edmonton, and Halifax. This second Afro-Caribbean immigration wave—those arriving between 1962 and 1971—got involved in negotiations and advocacy that brought changes to immigration policies and led to the establishment of the Ontario Human Rights Commission.[5]

By the mid-1970s, however, a wave of racist attacks in cities from coast to coast made it clear to newly arrived immigrant populations (and affirmed what African Canadians already knew) that public displays of diversity and tolerance had not yet trickled down to shift the racist beliefs of many white Canadians. In a Montreal speech in 1975, for example, Trudeau declared, "Racism is evident in this country."[6] In 1972, the racial unrest in the Nova Scotian town of Antigonish, home to St. Francis Xavier University, became so bad that it made national headlines. In an interview with *The Globe and Mail*, Pat Skinner, a council member of the Black United Front said, "There is no justice for black people here. They follow around behind you in stores to see what you are going to pick up. It's terrible. I stopped going out on Friday nights (when dances are held) because the kids drive around in cars calling dirty names at you."[7] Such reporting gave proof to the fact that while Canada was becoming a racially and ethnically diverse country, government discourse and symbolic gesturing was not going to be enough to eradicate racism. An American television program in 1977 even went so far as to describe Toronto as "a racial time-bomb."[8] Despite this, black people continued to immigrate to Toronto, Hamilton, Montreal, Calgary, and Edmonton, while cities such as Halifax, Vancouver, and London, Ontario, witnessed little West Indian immigration. By 1969, over twelve thousand Caribbean immigrants had entered Canada, most of whom went to Ontario, establishing a pattern that continues to this day.[9]

As the decade of the 1970s progressed, African American communities seemed to split along class lines. Mark Anthony Neal observes that "the Black Public Sphere began to exhibit early signs of deterioration" and that, "predicated on black middle-class flight, the demise of central cities, and the postindustrial transformation of urban economies, black identity—in other words Blackness—became largely mediated and thus determined by the mechanisms of mass consumer culture."[10] Conversely, black Canadians began to form coalitions and began to work towards consensus on key issues during the 1970s as emergent associations such as the Canadian Negro Women's Association (CANEWA) drew together highly skilled professionals, service-sector employees, black educators, and those still marginalized.[11] CANEWA remained relatively unknown until acclaimed author Lawrence Hill (son of Daniel G. Hill) told the organization's story in his 1996 book, *Women of Vision*. One of the presidents of CANEWA was Kathleen ("Kay") Livingstone; born in London, Ontario, on October 13, 1918, she was the daughter of James and Christina Jenkins, editors of the *Dawn of Tomorrow*,[12] and she also appeared on a commemorative Canada Post Stamp in 2018. In the forward to Hill's book, Rosemary Brown, the first black woman to become a member of a provincial legislature (she served as a member of the Legislative Assembly of British Columbia from 1979 to 1986) and the first woman to run for leadership of a federal political party recalled:

> As the organization's name indicates, and a reading of its history will reveal, the Association was born before the day of Black Power, before we chose to tell ourselves that "Black is Beautiful," or to call ourselves Black, African Canadian or Visible Minority. In fact, the organization was in many ways, years ahead of those movements. The Association recognized the importance of self-respect and self-esteem to Black people and set forth to build and encourage the development of both of these in its members and in the young people of the community. In doing so, it also built respect for the Black community in the wider community.[13]

While most CANEWA members were born in Canada (although a few had emigrated from the Caribbean and the United States) and active membership never exceeded forty women, CANEWA was one of the most dynamic and best-organized black organizations in Canada in the period from 1951 to 1976.[14] Such organizations helped arriving West Indian immigrants to settle and find community in Canada. By the mid-1970s, many of these immigrants formed part of a black middle-class in Toronto, and as a result, many families left the city's downtown for the suburbs, like my parents did.[15] This move to Toronto's suburbs (Scarborough, Etobicoke, North York, and East York) and eventually to Mississauga and Brampton to the west, Pickering, Ajax, and Whitby to the east, and Markham and Vaughan to the north, all of which constitute what became known as the Greater Toronto Area (GTA), meant that by the 1980s, black community was no longer centrally located downtown, as it had been for most of the twentieth century. The period between the 1970s and 1980s is the moment where black Canada, as we know it today, entered the dominant public sphere. Black beauty culture also formed a more central part of the pages of Toronto's West Indian-operated newspapers and products finally broke the colour barrier, appearing on department-store and drugstore shelves and in the pages of *Chatelaine*.

This chapter explores the advertising and editorial content of Toronto's *Contrast* newspaper and *Share* magazine. As noted in chapter 2, *Contrast* (1969–91), like the *News Observer* before it, promoted black beauty culture in Toronto, but also promoted the transnational entry of African American and white-owned black beauty companies into the country. As these firms entered the local and national marketplace (*Contrast* reported on developments in black communities from coast to coast) with products available for sale at mainstream retailers—department stores, drugstores, and black-owned beauty product shops—the strategies used to lure black women consumers changed. Since its debut, *Share* has focused almost exclusively on the GTA's Caribbean communities, and in its pages, a localized black beauty culture made up of hair salons, barbershops, and beauty product distributors also appeared. The weekly community periodical, published by Arnold A. Auguste, who came to Canada in 1970 from Trinidad and Tobago, hit newsstands on April 8, 1978, and it continues to this day.

This chapter argues that Toronto's black newspapers, while much smaller in scale than *Essence* and *Ebony*, did exactly what African American periodicals did during the 1970s and 1980s—promote black culture and black beauty to black readers—and they did so, in some cases, years before their African American counterparts. Where *Ebony* and *Essence* magazines were able to attract advertisers from corporate America, in 2017, acclaimed novelist and scholar Cecil Foster, who was an editor of *Contrast* in the 1970s, revealed that it was a day-to-day struggle for Alfred Hamilton, editor-in-chief, to find Canadian companies willing to advertise in the newspaper. "None of the banks, the car and insurance companies, the government agencies, media houses, and so forth, would take out an ad with the newspaper that prided itself as the voice of the Canadian black community," Foster writes, adding, "His message was that if blacks were perceived to be doing these everyday Canadian things, then it would follow that they would be viewed as part of a desirable market and courted in a medium that proudly represented them."[16] Hamilton's message finally began to pay off in the early 1970s as Canadian retailers began to view the newspaper as a viable outlet for the promotion of products geared toward black women (and men) consumers. Importantly, this chapter is not concerned with official corporate documents or the actual practices that created the corporate advertisements and retail strategies. Instead, its focus is on the textual and visual strategies used by corporations to cultivate black beauty culture in local media outlets, and the social and cultural factors that shaped the image of black beauty that emerged during the period. It explains how black beauty culture, which was a small niche market before the 1970s, entered Canada's mainstream retail sector, and how this entry shifted the image of black beauty in product advertising. It also probes the marketing strategies used by white-owned American companies as compared to those used by African American–owned firms to cultivate black Canadian women consumers.

For the first time in the 1970s, beauty firms actively sought black Canadian women customers like they did their African American counterparts. Black women also entered the catalogue pages of department stores, as products geared toward them were offered for sale at Eaton's, Hudson's Bay, and Simpson's, all of which placed advertisements in the pages of *Contrast* and *Share*. When a new black beauty product arrived at their various locations in Toronto, but also in Hamilton, Edmonton, Calgary, and Montreal, advertisements appeared in black Canadian newspapers. How and why did Canadian retailers actively seek black women as customers in the 1970s and 1980s? The first step toward cultivating black women consumers began with department stores and *Chatelaine*, both of which began to embrace the Afro aesthetic in the early 1970s. Prior to this, however, the pages of *Contrast* reveal how active newly arrived West Indians were in establishing businesses, beauty salons, and barbershops in the post-1967 period.

In September 1970, *Contrast* published a black business directory for the city of Toronto.[17] This directory listed the social clubs, restaurants, dentists, doctors, lawyers, and food markets owned and operated by blacks. It also provided a list of barbershops, beauty salons, and beauty supply shops; there were five barbershops, twelve beauty salons, and seven beauty supply shops. These businesses were primarily located on Bathurst Street, St. Clair Avenue West, Oakwood Avenue, Queen Street West, Ossington Avenue, Dupont Street, Davenport Road, and College Street. While Toronto was hardly New York or Chicago, in relation to the rest of Canada, black culture was visible in the city and there was an ever-growing presence of black businesses. In March 1970 for example, *Contrast* reported on the rise of black business ownership.[18] "Two years ago there were no black owned book stores, today there are three," the newspaper reported, adding, "Two years ago black people could only buy West Indian food stuffs at Gonsalves or at the Kensington Market. Today supermarkets are filling the need." The editorial underscores that by the early 1970s, black Canadians were increasingly a part of the socio-cultural and economic fabric of Toronto, not merely existing on its outskirts, as was the case in the early twentieth century. The pages of *Contrast* were also filled with editorials that let readers know that it was a West Indian newspaper, and that its politics paralleled those of Marcus Garvey's *Negro World*, the voice of the Universal Negro Improvement Association (UNIA) discussed in chapter 1. The UNIA was the first civil rights organization in Canada; it was also an outlet for community building and cultural expression, offering the first wave of West Indian immigrants (arriving between the 1910s and 1940s), who were well educated and literate, opportunities to become engaged in transnational pan-Africanist discussions. *Contrast*'s editorials took an unabashed pan-Africanist tone, tackling racism and the disenfranchisement of black people on Canadian soil.

Where the dominant press had focused on civil rights and racist violence south of the border in the late 1960s, as noted in chapter 2, *Contrast* was one of the only voices—if not the only voice—for black Canadians battling comparable instances of institutional racism in Canada in the early 1970s. For example, in an April 1970 editorial, *Contrast* reported on a CBC "fifteen-minute" special on black West Indian immigrants in Toronto. "The idea behind this type of program is to inform or educate the general public about the minority groups which exist in their midst and thereby create a climate of greater understanding and acceptance of those who are 'different,'" the newspaper reported. However, it concluded, these efforts "invariably fall short of achieving a truly educative function because the minority group itself is never allowed to be involved in the presentation of its own image; individuals are chosen at random, interviewed by a stranger with a microphone, manipulated like puppets by leading questions requiring quick answers, and generally pressured into doing their 'thing' before the cameras, much like a dancing bear being prodded to perform for an audience."[19] Importantly, Toni King found that *Ebony* "offered black women of the 1970s an opportunity to witness themselves negotiating new occupational terrain, while at the same time accommodating current mainstream ideologies of womanhood."[20] On one level, she writes further, "this format helped black women find a sense of solidarity in their collective image of themselves" but on another level, *Ebony* "was a vehicle for black aspirations of middle-class status, which often implies some level of assimilation."[21] *Contrast* did not brand itself as a "middle-class" periodical, but its editorial tone, similar to that of *Ebony*, emphasized the need for solidarity in the collective black experience.

The newspaper made it clear that it sought to reflect black Canada, and by doing so, to expose black people to the diversity within the varied communities. The newspaper's pages also reflected moderate, militant, and conservative thinking as it existed across the city, although its approach was often surprisingly direct. For example, when renowned Barbadian writer Austin Clarke (1934–2016) wrote for *Contrast* (he also served as managing editor for a few years), he not only encouraged young writers to write, he also urged black readers to engage in political action, such as marches against apartheid and speaking out against police brutality. In one representative editorial that appeared on October 1, 1970, Clarke wrote, "There is only a handful o' black head-nurses in all the horsepitals in Toronto; number two, you ever see a black reporter 'pon the Globe and Mail, or the Telly, or the Star?; number three, you ever see a black man interviewing anybody 'pon the CBC?; number four, any black policemen get make sargeant yet?; number five, a black waiter ever serve' you in a restaurant, in a bar, in a hotel, 'pon one o' them Air Canada planes, eh?"[22] His use of creolized Caribbean English reveals how close *Contrast* writers were with their audience—they spoke to them directly in a language they understood because they *were* them.

In December 1973, an editorial on shopping for a black doll in Toronto similarly spoke directly to readers about the day-to-day realities of being black in a city that was still predominantly white, and about the experience of patronizing department stores. It began with the following statement, "Shopping at Christmas time is admittedly a hassle. But searching for a black doll in the shops of Toronto is a whole exercise in frustration."[23] Because of the large concentration of black people living in the Annex's Bathurst and Bloor community, euphemistically known as "Blackhurst," the article's author, Liz Cromwell, believed that it would be a good place to start her search for a black doll. However, after stopping at Woolworths, the American discount retailer, she realized it would be difficult. When she arrived at Eaton's, Cromwell reported that there was one black doll named "Gloria" but a variety of other dolls, such as "Eskimo" dolls, "Dutch" dolls, and "Greek" dolls. This led her to conclude, "If we are going to open our doors and invite people to make their home among us, if Canada is to be the home of some black people, then the needs of these people must be

taken into account." The search for black dolls in 1970s Toronto is significant because, by the late 1960s, the American toy company Mattel tried to
respond to the Black Is Beautiful sentiment with a line of black dolls.

In 1967, Mattel premiered a black version of the Barbie doll called "Colored Francie." Although the Black Is Beautiful theme of both the civil
rights and Black Power movements may have suggested a ready market for
a beautiful black doll, Colored Francie did not sell well.[24] Cynthia Roberts
maintains that Colored Francie flopped because of her straight hair and
white features.[25] In 1968, Mattel took the doll off the market and replaced
her with a black doll called "Christie." Several other black dolls appeared
throughout the late 1960s and 1970s, including the "Julia" doll, modelled
after the TV character played by African American actress Diahann Car-
roll on the sitcom *Julia* (1968–71).[26] Yet in Canada, these dolls were not
available. Thus, while in the United States white-owned manufacturers
began to create products specifically geared toward African American consumers (however flawed their initial attempts might have been), in Canada, products geared toward black consumers were still mostly absent from
retail shelves. Black beauty products, however, changed all of this.

In May 1970, *Contrast* announced that two beauty salons, Azan's Beauty
World and Nouveau Femme, had teamed up to bring model Naomi Sims
to Toronto.[27] Dubbed "the world's top black model," Sims appeared at
the Royal York Hotel on May 17, and the following month, Sims, along
with two other black models, appeared in a full-page fashion spread in the
newspaper.[28] In August of that year, however, advertisements in the newspaper spoke to a lack of consensus on black cultural expressions. Placed
side by side on the page, one ad for Third World Books and Crafts promoted "Dashikies and African Fabrics... Specializing in Afro Asian Books
and Crafts,"[29] while another from a hairstylist proclaimed, "Let Mr. Stephen Straighten You Out... When You Feel The Urge To Be BEAUTIFUL
Call Me Anytime."[30] In the same issue, Harvey Gellman, Sales Manager
for Townecraft Industries, placed an advertisement for Afro wigs; under
the slogan, "Black Is Beautiful... With Kinky Hair," it continued, "No
more expense at the Beauty Parlour—Just Wash 'n Wear—Permanently
Kinky.... The only synthetic Afro wig in Canada that looks natural.... Also
available long wigs, short wigs, and 100% human hair pieces.... These wigs
are not sold in the stores but only in the comfort of your home."[31] From
Afros to hair straighteners to wigs, in the early 1970s, *Contrast* celebrated
the diversity of black cultural expression and its contradictions. Importantly, the popularity of the Afro coincided with "the soul aesthetic," an

amalgam of African cultural elements into a personal style and clothing, like the dashiki—a loose-fitting, brightly coloured tunic, originally from West Africa. The soul aesthetic was also part of Black Is Beautiful.

In February 1970, *Contrast* ran a full-page cover story on a "dasheiki party" organized by designer Toronto-born Ola Skanks, a dancer who was one of the first to bring traditional African dance to Canada in the 1960s. "Everyone sported an exclusive designed dasheiki and had a chance to sample an African dish," the article noted.[32] As William Van Deburg explains, "soul style was a type of in-group cultural cachet whose creators utilized clothing design, popular hair treatments, and even body language (stance, gait, method of greeting) as preferred mechanisms of authentication."[33] In keeping with Black Is Beautiful, beauty product manufacturers incorporated the soul aesthetic into their advertising campaigns. Johnson Products marketed the Afro Sheen product line using Swahili words and phrases in their ad campaigns: "Watu-Wazuri (Beautiful People) use Afro Sheen"; "Kama Baba, Kama Mwana" (like father, like son); Pamoja! (Together!); and "Kama Mama, Kama Binti (like mother, like daughter)." Between 1970 and 1975, Johnson Products ran a series of advertisements using these slogans in *Ebony* and *Essence*. Swahili is a Bantu language spoken in Tanzania, Burundi, Congo, Kenya, Mozambique, Rwanda, Somalia, South Africa, and Uganda. Thus, the fact that an African American company adopted Swahili for its slogan points to how Africa was being called upon for marketing purposes to help foster a consumer culture around the soul aesthetic. In the United States, a person could acquire a soul aesthetic without growing an Afro, but the political and intellectual savvy of those individuals who continued to "process" was often brought into question. In Toronto, there was not one "authentically" black aesthetic; as a result, *Contrast* did not equate soul style with a black political consciousness. At the same time, the year 1970 also marked the moment the Afro and black models entered the pages of *Chatelaine*.

In December of that year, a black model appeared in an Eveleen Dollery fashion spread.[34] Dollery, who passed away in 2011, worked as a fashion editor for three decades (1958–88) at *Chatelaine* and was a founding member of *Flare* (*Miss Chatelaine*). The model, who was dressed identical to her white counterpart, wore a large Afro (possibly a wig) and in another instance, her hair was straightened and pulled back. The only discernible markers that distinguished her from the white models were her dark skin and Afro. While the model's name is not listed, her appearance represents the first time a black model appeared in a *Chatelaine* photographic feature.

Just as an Afro made one's blackness hypervisible in the fashion world, dark-skinned models have historically been used to accentuate the *blackness* of blackness.[35] An example of this appeared in the work of 1980s Italian photographer Oliviero Toscani (b. 1942), who in the early 1990s drew upon the controversial image of black women as wet nurses in a clothing advertisement he created for the Italian clothing company Benetton. The advertisement featured a close-up of a white infant suckling the breast of a dark-skinned woman who wore a red Shetland Benetton sweater. In other advertisements, Toscani paired dark-skinned children with white children, an act that also accentuated the *blackness* of their blackness as both different and exotic in the same instance. As numerous African American scholars have pointed out, while "the aestheticization and commercialization of racial taboos in the advertising campaign generated shock, praise, and discomfort,"[36] it won more advertising awards than any other image in Benetton's advertising history.[37] When a second black model appeared in *Chatelaine* in October 1971, she was also a dark-skinned woman with an Afro.

Black models first began to appear on the cover pages of America's magazines in the late 1960s. Donyale Luna appeared on the cover of *UK Vogue* in March 1966; Naomi Sims appeared on the cover of *Ladies' Home Journal* in November 1968 and *Life* magazine in October 1969; Peggy Dillard appeared on the cover of *Mademoiselle* in March 1974; and Beverly Johnson became the first African American woman to appear on the cover of *Vogue* when she graced its front page in August 1974. While a comparable study has never been done in Canada, in my assessment of *Chatelaine* magazine since its inception in 1928, I found political figure Zanana Akande (b. 1937), the first black woman elected to the Legislative Assembly of Ontario, to be the first black woman to appear on the magazine's cover when she did so in 1991. In a feature about the groundbreaking number of women (eleven) in the New Democratic Party cabinet in Ontario that year, she appeared in a group shot alongside ten other women, all of whom were white.[38] The year before, M. NourbeSe Philip, the Trinidad-born Canadian poet, writer, and lawyer appeared in a six-page feature story about a protest she helped to organize in September 1989 in response to the Canadian Centre of PEN International's literary conference, at which only white authors were recognized.[39] In 1994 a second black woman, the Honourable Jean Augustine (b. 1937), the first black woman elected to the Parliament of Canada, was featured in a multi-page editorial written by the renowned black Canadian author Cecil Foster, who also wrote a series of black-focused articles for *Chatelaine* in the early 1990s.[40] Augustine helped to get Black History Month recognized as a national celebration when she brought the motion before Parliament in 1995. The first black Canadian model to appear in *Chatelaine* magazine did so in 1994 when Lana Ogilvie, who was born in Toronto, was featured in an advertisement for Cover-Girl lipstick. In the December issue, Ogilvie, who is light-skinned and is the first non-white model to be given a contract with CoverGirl, appeared alongside two white models in a campaign for CoverGirl's Luminesse Lipcolour Collection.[41]

While we do not know the names of the black models that appeared in *Chatelaine* in 1971, in chapter 4 I explain why Canada's beauty industry has never embraced racial diversity to the extent that modelling agencies have been forced to in the United States. In fact, the first black Canadian woman to appear alone on the cover of *Chatelaine* did not do so until 1999, when Gloria Rueben, the Toronto-born actress, who was starring on the hit television show *ER* at the time, was the subject of a six-page feature in the March issue.[42] In December of that year, Toronto-born R&B singer Deborah Cox became the second black woman to appear alone on a *Chatelaine* cover. Cox was the subject of a seven-page feature on her musical success stateside.[43] If African American models first graced the cover pages of women's magazines in the late 1960s, why did it take so long for this breakthrough to occur in Canada? While the racism in America's beauty and fashion industries is often placed under a spotlight, there has been little attention paid to how black women have, historically, been excluded from Canada's beauty and fashion industries. It was in the 1970s that black models also entered the pages of Eaton's catalogues for the first time.

In her examination of the history of women at Eaton's, Lorraine O'Donnell found that "through the medium of its covers... Eaton's proposed ways of seeing the female customers to whom it appealed, the country in which it operated, and itself: the meanings of all three were mutually constructed through this popular, powerful medium."[44] Like *Chatelaine*, Eaton's covers remained exclusively the domain of white women, men, and children. Throughout the 1970s, no black model (female or male) appeared on the department store's catalogue covers. However, in the Fall/Winter 1971 catalogue, for the first time, two black women appeared inside the catalogue, on separate pages. The first black model wore an Afro, and the second wore a straightened "Greek boy" (closely cropped) hairstyle. Black models appeared in the pages of Eaton's catalogues only between 1972 and 1976, the year the company ended its mail-order catalogue business. After the 1971 fashion spread in *Chatelaine*, another black model did not appear in that magazine until 1979, when an advertisement for the clothing line Cachet featured a black model.[45] By the end of the 1980s, black women remained absent from the magazine's cover; it is interesting to note, however, that throughout the 1980s black models were represented in American beauty advertisements in the pages of *Chatelaine*.

For example, in a full-page advertisement for Clairol's Claireese ammonia-free shampoo-in hair-colour product, placed on the inside cover of *Chatelaine*'s February 1982 issue, supermodel Beverly Johnson appeared alongside Cheryl Tiegs and three other models.[46] Between 1982 and 1989, black models appeared fewer than ten times in advertisements and/or fashion features in the magazine. A black model appeared in a Sears advertisement placed in the inside cover of the May 1982 issue, and in June 1986, a black model was featured by herself in a *Chatelaine* fashion spread titled "Black and White...Always Right."[47] The spread captured the model in four separate looks, but in each image, she was arrayed against a white background, she wore a white jacket, and her hair was straightened. But while images of black models were few and far between in Eaton's catalogues and *Chatelaine*'s pages, black beauty culture, specifically cosmetics and hair care products, entered department stores and drugstores during this period.

The year 1971 marked the first time that black beauty products were offered for sale at Eaton's and Simpson's, the two leading department stores in Canada at the time. Initially, when white-owned American firms entered the Canadian market, they relied upon the image of the Afro coupled with other Black Is Beautiful motifs to cultivate black women consumers. The Flori Roberts Company was the first black cosmetics firm to do so. Established in 1965 by Roberts, a white woman with an extensive background in the fashion industry, the company came to life because Roberts had noticed the problems faced by black models seeking desirable facial makeup.[48] In 1967, she became one of the first non-black entrepreneurs to enter the previously segregated black beauty market. Up until the early 1970s, black beauty products were sold almost exclusively at local black-owned mom-and-pop shops. When Roberts spoke to company executives and advertising representatives at an industry seminar in 1969, she told them that the history of neglect of black women's cosmetic needs required established white companies to develop separate product lines with different brand names.[49] In an April 1971 *Contrast* article, "Now Black Can Be More Beautiful," readers were introduced to Roberts's cosmetic products through both an advertisement and a feature article: "It is a fact that Black women have a proud, natural beauty and a graceful style which

is distinct and unique. At last there is an entire line of cosmetics catering to this unique style of Black women."[50] Alyce Stoney, a former modelling school director and self-dubbed black beauty expert, had travelled to
Toronto to introduce the Flori Roberts cosmetic collection. "Researched
for over a year and formulated with scientific data, the entire line is based
on the Melanin concept which revolves around the fact that it is the dark
pigment present in the skin that makes one complexion different from the
other," the article noted. "These colorings will be available at Eatons in
products that include a sheer liquid foundation in nine sepia shades, plus
an undertoner, facial-Do cremes to cover shadows, wrinkles, or blotches
and to reshape large unattractive features," the article added. For the first
time in "any local cosmetic department" a Flori Roberts trained beauty
consultant, Gloria Shreve, would be on hand full-time at Eaton's Queen
Street location in downtown Toronto to measure every skin tone, offer a
free introductory gift, and teach the principles of Melanin makeup to the
public. In an accompanying advertisement, a sketch of a black woman with
a perfectly coiffed, medium-length Afro and hoop earrings appeared. For
all intents and purposes, the Flori Roberts Company was a black beauty
firm. Even though a white woman owned the company, she developed
her products specifically with black women in mind, as opposed to José
Baraquiel Calva, discussed in chapter 2, whose Lustrasilk products were
originally intended for industrial purposes but were repurposed for use by
black women.

Roberts sought to improve black women's sense of self, not disparage
them into purchasing skin- or hair-altering products. Further, the Flori
Roberts Company did not simply jump on the Black Is Beautiful band-
wagon; black women consumers were its target market from the outset.
In June 1971, a dark-skinned black woman with a large Afro and earrings
featured in a Flori Roberts advertisement for the company's wig collection.
The following month, Roberts formally introduced the sale of Afro wigs at
Eaton's Queen Street location with the tagline, "It's a Natural, the Softest,
Silkiest Afro Stretch Wig Ever." The advertisement's copy read: "All Part of
the Flori Roberts' Way to be BLACK, BEAUTIFUL AND TOGETHER!!!"[51]
The fact that Flori Roberts also sold black hair wigs at Eaton's was not
coincidental. Eaton's had been in the wig business for years. Throughout
1968, for example, it regularly advertised its Wig Shop in the *Toronto Star*
and *Telegram*. In one representative advertisement in the *Star*, Eaton's proclaimed, "Change your hairdo as often as your mood!"[52] In the *Telegram*,
the company declared, "If you already own a wig or hairpiece from Eaton's

Fashion Wig Salon—no need to persuade you. But it's a great time to add to your collection! If not—there never was a better time to try one. Take...a wiglet to add height and body to your own. Or a full wig to keep at-the-ready for great evenings—or emergencies!"[53] (A "wiglet" is a small wig used to enhance a hairstyle.) Following Eaton's lead, in July 1971, Simpson's began to sell black beauty products. An advertisement for the white-owned company Posner declared that "Custom blends cosmetics for black complexions" were now available at Simpson's, in addition to Afro products; both lines were, as with Eaton's, available only at the Queen Street location in downtown Toronto.[54]

While Eaton's promoted the sale of black beauty products in *Contrast*, it did not focus on drawing black consumers into its stores, as it did in the case of white consumers. For example, in 1968 when Estée Lauder came to Canada, Eaton's proudly and loudly announced the cosmetic firm's arrival in the *Toronto Star*: "Now we are able to supply the exciting line of Estée Lauder cosmetics at both your favorite downtown stores. At Eaton's College Street, a bright new counter has been set up. An Estée Lauder cosmetician is at all stores to guide your selection."[55] Meanwhile, in the black beauty advertisements appearing in *Contrast*, Eaton's made no grand announcements. The department store's logo was strategically placed in print advertisements, but its voice, as a retailer, was absent. Although products from Helena Rubinstein, Max Factor, and Estée Lauder were sold not only at Eaton's Queen Street but also at Don Mills, Oshawa, Yorkdale, Shopper's World (Brampton), Hamilton, and Kitchener, black beauty products through the 1970s were available only at Eaton's Queen Street location in downtown Toronto. If you consider that many black Torontonians had relocated to the suburbs in the early 1970s, there was still a large segment of the black population in the GTA that did not have access to these products or had to travel great distances to purchase them. Ultimately, department stores might have been keen on black women consumers, but they kept their interest a "secret" from the general public. Products geared toward white women appeared in dominant media outlets as *products for everyone*, while black beauty products remained relegated to black newspapers, exclusively.

Throughout 1971, Flori Roberts continued her aggressive expansion into Toronto's black beauty market. In September of that year, the company held a "Black and Beautiful" workshop at Eaton's Queen Street location.[56] Tailored specifically for "dark skins," the promotional advertisement for the workshop read: "Find out the best treatments for your skin type....Even learn the basics of Hair and Wig Care. You'll watch a demonstration, then these experts will help you make up your own face, with individual instructions, complimentary samples and personal attention to special problems." Flori Roberts's marketing strategy was genius in that it carefully persuaded black women that their darker skin was beautiful, and that it could be improved (not "cured") using Flori Roberts cosmetics. In August 1971, the company also set up a booth at the annual Caribana festival to promote its products, which suggests that it was paying attention to the nuances of Toronto's black community and its growing West Indian population. Unlike Flori Roberts, when Johnson Products came to Canada, it took the efforts of a local beauty culturist, Beverly Mascoll, to get its products into department stores.

Mascoll was born in Halifax in 1942; she relocated to Toronto as a teenager. Her foray into the black beauty business began when she got a job as a receptionist at Toronto Barber and Beauty Supply. She quickly noticed that there was a major gap in Canada's beauty industry—a lack of black hair and skin care products. In 1970, she started her own business, Beverly Mascoll Ltd., and soon thereafter went to Chicago and convinced Johnson Products to make her the sole distributor of the company's Ultra Sheen products in Canada. Johnson Products would become the first African American–owned beauty firm to expand into Canada. In 1971, Mascoll, the largest distributor of black beauty products in Canada at the time, gave an interview to *Contrast* in which she said, "As a Black-owned company, the leader in the field, Johnson's growth and success was due to the fact that they always realized that the black consumer knows quality. Now we can have, in Canada, a black cosmetics line that is quality right and priced right."[57] In 1998, the Canadian government recognized Mascoll's entrepreneurial efforts when she was appointed as a Member of the Order of Canada. Sadly, Beverly Mascoll died from breast cancer in 2001, but her legacy remains. She singlehandedly turned a grassroots business into a lucrative company while creating a market for the large-scale distribution of black beauty products in Canada. In September 1971, Mascoll placed her first advertisement in *Contrast*. The advertisement noted that Johnson's Ultra Sheen product was available for purchase directly through Mascoll, who at this point was still selling the products out of her residence.[58]

By December 1972, Mascoll's business, incorporated as Mascoll Ltd., dubbing itself "Canada's Largest Distributor of Black Beauty Products," placed another advertisement in *Contract* with the tagline, "We knew Black was beautiful, long before it became popular."[59] In addition to Ultra Sheen, the company's distribution list had grown to include products from white-owned companies such as Posner, Hair Strate, Black Velvet, and others; and all of these products were available at the Simpson's Queen Street location. By 1975 other African American–owned cosmetic firms began to advertise in *Contrast*, including Monette Cosmetics, which posted an advertisement in February of that year for its line of over twelve products specifically formulated for black skin.[60] The advertisement also stated that the product had been "featured on the August [1974] cover of *Essence* magazine." In 1975, the largest black cosmetics firm at the time, John H. Johnson's Fashion Fair Cosmetics, also arrived in Canada. Fashion Fair Cosmetics, founded in 1973 by Johnson, the *Ebony* magazine publisher, was an outgrowth of the magazine and its popular *Ebony* Fashion Fair Show, which began in Chicago in 1958 as a travelling fashion show that showcased African American women.

Prior to the 1970s, white-owned cosmetics firms offered a limited range of product shades, often selling only those colours that suited the complexions of white women. Like Flori Roberts, this practice frustrated Johnson's wife, Eunice. When the Johnsons noticed that the Fashion Fair models had to blend cosmetics to match their skin tones, they approached cosmetics companies to create products for black women; after their attempts proved futile, they went into a laboratory and created Fashion Fair Cosmetics. Outside of Flori Roberts, white-owned cosmetic firms did not consider black women a viable market in the 1970s. In chapter 4, I explain how and why, by the 1990s, these same firms began to target black women (primarily Revlon and L'Oréal) with darker cosmetic shades. Before this shift occurred, however, Fashion Fair Cosmetics was the only black-focused product sold at high-end department stores such as Bloomingdale's in New York City, Marshall Field's in Chicago, and Neiman-Marcus in Dallas.[61] If you consider that Estée Lauder products appeared at Saks Fifth Avenue, Neiman-Marcus, Bloomingdale's, and Marshall Field's as early as the 1940s,[62] Johnson's entry into these stores was a very big deal. One reason why Johnson was able to get his products into such high-end stores was that he never aligned Fashion Fair with Black Is Beautiful, the Afro, or Black Power.

As Susannah Walker observes, "Fashion Fair ads tended to mimic the celebrity-studded articles common in the parent company's magazines."[63] A full-page advertisement for Fashion Fair Cosmetics appearing in *Contrast* in December 1975 featured three women—one white, one Asian, and one black woman (in that order, from left to right)—with similar skin tones and straightened hair. Unlike Flori Roberts' products, which were available at Eaton's and Simpson's Queen Street locations only, Fashion

Fair Cosmetics became the first black beauty product to be sold at Eaton's Queen Street, Eaton's Yorkdale (in the city's north end), and at the department store's Hamilton location. "It's the difference that delights," the advertisement read; "Fashion Fair cosmetics from EATON'S can help bring out *your* individual beauty."[64] The advertising copy then explained why Fashion Fair was "every woman's cosmetics": "Fashion Fair is a welcome new beauty preparation created especially for Black, Oriental or brunette complexions. It's rich in the colours needed to make the most of your skin; yet it is not overpowering. The look is healthy and radiant, but most of all, natural....Fashion Fair lets you be beautiful by being yourself!" Given Johnson's ties to the fashion industry, where political statements became mere fashion aesthetics, there was no hint of Black Power in Fashion Fair advertising, and as a result, high-end retailers found the product "acceptable" to include into their offerings.

Style as resistance becomes commodified as chic when, as Danae Clark notes, "it leaves the political realm and enters the fashion world. This simultaneously diffuses the political edge of style. Resistant trends [such as wearing an Afro] become restyled as high-priced fashion"[65] Importantly, by the mid-1970s, Afros and Black Is Beautiful were increasingly depoliticized fashion aesthetics adopted by beauty companies, but as part of the soul aesthetic, both still had the power to cultivate a sense of collective black pride. Fashion Fair entered the mainstream fashion world by rejecting the Afro and all its African-inspired sentiment; conversely, when the African American–owned firm Barbara Walden Cosmetics came to Canada, it chose drugstores and discount stores for its products, and Black Is Beautiful was its brand. Since brands refer not primarily to the product, but to the context of consumption, they stand for a specific way of using the object, a propertied form of life to be realized in consumption;[66] Walden Cosmetics *really* spoke to the everyday black woman in ways that Fashion Fair, while high-quality products, did not. In an article in *Contrast* in April 1975, Walden, a former dancer and actress, explained that she first launched her products in 1960 and, after sales "boomed all across the United States," she decided to bring her Black-Is-Beautiful-themed products to Canada.[67]

Like Eunice Johnson, Walden had noticed that, on film sets and in photographs, her skin would lose its tone after she applied makeup made for white women. "In exasperation she sought a chemist's help and together they developed a formula to meet her particular skin problems," *Contrast* reported. "I've been black all my life and I always felt beautiful....It's just sad that it has taken so long for black women to become proud of their looks and to really believe that black is beautiful," said Walden in the interview. A week prior, Walden Cosmetics, distributed in Toronto by Sonjia Chin, placed an advertisement in *Contrast* explaining to readers that not only would Barbara Walden be available for a "meet and greet" in the city but the company's cosmetics were also uniquely tailored for *them*:

> Because no matter how light or dark, there is an orange, or sometimes a blue undertone to black skin. That's why makeup created for the pink undertones of the Caucasian skin can never be right for the black. Also there are more oil glans in the black skin, which make water base or matte finish foundations unsuitable. Barbara Walden makeup preparations are made with natural oils and they're also transparent to let the warm skin tones glow through.[68]

Following in the tradition of Madam C. J. Walker, Walden wanted to uplift black women's self-esteem. Thus, instead of pitting a light-skinned woman against a dark-skinned woman, she focused on the commonality of the problem—finding the right cosmetic shades for *all* shades of blackness. Even Fashion Fair had been guilty of reproducing the binary juxtaposition between lighter skin and darker skin. In a May 1976 advertisement for instance, the company used the tagline "Fashion Fair for the dark skinned woman" but the advertising text immediately aligned this beauty with that of a light-skinned woman. "Black is beautiful," the advertisement asserted, adding "as is Oriental, brunette and even deeply sun-tanned skin."[69] In comparison, when Walden Cosmetics entered Towers Department store, a discount retailer at Jane Finch Mall in Toronto's northwest end in May 1976, the company used the slogan, "Make Up Just Right For You," without drawing a distinction between darker and lighter skin tones.[70] Walden's emphasis on the beauty of dark skin without a lighter skin comparison held significant meaning, especially at a time when advertisements for skin-bleaching products still appeared in black media. In February 1972, the skin-bleaching firm Nadinola placed its first advertisement in *Contrast*.[71] While the advertisement did not include an image, and the product was available only through home delivery via a small network of distributors in Toronto, Ottawa, St. Catharines, and Montreal, it marked the beginning of skin-bleaching advertisements appearing in the newspaper's pages.

In the early 1970s, skin-bleaching products still appeared regularly in *Ebony* and *Essence* (the latter calling itself "The Magazine for Today's Black Woman"). One representative advertisement in November 1972 proclaimed,

"Nadinola beauty creams are specially formulated for you."[72] The ad also noted that the product contained hydroquinone, a skin-lightening agent that specifically targeted dark areas of the skin. In recent years, studies have shown that, while hydroquinone does lighten the skin, it does so by killing pigment cells and is highly toxic. At this point in the product's use, however, the term hydroquinone likely reassured consumers that it was "scientifically" formulated and therefore safe. By the 1980s, other companies began to advertise their skin-bleaching products in Canada, such as Dr. Fred Palmer, which claimed that its products possessed special gifts, invented by "secret formulas." In one representative advertisement in *Contrast*, the company promoted a facial soap and skin whitener: "Dr. Fred Palmer's SKIN WHITENER, an exclusive formula, will help give you a lovelier complexion. Your skin will be lighter and smoother and seem to glow as it succinctly comes alive! A pleasant, easy way to a soft, lovely and glowing skin…beauty cream that works to produce a clearer, lighter, brighter complexion."[73] Despite Black Is Beautiful, skin-bleaching products never waned in popularity throughout the 1960s and 1970s. By the early 1980s, other skin-bleaching creams, such as Ambi Fade Cream, which began to advertise in *Ebony* in the mid-1970s, hit the Canadian market.

In one representative advertisement from the October 1975 issue of *Ebony*, Ambi introduced itself to African American readers: "Welcome to AMBI's world of beauty.…AMBI helps clear your complexion leaving it radiantly alive and more naturally clear. AMBI leaves your skin looking more evenly toned, lovelier, soft and glowing. Blotches and ashiness seem to fade away."[74] In a June 1983 advertisement in *Share*, the company's slogan became, "Show-off the natural you…with Ambi skin toning cream."[75] Significantly, Ambi never branded its product as a skin whitener; instead, it emphasized the need for a clearer complexion. According to one regular user, many black women bought skin whiteners not to look white but to lighten their freckles and smooth out dark spots.[76] With respect to Nadinola, unlike its advertisements in *Ebony* in the 1940s, 1950s, and 1960s, which had celebrated the "Brownskin" beauty, by the 1980s, the company refrained from placing an emphasis on skin colour. Instead, its skin-bleaching creams became age-defying products. In one representative advertisement in *Share* in February 1985, the company's tagline read: "Smoother, Youthful-looking Skin All Over in Just Minutes a Day."[77] When I visited a black beauty store near Dufferin and Bloor Streets in Toronto in 2013, I counted nine skin-bleaching creams on the store's shelves—Dr. Clear, Dr. Fred Summit (formerly Dr. Fred Palmer), Nadinola, Ambi, Venus de

Milo, Carotone, Dermaclair, Sure White, and Palmers. Since the late 1970s, chemical relaxers have also appeared in the advertising pages of not only *Contrast*, but, since its appearance in 1978, *Share* as well. Importantly, the widespread use of chemical relaxers would not have been possible without a tight-knit network of local hair salons. Since the late 1960s, Toronto's West Indian community has thrived in part because of hair care businesses specializing not only in the latest hairstyles but also in the use of new chemical hair products.

Initially, black hair salons in Toronto almost exclusively offered thermal (hot-comb) hair straightening, salons such as Kemeel Azan's Beauty World, which opened in 1968, and Mells Hair Dressing, which posted an advertisement in the *News Observer* for the salon at Yonge and Dundas in December 1967. An advertisement for Phyllis' Authentic Hair Styles on Vaughan Road (at Oakwood) appeared in January 1968, and in April of that year, Rose's Beauty Salon on Oakwood Avenue, also advertised thermal hair straightening services. The latter also offered wig services. By the 1970s, however, Afro hairstyling became part of the repertoire of most black salons in Toronto. In 1973, for instance, Azan's Beauty World, which had vehemently resisted the Afro back in 1968, openly embraced the style. In November of that year, the salon posted an advertisement in *Contrast* that read, "Living Black—From the Afro to the Cornrow."[78] In April 1970, *Contrast* also reported on the one-month anniversary of Chalet Beauty Bar, a beauty salon operated by Jamaican-born Dorothy Flint.[79] Located at Queen Street East near Coxwell Avenue, a predominantly white neighbourhood at the time, Flint derived 75 percent of her business from white clientele. Where, by the mid-1960s, beauty salons in urban business districts in the United States increasingly integrated, with about one-quarter of black beauticians working in white-owned shops or on white customers,[80] in Canada, most black beauty salons were in predominantly white communities. As the black population was largely dispersed, there was no critical mass that would have justified exclusively servicing a black clientele. As such, black hairdressers who serviced white customers were not an anomaly; if a business were to survive it had to cater to all. Beauty schools, however, did not historically seek out black women. In keeping with the sea of change that swept across Toronto in the 1970s, that too began to change.

In 1928, Marvel Beauty School first advertised in the *Globe* that its Yonge Street location (opposite the Pantages Theatre) in Toronto was seeking hairdressers; by 1947, Marvel had operations on Bloor Street West in Toronto, and in Bramalea, Hamilton, and Ottawa.[81] As noted in chapter

2, Marvel openly denied black women access to their training schools in the 1940s, but by the early 1970s beauty schools actively sought to expand their black enrolment. In 1972, for instance, Marvel advertised its training for black hairstylists in *Contrast*; in an advertisement in September of that year, the school proclaimed, "It takes a SPECIAL talent to become a BLACK HAIR STYLIST.... Few hair stylists have the skill to work properly with black hair and white hair. A true styling specialist can achieve the sensational natural look in both. That specialist should be *you*. Marvel Schools is the only Beauty School in Canada teaching the professional level in both. You'll learn the art of temporary pressing, thermal setting and permanent hair straightening."[82] It is important to note that Marvel did not provide training in natural hairstyling; instead, it valorized the practice of hair straightening as the only technique for the handling of black hair. This is significant because, by the end of the decade, the chemical relaxer would return full force, marking the end of the Afro and the beginning of a *new* black beauty ideal. Toronto's black hair salons played pivotal roles in transitioning customers from wearing their hair in Afros to using chemical straightening products.

While hairdressers had used hair-straightening products since the 1960s, the first chemical hair-straightening products advertised in *Contrast* for sale in the city appeared in the early 1970s. In 1974, for example, Revlon's French Perm "no-base" chemical relaxer was offered for sale at Canadian drugstores.[83] The use of the term "no-base" was a strategy to minimize the product's potentially harmful effects by focusing on its ease of application; the health effects of using chemical relaxers were ignored, then minimized throughout the 1970s and 1980s. Instead, companies emphasized the low-maintenance appeal of relaxing one's hair. Where "base" relaxers required a person to coat their entire scalp with a protective cream prior to applying the chemical relaxer, "no-base" relaxers had a protective cream built into the relaxer that settled onto the scalp. Thus, Revlon's French Perm was a product that made the process of chemical relaxing easier. At the same time, when the company entered Canada's black beauty market, it continued the historical practice of white-owned companies masking their ownership of a black hair care product. Instead of using its trademarked company name, at first, Revlon's relaxers simply used the product name, French Perm. In April 1974, for instance, the company informed *Contrast* readers that French Perm No-Base Creme Relaxer, distributed locally by Ebony Eye Beauty Supplies, was available at several beauty salons located on Eglinton Avenue West.[84] Two months later, an Ebony Eye Beauty Supplies advertisement described the product as "French Perm ... The No-Jive, No-Base."[85] If one did not know that Revlon was the manufacturer of French Perm, one would think it was a black-owned product. The company's name did not appear anywhere in both advertisements. In May of that year, Royal Crown also promoted the sale of its no-base relaxer at "most food and drug stores"[86] in Toronto. In the early 1970s, the vast majority of Toronto's black hair salons were located in the Eglinton West community. Euphemistically known as "Little Jamaica" (although the neighbourhood's inhabitants range from across the Caribbean), Eglinton West stretches from Marlee Avenue to Dufferin Street; as the New York–based urban magazine *Fader* described in a 2016 feature, "[It's] the 'Harlem' of Toronto as it was and still is a major pulse for the Caribbean diaspora, as well as an economic hub for black Canadian businesses."[87]

Today, this stretch is still home to dozens of black hair salons and barbershops, such as Glamour Cuts Hair Design, Monica's Cosmetic Supplies, and Just Incredible!, which have been servicing a majority black clientele for decades. However, beginning in 2014, the construction of the Eglinton Crosstown, a new subway line, resulted in the closure of many of these businesses, and at the same time, many black businesses owners, in the city's most iconic West Indian neighbourhood, left the area permanently. In many ways, the lack of investment in black beauty culture from mainstream media parallels the lack of investment in black communities from municipal governments. But what is so inspiring about these businesses is that they do not thrive because of large-scale media promotion; they exist and continue to exist because of word of mouth and small-scale promotion in black communities. In the early 1970s, newspapers like *Contrast* understood the important role local black media could play in this regard.

In June of 1974, Ebony Eye Beauty Supplies informed *Contrast* readers that hair salons on Eglinton Avenue West, St. Clair Avenue West, and Dufferin Street were now using Revlon's French Perm.[88] In November 1975, when Eaton's placed an advertisement for a chemical relaxer treatment in *Contrast* it marked the decline of the retailer promoting Afro products in the newspaper. "For today's contemporary young woman, here's a great way to be first in hair fashion—and it won't cost you a penny," the advertisement read, adding that "Walter Fountaine, internationally known fashion and technical director for Glemby International, is coming to town—with a brand new technique called 'Defrisage' ... A contemporary method of relaxing hair to form its own curl pattern."[89] The advertisement also featured a light-skinned woman wearing the new style with a caption, "We'd

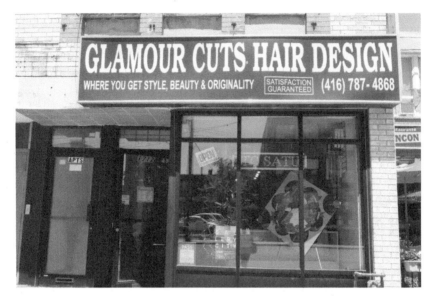

Figure 13a. Glamour Cuts Hair Design, Eglinton Avenue West, Toronto, Ontario, 2018. Photograph by author.

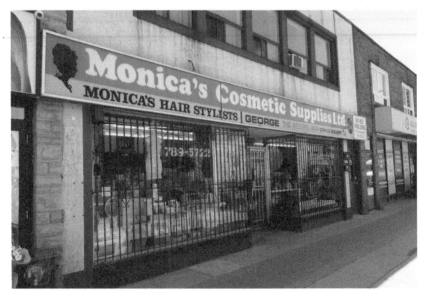

Figure 13b. Monica's Cosmetic Supplies, Eglinton Avenue West, Toronto, Ontario, 2018. Photograph by author.

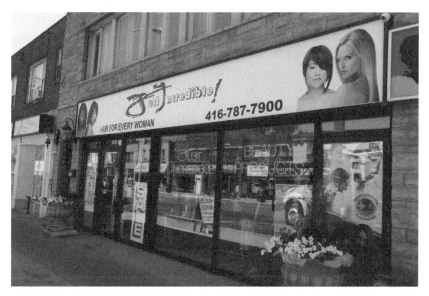

Figure 13c. Just Incredible!, Eglinton Avenue West, Toronto, Ontario, 2018. Photograph by author.

Like to Use Your Head." A few weeks later, Eaton's added "Defrisage" to its salon repertoire at its Queen Street, College Street, Yorkdale, Sherway Gardens, Don Mills, Bramelea, and Oshawa locations. "Different heads need different care and Eaton's 'Hairworks' has the answer," the advertisement read. "After a soothing shampoo, trained specialists smooth your hair with a new relaxer technique—Defrisage press-and-curl—and your hair emerges sleek and satiny. Then talented fingers snip and shape it into just the right style...and it's blown dry into a look you'll live happily with."[90]

In May 1976, Johnson Products, in co-operation with Marvel Beauty School, held one of the first chemical relaxer demonstrations in Toronto. According to *Contrast*'s reporting, a large number of hairstylists gathered at Yonge and Bloor in the city's core to hear advice from Marcia Glenn, a representative of Johnson Products in Chicago.[91] The newspaper may have continued to promote Black Is Beautiful, as in a September 1972 feature called, "Headwrapping Made Easy" that instructed readers on how to wrap their hair in a traditional African style,[92] but as the decade progressed, the advertising imagery of American-owned beauty companies appearing in the newspaper began to increasingly privilege straightened hair. One of the last advertisements to make prominent use of the Afro appeared in a July 1974 Flori Roberts advertisement in *Contrast*; it featured a sketch of a dark-skinned woman with full lips and an exceedingly large Afro. In her 1977 single, "Yu-ma/Go Away Little Boy," soul singer Marlena Shaw sang about Afro Sheen and Black Is Beautiful. By spring of that year, however, the Afro was unequivocally out, and the chemical relaxer was in. From thereon companies began to actively pursue strategies to expand the sale and use of the chemical relaxer across North America.

In May 1977, for example, one of the largest chemical-relaxer demonstrations took place in Toronto at the Westbury Hotel, at 475 Yonge Street, one block north of Carlton Street. *Contract* dubbed the Beverly Mascoll-organized event as a "Hair Relaxing and Mind-Blowing All in One Show."[93] The leading hair care firms—Revlon, Johnson Products, and Clairol—all appeared at the show. The demonstration was called "Yesterday, Today, and Tomorrow" and over two hundred people attended. According to *Contrast*'s reporting, "[The show] combined demonstrations in the new techniques of 'hair-relaxing,' and the latest examples of the new range of hair colouring open to Black people with a dazzling fashion parade." Mascoll introduced the hair show by telling the audience that ten years prior "few black women wore make-up—a fact which indicates the great strides which have been made by Black entrepreneurs in their efforts to bring the 'business' of beauty to the heart of beauty, the Black woman of today." Revlon also launched its Realistic relaxer at this hair show, which was purported to be "gentler" than previous products. Alongside Avril Spence, a contestant in the 1977 Miss Black Ontario beauty pageant, Bill Madison, Vice-President of Revlon-Realistic, demonstrated how to use the new chemical product. Madison was followed by the husband-and-wife team of Bill and Phyllis Broome from Johnson Products, who "willingly gave away some of their own trade secrets as they demonstrated the Afro-Sheen range of hair products from Johnson's," the newspaper reported. Tonya Lee Williams, best known for her role as Dr. Olivia Barber Winters on the American soap opera *The Young and the Restless*, was the first black women to be crowned Miss Black Ontario in 1977; the then 18-year-old Williams was chosen as Miss Oshawa and then became Miss Black Ontario at the pageant, which was held at the Royal York Hotel in downtown Toronto. In her publicity photograph, Williams, who was born in England but raised in Oshawa, Ontario, wore a short-cropped, straightened hairdo.

The 1977 black hair show was essentially a coming-out party for American companies and their newly formulated relaxers. It also marked the historical moment when chemical hair straightening became the cornerstone of black hair care. Product advertising from 1977 onward positioned the chemical product as "safe" while also equating hair straightening with a new kind of black woman. Straightened hair signalled a form of "feminine" black beauty that was also "sexy"; conversely, natural black hair—that is, tightly coiled hair—became an undesirable "masculine" look. From 1977 onward, advertising consistently affirmed this shift. In May of that year, for example, an Eaton's Fashion Fair advertisement for a new product line called "Sophisticated Lady" appeared in *Contrast*.[94] It featured a black model with chemically relaxed hair. The model's eyes gaze outwardly in a seductive pose and her bare shoulder is the focal point. The "sophisticated lady," the advertisement implied, was a woman who straightened her hair. The model invited a heterosexual *to-be-looked-at-ness* in which her desirability was made possible *because* of her long, flowing, straight hair.

In her iconic essay, "Visual Pleasure and Narrative Cinema," Laura Mulvey argues that white women in film were simultaneously looked at and displayed, with their appearance coded for strong visual and erotic impact so that they could be said to connote *to-be-looked-at-ness*."[95] She writes further that woman stood "in patriarchal culture as a signifier for the male other, bound by a symbolic order in which man can live out his fantasies and obsessions through linguistic command by imposing them on the silent image of woman still tied to her place as bearer, not maker, of meaning."[96] Several feminist writers have astutely pointed out that race and gender complicate Mulvey's theory. As Jane Gaines notes, "The notion of patriarchy is most obtuse when it disregards the position white women occupy over black men as well as black women."[97] The *to-be-looked-at-ness* of chemical-relaxer advertisements did not work the same way that hair care ads featuring the Afro had. Chemical-relaxer advertising constructed an image of "black woman-as-spectacle," as passive (i.e., feminine) and male-seeking (i.e., the bearer, not maker, of meaning), shifting the symbolism of the Afro, which from then on denoted an aggressive (i.e., masculine) form of black womanhood and connoted a lack of sexual attractiveness as far as the male (black) gaze was concerned. In October 1977 when the African American–owned Pro-Line Corporation, founded in 1970 by entrepreneur Comer Cottrell, placed an advertisement in *Contrast* for its Hair Food and Kiddie Kit relaxer for children, the advertising copy read, "Deep feelings create special occasions for you to look good. Beautiful luxurious hair requires the best Pro-Line Hair Food."[98] The advertising effectively equated straightened hair with the act of "appearing" and "being seen"; much like in the 1920s, when black women had faced a particular burden of *appearing*—that is, of deploying their own status as spectacular objects and as representations of a collective—chemical-relaxer advertising in the late 1970s equated "appearing" and "being seen" with new forms of black consumerism.

From today's vantage point, these advertisements reveal a tension between the representation of one's self and that of the collective. Chemical relaxers that targeted young black girls sought to cultivate the idea that straightening one's hair was a rite of passage into *true* womanhood. The chemicals in "kiddie relaxers" may have been less harsh than relaxers geared toward adult women, but the products did (and continue to) contain the caustic compound lye. Shauntae Brown White, in her analysis of the Motions for Kids comic book, *The Big Girl's Chair*, found that the goal of the comic book was to sell chemical-relaxer products to mothers and young girls. Within the story, she argues, the reader learns the benefits of the products (it is mild, it feels good, it smells nice, there is a colour change that signals that the relaxer is not completely washed out of the hair), which are all tucked into the story.[99] White also observes that natural hair was equated with a lack of progress and with the "dark ages."

In 1977, *Black Enterprise* (*BE*), the business magazine geared toward African Americans, listed Pro-Line and Johnson Products on its *BE*100, a list of the hundred largest black-owned firms.[100] Even though these companies created images that evoked a sexually available stereotype of black womanhood, they still became emblems of black business success. Back in the 1920s and 1930s, most African American photographers had favoured models that approximated a white European standard of beauty, especially straightened hair. As Deborah Willis and Carla Williams note, "their stock, soft-core imagery with an ethnic spin was created for the audience it represented and it perpetuated the ideal of black female beauty that closely resembled a white body."[101] Similarly, African American beauty firms in the late 1970s perpetuated a stock characterization of black womanhood that closely resembled a white body: one with long, flowing straight hair. For most black women, this aesthetic was almost impossible to achieve without the use of a chemical product. Therefore, it should have been of no surprise to Johnson Products and Pro-Line that, by 1978, both firms would face tough competition from white-owned companies, especially Revlon. One of the major reasons why white-owned companies successfully made inroads into the black hair care market was due to the industry-wide return of the cultivation of an image of black beauty that approximated a white standard of beauty.

Advertisements for hair straighteners in the late nineteenth and early twentieth centuries had relied on techniques that disparaged African features—often referring to black women's hair as "kinky," "ugly," or "unruly" and dark skin connected to a dark past while a prosperous future depended on a brighter and lighter skin tone. By the late 1970s, this juxtaposition disappeared through the seeming erasure of natural black hair and dark skin altogether. Straightened hair and light skin became the dominant image of black beauty, and in turn, dark skin and natural black hair ceased to exist as symbolic representations of Black Is Beautiful. Critics of turn-of-the-twentieth-century black beauty culturists claimed they exploited black women's insecurities, but the argument can be made that chemical relaxer firms in the late 1970s similarly exploited black women's insecurities. By the end of that decade, white-owned companies gained more control of the black hair care market by employing strategies first used by African American–owned firms like Johnson Products to woo black women consumers into chemically straightening their hair. In fact, one can trace the eventual loss of control of the black hair care market by African American firms to events that took place in 1975.

That year, the Federal Trade Commission (FTC) forced Johnson Products to sign a consent decree acknowledging safety problems with its Ultra Sheen Permanent Creme Relaxer, which according to the FTC contained sodium hydroxide (lye), a chemical that could cause hair loss and eye and skin damage. The FTC mandated that Johnson Products place a special warning for consumers on all its chemical relaxers that improper use could result in eye and skin damage.[102] The company agreed to the consent decree because it was under the impression that its competitors, most notably Revlon, would also be forced to follow suit. Instead, Revlon was not required to place a warning on its advertising and relaxer products until approximately two years later.[103] In the meantime, black consumers were given the impression that Revlon's French Perm and Realistic relaxers were safer than Johnson's Ultra Sheen relaxer, despite the fact that Revlon's relaxers also contained lye.[104] Outwardly, this decision by the FTC gave the appearance that the United States government was involved in a strategy to limit African American business development, especially in the context of a decade marked by white-owned companies' increased control of the black beauty market.

By the 1980s, Revlon and numerous other white-owned beauty firms began to dominate the chemical-relaxer market, either through product innovation or the acquisition of African American–owned companies. In response to firms like Revlon, some African Americans began to speak out against what they felt was an unequal playing field. In November 1986, for example, *Share* ran a story about a group of black hairstylists in Ontario who were discussing the Reverend Jesse Jackson's call to members of the African American community to boycott all Revlon's products. *Share's* reporter, Peter Scott, noted that in an article a month prior in the *Chicago Daily Defender*, Jackson had urged African Americans not to buy products from the company until it agreed to pull "its business out of South Africa and develop better relations with black America." In the opinion of Jackson and others, Revlon was "stealing business away from black companies."[105] Jackson's claims might have been true but he, and others like him, continued to ignore the damaging effects of long-term use of chemical relaxers. They also ignored the ways in which white-owned and African American–owned companies alike had once again, as was the case before Black Is Beautiful, valorized the light-skinned, straight-haired woman as emblematic of black beauty.

Following the Johnson decree and Revlon's growing presence in the black hair care market, many African American entrepreneurs began to fear that they were losing their grip on an industry they had created. It did not help that some black hairdressers publicly expressed a preference for Revlon's products over Johnson's products. In 1980, for instance, Barbara Ruffin, vice-president of Black Hair Is, told *BE* that Revlon's products were superior to Johnson's products. "It would not be fair to my customers to use a product just because a black made it," she told the magazine.[106] In the *BE* article, Irving J. Bottner, president of Revlon's Professional Products (salon) division is quoted as saying that the company had sold over seventeen million units of relaxer in 1978 and salon sales had risen 250 percent since 1975.[107] In chapter 4, I explain how, by the 1990s, the vast majority of the African American–owned beauty firms, including Johnson Products and Pro-line, had been acquired by Revlon and other white-owned companies such as L'Oréal, which introduced its own line of chemical relaxers called Radiance.

With respect to the black cosmetics market, through the 1970s, it was still nearly five times larger than the black hair care market, and as a result, Fashion Fair Cosmetics remained one of the only profitable African American–owned beauty companies, with products reportedly in over eight hundred department stores across the United States and Canada.[108] After the FTC ruling, however, the battle for control of the black hair care market intensified as firms feverishly worked to find ways to minimize the damaging effects of their products on the hair and scalp. Carson Products, founded in 1951 by African American Abram Minis, a native of Savannah, Georgia, was one of the first companies to do so. Carson Products first appeared in Canada when the company placed an advertisement for its Sta-Sof-Fro product in *Share* in April 1978.[109] Carson was also the first chemical-relaxer firm to use product labelling to convince users of the "safety" of relaxing their hair. Carson introduced a line of hair colour formulated specifically for black women in the early 1970s, but by 1978, it had also developed one of the first "no-lye" relaxers available at retail. On the heels of the FTC ruling against Johnson Products, Carson introduced Dark & Lovely, and while Sta-Sof-Fro for natural hair remained a top seller, the no-lye Dark & Lovely soon became Carson's flagship product.

The first Dark & Lovely advertisement in Canada appeared as a full-page spread on the inside cover of *Share* in July 1978.[110] The advertisement alerted readers that for the first time, they could purchase Dark & Lovely not only at beauty salons in Toronto but also in Hamilton, Edmonton, and Calgary. The black population in Alberta had been growing since the 1970s, and while the numbers paled in comparison to Toronto, Hamilton, and Montreal, the number of blacks in Alberta jumped from .09 percent in 1971 to roughly 1.5 percent by 1981.[111] According to a 1981 feature about black Calgary in *Contrast*, "In 1960 you couldn't find black hair products to save your life, but you could find a real community feeling among the people. Today, with approximately 7,500 blacks making their homes in Calgary, you can buy the things you need but the community feeling is gone."[112] This loss of community, the feature explained, was due to the diversification of both the constituents and the physical location of the black community, which now included people from "the West Indies, Africa, the United States and Canada" and was scattered with "Calgary's suburban spread" over an area of thirty or forty miles. This firsthand account of black Calgary points to the fact that while histories of black Canada have mostly focused on black populations in Ontario, Quebec, and Nova Scotia, there are a great many stories about blackness in Western Canada that have yet to be fully explored. For example, from the early 1900s to the 1960s, the Vancouver neighbourhood of Strathcona, also known as "Hogan's Alley" was home to the city's first and only black community. Hogan's Alley and the surrounding area was an ethnically diverse neighbourhood during this era—much like Toronto's "The Ward"—and was home not only to Italian, Chinese, and other immigrant groups, but also black families, black businesses, and Vancouver's only black church, the African Methodist Episcopal Fountain Chapel. Although it is the first and last neighbourhood in Vancouver with a substantial, concentrated black population, there has been little written about black life and black entrepreneurship in Hogan's Alley. While it is beyond the scope of this book, Hogan's Alley is yet another example of a black Canadian story that has scarcely been told.

Just as the 1980s marked a turning point in the growth and gentrification of black communities across the country, it also marked a moment when the government of Canada began to place advertisements in *Share* in promotion of multiculturalism, as policy but also as a national brand. The first of these advertisements appeared in 1979. In February and April of that year, the government of Canada ran an elaborate campaign in the magazine's pages that began, "All Canadians are not alike. Vive la différence!" and continued, "Canada is a unified nation made up of people from all corners of the world. It is a marvellous mosaic of peoples whose diverse cultural roots and values are uniquely united into one national family, living together in peace, understanding, and a spirit of freedom. The fact that all Canadians are not alike gives us our diversity. It's a rich diversity that allows each Canadian the freedom to be different...equal."[113] Multiculturalism, the ad continued, "both reflects and responds to this Canadian reality." Signed by the Honourable Norman Cafik, Canada's first Minister of State for Multiculturalism, the advertisement included the slogan, "Multiculturalism: unity through human understanding." Others advertisement included the tagline, "There's No Such Thing as Being More or Less Canadian."[114] "In our country," the February 1979 ad copy stated, "a Canadian is a *Canadian*, regardless of his or her background...regardless of whether they were born in Canada or immigrated here. In Canada, we respect each person as an individual. We respect the individual's race, cultural roots, religious and spiritual values....All Canadians are *equal*. There is no such thing as being more or less Canadian...thanks to our policy on Multiculturalism."

While variations on this advertising campaign appeared in *Share* between 1980 and 1988, the acknowledgment of multiculturalism in the Canadian Charter of Rights and Freedoms in 1982, the formalization of the Canadian Multiculturalism Act in 1988, and the passage of the Employment Equity Act (1986/1995) all helped to entrench widely held beliefs in the ethos of diversity *as* Canadian. After all, it is our policy of multiculturalism that distinguishes Canada from the United States. By promoting multiculturalism to black readers of *Share*, the government (knowingly or not) helped to construct the notion that black people were all newly arrived immigrants, rather than the multi-generational Canadians that many were. This framing of black *as* immigrant, which has continued since the late 1980s, has placed a symbolic veil of erasure over historical black communities in Western Canada, the Maritimes, and small towns throughout Ontario. At the same time, the protection of cultural rights in Canada has meant that, even allowing for the smaller Canadian population, there have been proportionately fewer cases involving discrimination as it relates to black cultural practices, such as hair, than in the United States. However, as discussed in chapter 5, in recent years, black women have been at the centre of hair discrimination in Toronto, Montreal, and elsewhere across the country. The first hair case to make headlines in the United States occurred in 1969 when Deborah Renwick, an African American flight attendant for United Airlines was fired after three years of employment because she wore a natural hairstyle rather than straightening her hair.[115] Airline officials considered Renwick's short Afro, about three inches from her head, "inappropriate." In 1981, when American Airlines fired ticket agent Renee Rogers for wearing cornrows, she filed a discrimination suit against the company, challenging its policy prohibiting employees from wearing an all-braided hairstyle. Rogers claimed that American Airlines' grooming policy violated the Civil Rights Act of 1964 because the policy discriminated against her as a woman, but also as a black woman. In effect, her claim was based on both racial and sex discrimination.

The US Federal District Court of New York rejected Rogers's claim that the style evoked her African heritage, observing that her wearing of the hairstyle came after the release of the 1979 film *10*.[116] At the height of the Afro's popularity in the early 1970s, cornrows and braids emerged as alternatives for women who felt Afros were too commercial and not authentically "African." In March 1980, *Share* ran an editorial titled "African Braids Are In This Summer." The article, written by one of Eaton's Hairworks' black stylists, informed readers that braiding was once a casual hairstyle, but that it had since become a trend: "It has been shunned and still is, by many who cannot appreciate the beauty, the art, and message that each individual strand of hair carries ... a message of strength, beauty and wonder," *Share* reported.[117] African American singers such as Peaches (of the group Peaches and Herb) and Patrice Rushen had worn braids, but in the mainstream media (and in some black circles) braids officially became a trend when the blonde-haired, blue-eyed Bo Derek wore her hair in cornrows in *10*. By 1980, in the pages of *Time* and *Newsweek* and in the lexicon of American mainstream culture, cornrows *became* "Bo Braids." Even though hair braiding was rooted in African cultures and several African

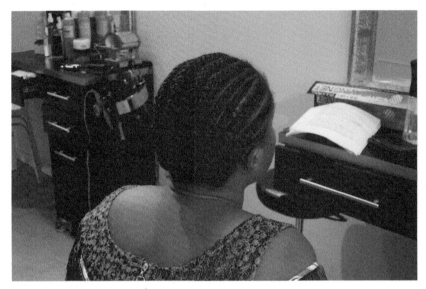

Figure 14. Cornrows hairstyle, Glamour Cuts Hair Design, Eglinton Avenue West, Toronto, Ontario, 2018. Photograph by author.

American actresses had worn the style on television—most notably, Cicely Tyson in the television drama series *East Side, West Side* (1963–64)—there were seldom any photographs or articles written about black women who cornrowed their hair. As far as the mainstream media were concerned, Derek was, effectively, the creator of the hairstyle, which, for many black women, added insult to injury.

In the 1960s and 1970s when black women first wore beaded braids and/or cornrows as an expression of their African heritage, this was not an accepted practice. Singer Roberta Flack, who had worn her hair braided for years, expressed some anger over the "Bo Braids" phenomenon. As Flack told *The Christian Science Monitor* in 1980, "Black women were wearing cornrows long before Bo Derek." "I took issue that they made such a big thing about Bo Derek and cornrows," Flack continued. "I can see this Bo Derek doll going out, the '10' doll, with braids. And they'll make a zillion dollars off it."[118] Following Derek's popularization of the style, white women were suddenly given liberty to once again appropriate the Other, as the style quickly swept across the mainstream hair care industry. Places such as Le Braids Cherie—a braids-only salon—opened in Hollywood, specifically catering to the new look. New York City's Pierre Mitchell Salon charged five hundred dollars to braid white women's hair and add accessories like semiprecious stones; white women looking to spend less could go to a beauty salon in Harlem to get cornrows.[119]

While in the 1960s and 1970s several non-black celebrities such as Barbra Streisand had adopted the Afro hairstyle, and Macy's sold Afro wigs in various colours,[120] the adoption of cornrows by white women was different. On the surface, it appeared that whites were taking their beauty cues from black culture, but the appropriation of the hairstyle was mostly superficial and had very little to do with black culture. When the court dismissed Rogers's argument that Bo Derek had not popularized cornrows and that it was a style worn by black women that was reflective of cultural and historical meaning,[121] the dismissal helped to disavow the style as being unequivocally rooted in black cultures and communities. As Susan Bordo asserts, with Bo Derek, and by extension all white women who wore cornrows, there was a privilege that was "so unimpeachably white as to permit an exotic touch of 'otherness' with no danger of racial contamination."[122] When Bo Derek wore cornrows, it was viewed as a normalizing feminine practice, but when black women did the same, the practice was regarded as mimetic. Eventually white women discarded the hairstyle almost as quickly as they had picked it up. For black women, however, wearing one's hair in cornrows—especially in the workplace—opened the door for a punitive response from white employers.

Throughout the 1980s, other African American women would be fired for wearing their hair in braids and/or cornrows. In 1987, Pamela Walker, a full-time teacher and doctoral student at the University of Illinois at Chicago, was fired from her part-time job at the Chicago Regency Hyatt for wearing cornrows; and a year later, the Marriott Hotel in Washington, DC, sent home part-time employee Pamela Mitchell because she wore her hair, in their words, in an "extreme, cornrowed hairstyle."[123] Two months later, a supervisor at the Hyatt Regency Crystal City, also in Washington, DC, told Cheryl Tatum, a thirty-seven-year-old restaurant cashier, to pull her braids into a bun to comply with the company's dress code. After she complied, the personnel director told her to take out the braids once again because the Hyatt prohibited "extreme and unusual hairstyles."[124] These cases help to explain why black women continued to use chemical relaxers in the 1980s, and why the appeals by companies about the safety of these products grew more overt. If a black woman could be punished for wearing a "natural" hairdo, using a chemical relaxer, especially one branded as "safe," would seem like the best option available to her.

When the first Dark & Lovely advertisement appeared in *Share* in 1978, it provided a detailed explanation of how to use the chemical product, including the following notice: "No base formula—one strength beautifully relaxes all hair textures. Gentle enough for colour treated hair. (DO NOT USE ON BLEACHED HAIR.) DOES NOT CONTAIN SODIUM HYDROXIDE (Caustic Soda—Lye)." Black women had commonly complained about damaged hair and burnt scalps from the use of chemical products; as such, in addition to these disclaimers, from the late 1970s onward, chemical relaxer companies also instructed users to "follow directions carefully to avoid hair loss, scalp and eye injury." The Dark & Lovely copy explained that Carson Products had conducted "interviews at beauty counters, in homes and beauty salons" with black women to find out what they wanted and did not want in a hair relaxer; these women said:

1 The product *must* work—it *must* relax the hair.
2 It should not irritate or burn the scalp.
3 It shouldn't break the hair or cause hair loss.
4 It should produce permanent results: the hair shouldn't revert.
5 It shouldn't have that caustic smell.[125]

In September 1978, a Carson Products demonstration for Dark & Lovely took place at a Shoppers Drug Mart in northwest Toronto. With a headline that read, "No Burns, Hair Product Claims," the *Share* article marked the first time that black beauty products were sold by the drugstore chain, which was founded by Romanian-born pharmacist Murray Koffler in 1962.

"In its promotional material Carson Products, the makers of Dark & Lovely hair preparations, claim beautiful hair is the result of good nutrition, adequate exercise, enough sleep and proper basic care," *Share*'s Jules Elder explained. "While some of the most popular relaxers contain lye which burns the hair and irritates the scalp, the Dark & Lovely product which does not contain soda or lye, is claimed to have proven in tests that it is less irritating," the article added.[126] A Shopper's Drug Mart Calgary advertisement, appearing in *Contrast* in November 1987, offered for sale not only Dark & Lovely but also Sta-Sof-Fro, Ultra Sheen, Lustrasilk, Ambi, and other hair care products that would come to the marketplace in the 1980s, such as T.C.B. and Blue Magic.[127] This suggests that by the late 1980s, the use of not only chemical relaxers but also skin-whitening creams was common practice in black communities in Alberta, as well. Dark & Lovely's safety claims had grown increasingly more convincing throughout the 1970s.

In a representative advertisement in *Share* in April 1979, for instance, the company declared that Dark & Lovely was "guaranteed less burning than other leading relaxers."[128] The copy then asked a series of questions, followed by detailed answers. The questions included "How does a relaxer work?" "Isn't relaxing harmful to the hair?" "Aren't relaxers pretty much all alike?" and "How is Dark & Lovely different?" With respect to the claim that Dark & Lovely caused "less irritation and burning," the company was asked how they could prove it. "First of all with animals," the advertisement read, adding:

> In independent laboratory tests, Dark & Lovely produced far less swelling and reddening [less than half as much] than the mild formulas of leading lye based relaxer. Then we supplied an independent laboratory with Dark & Lovely, Ultra Sheen and Revlon Realistic for testing on human volunteers. The products were coded so the technicians would not know which product was being applied to individual test areas. Each product was applied to its own test area on each of 100 persons. Each person was asked to comment on any burning sensation at the test sites. The areas were also closely examined by laboratory personnel.

Not surprisingly, the copy said that Johnson Products' Ultra Sheen caused the greatest number of irritations and/or burning sensations, Revlon's Realistic placed second, and Dark & Lovely caused the fewest burns and/or scalp irritations. Carson Products essentially affirmed the fact that while a chemical relaxer did cause some degree of burn, the burning was a "natural" part of the process, and at least Dark & Lovely was the "safest" option. By the end of 1979, Dark & Lovely, which was available across Canada via local distributors in Toronto, Ottawa, Montreal, Winnipeg, and Edmonton, was reportedly "the largest selling complete line of hair products for the black woman" and the product was described as "a beautiful way to relax your kind of hair."[129] When I got my first relaxer at the age of fourteen, I vividly remember choosing Dark & Lovely because I believed that it was "safer" than other products. Undoubtedly, thousands of other black women and girls also used this product because of its safety claims. As Sut Jhally notes, advertisements "have to move us in some way, make us think or react; they have to pull at our emotions, desires and dreams; they have to engage the audience actively in some thought process that will, advertisers hope, lead to the purchase of their product in the marketplace."[130] The power of

Carson's advertising had spoken. Chemical relaxers *became* "safe"; black women consumers had no reason to assume that they were not. However, these companies were selling a bag of lies about the caustic nature of no-lye versus lye relaxers.

The main, active ingredient in a no-lye relaxer is calcium hydroxide or guanidine hydroxide. Although the pH of a no-lye relaxer is typically lower than lye-based products, no-lye relaxers are often associated with dryer hair due to potential calcium buildup. The only potential benefit of a no-lye relaxer is that it is milder on the scalp at the time of application; in the long-term, a no-lye relaxer still has the effect of damaging the hair follicle. Both types of relaxers contain ingredients that work by breaking chemical bonds of the hair, and each will eventually cause some damage to the hair. Therefore, women who use chemical relaxers also use a myriad of products to keep the hair moisturized to avoid excessive dryness of the scalp. Over the years, the US Food and Drug Administration (FDA) has received complaints about scalp irritation and hair breakage related to both lye and no-lye relaxers. The FDA has a page on its website that warns consumers about the use of hair dyes and hair relaxers. Comparatively, Health Canada has never issued any warnings about chemical relaxers, though it has advised against keratin treatments also known as "Brazilian straightening."

In 2010, Health Canada warned the public that some professional keratin hair-smoothing solutions had been found to contain levels of formaldehyde (a known carcinogen) above regulated limits. The CBC reported that, as of 2010, formaldehyde was permitted as a preservative in cosmetics at levels no higher than 0.2 percent, but Health Canada had found ten products that contained levels higher than allowed, ranging from 1.8 percent to 7 percent.[131] The products were available at salons across Canada and were not generally available directly to consumers, but Health Canada had received complaints of burning eyes, nose, and throat, breathing difficulties, and one report of hair loss. In 2011, eleven more keratin hair-smoothing solutions were found to contain formaldehyde levels above Health Canada's limit.[132] A keratin straightening treatment is a semi-permanent hair-smoothing system that targets the cuticle, or the outside layer, of the hair. In an article in *Bazaar* in 2016, David Babaii, a celebrity hairstylist in Los Angeles explained the process: "It deposits a liquid version of the protein keratin that your hair is made up of along with a chemical preservative—this is then blown dried directly into the hair followed by flat ironing the strand into a straight position."[133] While the dangers of keratin, used primarily by women not of African descent, have caught the attention of Canada's dominant media and that of women's magazines in the United States, the dangers of chemical relaxers, used primarily by black women, have been all but ignored by these same outlets. This lack of media focus and governmental attention speaks to the ways in which institutional discourses about health and product awareness ignore black women even as there is growing health research pointing to the harm chemical products cause to the scalp and body.

In 2003, dermatological researcher Amy McMichael found a causal link between hair shaft dryness, increased fragility of the hair cuticle, and chemical relaxers, which is why users are required to treat their hair with oils and other products: that is, to a great extent, to lessen the potentially damaging effects of the chemicals on the hair.[134] Hair studies in South Africa have found that chemical relaxers are used by more than two-thirds of African women to straighten their hair, and that relaxed hair lengths were found to be much shorter than non-relaxed hair, suggesting increased fragility.[135] A published 2011 study in the *American Journal of Epidemiology* was one of the first to link chemical relaxers with an increased risk of uterine leiomyomata (also known as uterine fibroids) in black women.[136] In this study, scientists followed more than twenty-three thousand premenopausal black American women from 1997 to 2009 and found that there was a two to three times higher rate of fibroids among black women that may be linked to chemical exposure through scalp lesions and burns resulting from chemical relaxers.

When researchers at Wake Forest Baptist Medical Center in North Carolina sampled 103 black women from the area in 2013, they found that about a third exercised less simply because they were concerned it would jeopardize their (chemically relaxed) hair.[137] A 2009 national study in the United States that was repeated in 2017 further indicated that an estimated 70 percent of white women and between 80 and 90 percent of African American women will develop uterine fibroids by the age of fifty; and while Central Centrifugal Cicatricial Alopecia (CCCA) is likely underdiagnosed, some estimates report a prevalence of rates as high as 17 percent of black women having this condition, which was the most common type of scarring hair loss found in African American women.[138] CCCA, sometimes referred to as "hot comb alopecia," is a permanent form of hair loss that begins at the central scalp. While for many years there was no conclusive evidence that relaxers or hot combs caused CCCA, a 2011 study published in *JAMA Dermatology* (formerly *Archives of Dermatology*) suggested that hair-grooming practices that cause traction, such as hair weaves and braids, may contribute to the development of CCCA.[139]

In 2018, a study published in *Environmental Research* that also made international headlines found that hair care products used primarily by black women in the United States contain a variety of chemicals that have been linked to asthma, hormone disruptions, and even cancer. After analyzing eighteen commonly used hair cosmetics such as chemical relaxers, root stimulators, and anti-frizz products, researchers detected sixty-six chemicals with potentially toxic effects, and eight in ten of the products studied contained parabens and phthalates, which are known endocrine disruptors—substances that disturb the body's hormone balance.[140] Regular exposure to phthalates is thought to cause early puberty and preterm births; as well, researchers found that compounds associated with obesity and a higher risk of breast cancer were present in 30 percent of the hair treatments they analyzed. The scientific evidence in the twenty-first century continues to affirm that black women are more likely than white or Hispanic women to suffer from hormonal diseases that are exacerbated by substances that disrupt hormonal balance; a 2016 study showed that black women in the United States have higher concentrations of such chemicals in their bodies than do women from other ethnicities.[141]

In the late 1970s, before dermatologists and health researchers paid any attention to hair-straightening treatments, chemical relaxers became the most commonly used product among black women. As previously noted, even though no-lye relaxers still contained a chemical compound that was just as damaging as lye relaxers, when Carson Products marketed Dark & Lovely as "safe," the result was big profits. With respect to Johnson Products, though the company had taken a hit in 1975 after the FTC decree, dropping in market share from 60 percent to 40 percent,[142] by 1980, it was aggressively attempting to reclaim its place atop the chemical relaxer market. At the Sheraton Centre in downtown Toronto in April of that year, the company unveiled its new no-lye relaxer, Ultra Sheen Precise TM Conditioning.[143]

According to *Contrast*'s reporting, the Precise relaxer was the first product to combine relaxing and conditioning in one step: "No one has ever been able to combine a relaxer and conditioner into one product, though some of the most sophisticated laboratories in the country have been working on it for years," said George E. Johnson to *Contrast*. "We've gone into salons and talked to stylists. We've gone into the streets and talked to Black women.... Other relaxers, both professional and retail, are effective straighteners but they tend to leave hair dry and brittle, with split ends.... Precise changes all that," Johnson added. In the same issue, a full-page advertisement for Johnson's Ultra Sheen Permanent Creme Relaxer appeared. The advertisement featured a light-skinned black woman with coiffed straightened hair, one hand resting on her bare shoulder; the caption read, "Because you're ultra special." When another advertisement from Johnson Products appeared in August 1980, the copy included the words "scientific," as Carson Products had done, undoubtedly to downplay the products' caustic nature. Emphasizing that the product was available only through licensed hair salons, the advertising copy read, "an incredible scientific breakthrough in hair relaxers. Developed after years of research, this fabulous product is the only one of its kind. The first relaxer that relaxes and conditions your hair in just one step and actually makes your hair look healthier."[144] In May 1981, Johnson Products renamed its Precise Relaxer "Gentle-Treatment" and added a "contains no sodium hydroxide (lye)" notice to all its advertisements. Since the early 1980s, all chemical relaxers sold at retail contain a warning of their potential to cause burns to the scalp and/or face, but there are no such warnings about the full range of chemicals (some listed under vague descriptions such as "fragrances") in many of these products.

Where, by the early 1980s, the chemical relaxer would become the industry standard, another chemical product briefly challenged its popularity. Known as the "Jheri Curl," it was also called the "Is Curl," "Jerry Curl" or "Jeri Curl." Companies marketed the Jheri Curl as a "low-maintenance" curly style, an alternative to the chemical relaxer. As Judy Davis explains, the style did not require the use of hot curlers or rollers for daily styling, and the curly texture was achieved via a two-step process: "an ammonium thioglycolate base used to straighten the natural hair followed by a roller set doused with a second chemical solution to create permanent curls. The style is thereafter maintained by liberal daily applications of a curl activator or moisturizing product."[145] It was Jheri Redding, a white, Illinois-born farmer turned hair care entrepreneur, who invented the chemical process to convert straight hair into curly hair and produce the original "curly perm" (as it was also known). Importantly, Redding's invention was not intended for coarse-textured hair; it was originally formulated for naturally straight hair.[146]

Willie Lee Morrow, author of the 1973 book *400 Years without a Comb* and creator of the plastic Afro pick, had been working on a chemical process to turn "kinky" hair curly since 1966.[147] Following Redding's invention, in

1977, Morrow changed the name of his company from the Tomorrow Curl to the California Curl, and the style began to take off. In the late 1970s, numerous Jheri Curl products hit the market, all of which used a different brand name. The African American–owned SoftSheen, founded in Chicago in 1964 by Edward and Bettiann Gardner, marketed a Care Free Curl product; Pro-Line had Curly Kit; Johnson Products sold Classy Curl; and Carson Products' Sta-Sof-Fro was also used to maintain a Jheri Curl. In March 1980, Eaton's made the Jheri Curl its highest priority, placing an ad in *Share* that gave a 20 percent discount on all relaxer perms, including the "exciting new 'Is Curl' (Jerry Curl)." The caption read, "'Is' . . . it's the right chemistry. More than a look, it's a let-go, laid-back feeling. In fact, a whole new no-fuss life for black hair. Leaves the shine behind. Makes hair easier to manage. You'll love it!"[148]

The supposed low maintenance claims of Jheri Curl products appealed to those who were looking for an alternative to using a chemical relaxer, which was quite labour intensive. However, the product contained similarly harsh chemicals and, if the hair was not cared for, left the hair just as brittle and dry. The style was also very expensive to maintain because it required a chemical process to start but also the daily excessive use of multiple products, from curl activator sprays to oils and moisturizers. Within months of the Jheri Curl's arrival, African American celebrities adopted the style, from the Jackson Five to New Edition, from Nikolas Ashford and Lionel Ritchie to actress Debbie Allen—all sported the new look. Unlike styles that depended upon chemical relaxers, which were primarily used by black women, both men and women wore the Jheri Curl. Part of the reason why men were attracted to the Jheri Curl was because it did not require curlers and irons, which were costly, time consuming, and historically coded as feminine beauty aids. When Michael Jackson was injured filming a Pepsi commercial on January 27, 1984, the hairstyle gained a lot of negative publicity. During a pyrotechnic stunt, sparks came in contact with Jackson's Jheri Curl, which was coated with curl activator, causing extensive burns to his hair and scalp. While many users suffered no ill effects with the style, some did encounter problems, including hair breakage and thinning.[149] By the end of 1984, the Jheri Curl had lost its lustre, and chemical relaxers once again became the dominant chemical hair product for sale at retail.

In Eddie Murphy's *Coming to America* (1988), the character of Darryl Jenks (played by Eriq La Salle) was a model and heir to his family's company, producers of "Soul Glo," a Jheri Curl-like product. The film parodied the fact that a Jheri Curl needed to be worn wet with activator products and in many cases the excessive wetness of the hair stained pillowcases, couches, and other fabrics. Because the Jheri Curl had declined in popularity after Jackson's burns, when it appeared in *Coming to America* four years later, the style was represented as a joke. It had become one. The product-intensive nature of the style, however, had catapulted African American–owned companies SoftSheen, Carson, and Pro-Line, to the top of the black hair care market. This reign would come crashing down in the 1990s when a frenzy of mergers and acquisitions—spurred on by the growth of white-owned beauty companies and the interest of consumer brand conglomerates in black women consumers—would see nearly all the major African American–owned black beauty companies bought and sold.

As global, multinational companies gained control of black hair care and cosmetics firms in the 1990s, black beauty aesthetics in advertisements shifted. The ownership and control of the black beauty market by global conglomerates also made the transnational linkages between advertising, consumers, and representation even more central to the question of beauty than ever before. At the same time, black women (such as Halle Berry, Veronica Webb, and Tyra Banks) became the "faces" of global beauty brands, and diversity was increasingly used as a marketing strategy to attract more black women consumers. American magazines and advertisers began to perceive "multiculturalism" as a fashion aesthetic. For example, in February 1989, *Vogue* loudly proclaimed, "Everybody's all-American," and "The face of American beauty has changed to reflect the nation's ethnic diversity."[150] In the next chapter, I explore three overarching questions. First, where and how did this new "multicultural" beauty appear in Canada? Second, as white-owned conglomerates acquired African American–owned beauty product firms, how did advertisements for black beauty products in the pages of *Contrast* and *Share* change? And third, why did it become important for white-owned conglomerates to hide their ownership of African American beauty brands behind "black" product labelling and imagery? In the 1990s, these questions became fundamental to the beauty culture industry's transnational, global expansion—not only into Canada, but into the Caribbean and Africa, as well.

CHAPTER FOUR

GLOBAL CONGLOMERATES TAKE OVER BLACK BEAUTY CULTURE: THE ETHNICALLY AMBIGUOUS, "MULTICULTURAL" 1990S AND 2000S

In the early 1970s, the three leading beauty firms in the United States were Estée Lauder, Avon, and Revlon, and each had different strategies for success. Avon, with US$1 billion in sales, was still selling products with its door-to-door strategy; Revlon distributed its high-end lines through department stores but also through drugstores and other mass-market outlets, which accounted for its US$506 million in annual sales; and Estée Lauder targeted the department stores and specialty stores for its high-end products.[1] By 1978, the cosmetics and hair care products industry was valued at US$7 billion in the United States.[2] With respect to black beauty culture, Johnson Products, with its Ultra Sheen and Afro Sheen product lines, held 30 to 40 percent of the estimated US$120 million yearly black hair care market.[3] The other leading African American–owned beauty firm, Fashion Fair, with annual sales of its cosmetic line conjectured to be in the range of US$25 million, was in tight competition against white-owned Flori Roberts and Revlon with its "Polished Amber" line, whose sales doubled year over year throughout the 1970s.[4] In an August 1978 feature in *Black Enterprise (BE)*, the African American business magazine estimated that African Americans spent US$750 million annually for toiletries, cosmetics, and hair care products.[5] Pro-Line and Barbara Walden Cosmetics still held their ground, Pro-Line with US$7 million a year in hair care product sales and Walden with US$1 million for their skin care product and fragrances.

:r, as a Barbara Walden executive admitted to *BE* at the time, the
. American–owned company was struggling, despite the fact that
lucts were in some of the top department stores in New York City,
Atlanta, Chicago, and Los Angeles.[6] That same year, *BE* also observed that
"[In 1968], when the Afro hairstyle was the order of the day and the Avon
lady was invariably white, the black beauty care market was virtually dominated by black manufacturers."[7] Over the course of the 1970s, however, black
beauty products entered the mainstream retail sector (department stores
and drugstores) and by the 1990s, white-owned conglomerates slowly and
steadily acquired black-owned firms. With this control, black beauty culture
remained "black" on the outside (i.e., its product labelling and branding)
but on the inside, black beauty culture was primarily controlled by the
same white-owned firms that had virtually ignored black consumers twenty
years earlier.

In a 1998 article in *BE* titled "Hair Care Firms Get Ownership Makeover," the magazine declared that the battle over the black hair care market
between white-owned firms—which included companies such as Unilever, Procter & Gamble, and Johnson & Johnson—and African American
firms had just begun.[8] In June of that year, Revlon acquired African Pride,
and with it gained 10 percent control of the black beauty product market.[9] In September, L'Oréal also acquired SoftSheen, gaining control of
the brands Optimum, Mizani and Wave Nouveau. SoftSheen, which had a
reported US$95 million in sales that year, was the industry leader in both
the retail and salon categories.[10] In 2000, in an effort to expand its reach in
the black hair care market, L'Oréal opened a multimillion-dollar research
and development laboratory in Chicago called the "L'Oréal Institute for
Ethnic Hair and Skin Research." The company claimed that it was the first
lab to focus specifically on the study of "ethnic" skin and hair. In 2000, the
Colomer family, together with the investment company CVC, purchased
Revlon's Professional Products division. This division included several
chemical relaxer lines (Creme of Nature, Realistic, and Fabu-laxer) that are
today sold through Colomer USA, which is based in Jacksonville, Florida.
Colomer was created in 1933 by Spaniard José Colomer Ametller who,
upon his return to Spain after a period in Paris, trained as a hairdresser and
created the company. With the Colomer family's purchase of Revlon's Professional Products division, the Barcelona-based firm became the Colomer
Group. Revlon first entered the black hair care market in the 1960s when
't acquired the African American–owned company Deluxol. While the
ïpany initially advertised under the Deluxol name, it soon abandoned

that strategy and began to use its own name. In so doing, it employed the same marketing strategy as that of African American–owned firms, most notably Johnson Products, which had lost 50 percent of its market share to Revlon after the 1975 Federal Trade Commission decree that required the company to affix a warning to its chemical relaxers.[11]

In 1998, Carson Products was the only African American–owned beauty products firm to make any acquisitions. It bought Johnson Products from the Miami-based IVAX Corporation for US$70 million; IVAX had acquired Johnson Products back in 1993 in a transaction valued at between US$61 million and US$73 million at the time. In 1993, Johnson Products was still the largest African American–owned company.[12] In addition to its existing brands Dark & Lovely, Excelle, and Beautiful Beginnings, after its acquisition of Johnson Products, Carson gained control of Gentle Treatment, Ultra Sheen, Afro Sheen and the Classic Curl lines. Just two years later, however, L'Oréal acquired Carson Products, creating the SoftSheen-Carson division, which included the aforementioned brands, in addition to the Precise relaxer and Let's Jam hair oils.[13] In 1999, Alberto-Culver acquired the African American–owned Pro-Line, gaining control of Soft & Beautiful, Just For Me, TCB (Taking Care of Business), and Motions chemical relaxer brands.[14] Alberto-Culver, founded in Illinois in 1955 by Leonard H. Lavin, also owned VO5, St. Ives (skin care products), and TRESemmé shampoo. With the acquisition of Pro-Line, Alberto-Culver became the second largest black hair care firm, behind L'Oréal.[15] Together, TCB and Motions accounted for more than US$50 million in global sales.[16] In 2010, however, the Dutch consumer-goods company Unilever acquired Alberto-Culver for US$3.7 billion, making Unilever one of the largest owners of black beauty brands.[17] After L'Oréal bought Carson, Proctor & Gamble (P&G), the Cincinnati-based multinational consumer goods company, purchased Johnson Products. In March 2009, however, an African American–owned holding company headed by Eric and Renee Brown, the son-in-law and daughter of former Pro-Line CEO Commer Cottrell, bought Johnson Products, repositioning the company once again as an African American–owned firm.[18] In 2003, P&G expanded into the foreign hair-colouring market when it acquired Wella, a German-based hair-colouring and fragrance business for US$7 billion.[19] The company first entered the hair dye business in 2001 when it acquired Clairol, a division of the New York–based pharmaceutical giant Bristol-Myers Squibb (BMS).[20] According to market research firm A. C. Nielsen, at the time Clairol had control of 39 percent of the US hair-colouring market, with L'Oréal controlling 50 percent.[21]

With respect to black cosmetics, in 1989 there were four cosmetics firms owned by African American women. These were Barbara Walden Cosmetics; Naomi Sims Beauty Products (founded in 1985 by the former model); Paris-based Gazelle International (founded in 1983 by Patricia A. French and chemist Amale Ayad, it first operated as a salon in Dakar, Senegal, before launching in France in 1986 and America in 1987); and Juin Rachele Cosmetics (founded in Houston in 1986 by former Max Factor executive Juin Rachele Cooper and her husband Patrick D. Cooper).[22] Alongside Fashion Fair and Flori Roberts, these women vied for a percentage of the upscale black cosmetics market. While Naomi Sims, Gazelle, and Juin Rachele products were available in stores such as Saks Fifth Avenue, Nordstrom, Macy's, and the Milwaukee-headquartered Carson Pirie Scott, these lines were also sold in Canada, Europe, and the Caribbean.[23] In 1994, Somali-born supermodel Iman also launched a cosmetics line. Today, Iman Cosmetics can be found in the United States, the United Kingdom, France, Brazil, Africa, and the Caribbean. In Canada, the products were sold at independent beauty supply shops and at Sears until the department store filed for bankruptcy in June 2017, closing twenty full-line locations across the country. By the 1990s, however, black-owned cosmetics firms also faced tough competition from global conglomerates. After 1990 US census data revealed that one in four American women described themselves as non-white, white-owned beauty companies pursued the black skin care market with separate distribution networks and advertising strategies. The 1990 census figures also showed that, of the African American population of nearly 30 million (29,986,060, according to 1990 census figures), African American women were younger (30 percent were in the prime purchasing age range of eighteen to thirty-four), better educated, and more affluent than in prior generations.[24] Thus, black women became a sought-after segment of the cosmetics market, in addition to the hair care products market. Further, the African American population in the early 1990s was also growing at twice the rate of its white counterpart. With this information, large conglomerates began to conduct market research on black consumers to gain deeper insight into how to reach this largely ignored segment of the beauty market.

The market research firm Business Trends Analysts Inc. found that, although African Americans constituted 12 to 13 percent of the US population in 1989, black women spent three times more per capita than white women on cosmetics and toiletries, and total black spending on personal care products (cosmetics, skin care, fragrance, and hair care) was projected to grow an average of 10 percent each year through 1995.[25] Throughout the 1990s, white-owned firms began to expand their cosmetics blends to include darker shades in order to tap into this previously ignored segment of the cosmetics market—black women. Historically, cosmetic firms offered a range of foundation colours that suited the complexions of white women. As Kathy Peiss notes, when advertising executives for CoverGirl were interviewed in 1991, "[they] voiced discomfort about discussing the racial implications of the look they had created, a look they knew had alienated a number of black consumers."[26] That same year, Maybelline (acquired by L'Oréal in 1996) made its first foray into the sector when it introduced its Shades of You line of cosmetics, which had an expanded range of foundation tints. CoverGirl (acquired by P&G in 1989) launched its Queen Collection in 1991, and in an attempt to compete with Maybelline and CoverGirl, Revlon followed suit with Darker Tones of Almay in 1991, and then in 1992, its ColorStyle Cosmetics.[27] When Estée Lauder launched its Prescriptive All Skins line in 1991, with an unprecedented range of 115 custom-blended shades, and expanded its Clinique brand with the Color Deep line, the company, along with the aforementioned, established a black consumer division. Estée Lauder's Prescriptive All Skins, which offered over a hundred makeup shades, reportedly attracted nearly 50,000 new black customers during its first year.[28]

Although white-owned cosmetic firms had established cosmetics lines by cultivating an image that linked their products with upper-class white women, black women were now on the radar. Prior to 1991, there were only seven brands tailored toward black women's skin tones, and African Americans owned six of them: Naomi Sims, Gazelle, Juin Rachele, Barbara Walden, Zuri Cosmetics, and Fashion Fair.[29] After 1991, there was a growing awareness of black women's spending power and as a result, black women consumers became a key segment for global conglomerates. Significantly, the 1990s also witnessed a mergers and acquisitions frenzy in Canada that shifted the retail landscape and the sale of black beauty products. Back in the early 1970s when Flori Roberts brought her products to Canada, they were from the start exclusively sold at separate department-store counters. By the 1980s, when black beauty products entered Canada's mainstream retail sector, *Contrast* was still reporting on such developments. In May 1982, for example, the newspaper informed readers that Flori Roberts, a white woman dubbed "the Queen of Cosmetics," had travelled to the city the week prior to launch the Flori Roberts Line at Simpson's.[30] (As discussed in chapter 3, Flori Roberts Inc. was an international cosmetics firm with over seven hundred outlets throughout the United States, England, Africa, Canada, the Caribbean, and the West Indies.) "Mrs. Roberts, a white woman," the *Contrast* report began, "became aware of the special beauty needs that existed for dark skinned women after overhearing the conversation of two black models 17 years ago while working as a fashion promoter for Dow Chemical's Textile Fibers Division," adding, "She learned that the black model's [*sic*] were frustrated over having to blend several shades together to get the colors that they wanted." During this same period, Honest Ed's, the Toronto discount store formerly located at Bloor and Bathurst Streets, also added the Dark & Lovely relaxer to its black beauty offerings.[31] Given that the Bloor and Bathurst neighbourhood (dubbed "Blackhurst") in Toronto was a hub for black community for over a century—not only for West Indian immigrants but also for black businesses such as Mascoll's Beauty Supplies—there would have been a local market for the sale of such products in this part of the city, which was also home to *Contrast* until it ceased publication in 1991.

In 1996, Hudson's Bay began to sell Fashion Fair cosmetics. Since the late 1970s, Hudson's Bay had steadily increased its presence in Canada, becoming the country's top department store. In 1978, it took over the Simpson's chain, and by the end of the 1980s, all Simpson's stores outside of Toronto had been converted to Hudson's Bay stores. In 1991, the last Simpson's store, its Toronto flagship in the city's downtown core, was converted into the flagship Hudson's Bay store and all remaining Simpson's operations were folded into the company. The first advertisement for the sale of Fashion Fair Cosmetics at Hudson's Bay appeared in *Share* magazine in February 1996. Prior to this, Fashion Fair Cosmetics had been available for purchase exclusively at Eaton's and Simpson's. Since the early 2000s, black hair care products have also become readily available at Walmart (which came to Canada in 1994), Shoppers Drug Mart, and more recently, Rexall in Ontario. According to a report in *The Globe and Mail*, Rexall's parent company, Katz Group, which operated more than 460 Rexall and Rexall Pharma Plus locations across Canada, sold the firm in 2016 to the San Francisco–based health-care-services giant McKesson,[32] which also owns IDA and Guardian pharmacies across the country. In Western Canada, black beauty products are sold at London Drugs, which operates seventy-eight stores throughout Manitoba, Saskatchewan, Alberta, and British Columbia. In Quebec, black beauty products are sold at Uniprix pharmacies, Jean Coutu, and Pharma Prix in addition to Walmart. In Atlantic Canada, in addition to Jean Coutu and Pharmasave, the Lawtons pharmacy network has seventy-nine stand-alone stores, some of which also sell black beauty products.

The white takeover of the black beauty industry ultimately brought appeals for more ethnic and racial diversity in advertising. Multiculturalism as *brand* became a marketing tool used by these firms to appear more inclusive than they had been in the past. However, these companies continued to perpetuate the ideal of lighter skin and/or straighter hair as more beautiful than darker skin and/or natural hair. This chapter argues that ownership changes in the black beauty culture industry have done more than just increase the availability of products sold at retail. As global conglomerates gained control of a market that was, before the 1990s, controlled by African American–owned companies, the advertising imagery for skin care and hair care products has changed. By removing the word "black" from beauty advertising geared toward black women and replacing it with the word "ethnic" or "multicultural," the new standard of black beauty created in the 1990s has had a lasting impact on the beauty culture industry.

This chapter also argues that the global expansion of the black beauty culture industry in the 1990s must be understood through a transnational framework with respect to consumer culture. This definition of transnationalism is not concerned with migration or the movement of bodies across borders and within the nation-state; instead, it calls our attention to the circulation of media, products, and aesthetic practices and the ways in which a globalizing African American culture helped to shape and create distinctly *Americanized* forms of blackness that have, since the 1990s, *become* the global "look" for black beauty. In her writing about Mattel Corporation and the transnational movement of Barbie into India in the 1980s and 1990s, Inderpal Grewal asserts that "since market segmentation in the United States has used gender, race, and ethnicity, and multiculturalism to sell products, and since products cross national boundaries, multiculturalism has also become transnationalized through global marketing practices by transnational corporations based in the United States."[33] In a June 2013 article in the *Harvard Business Review*, for instance, titled "L'Oréal Masters Multiculturalism," Hae-Jung Hong and Yves Doz reported that, since the late 1990s, L'Oréal Paris has placed executives from mixed cultural backgrounds in its most critical activity: new-product development.[34] The authors note that in 2012, the company's sales grew in the Asia Pacific region by 18.4 percent and in Africa and the Middle East by 17.6 percent, without significant acquisitions, because of the product development from its team of "multiculturals," the company's most critical source of competitive advantage. Today, global conglomerates continue to use strategies of inclusion to woo black women consumers, and while on the surface the appearance of dark-skinned black women with natural hair in advertisements for global beauty brands or on the cover pages of fashion magazines such as *Vogue* appear to be a step in the right direction, such imagery contains new sets of concerns about the ways in which a globalizing American beauty culture can influence not just the sale and distribution of products, but identity formation as well.

In 1998, Kathy Peiss astutely observed that "the multicultural look, and the self-congratulatory tone of its promotion, has been censured...as a new form of exploitation masquerading as inclusion"[35] and quoted bell hooks, who stated that the commercial media was "cynically depict[ing] racial diversity to profit from a liberal image."[36] It is important to remember that even with unprecedented inclusion in the mainstream beauty culture, black women did not control the terms of their representation. Models with light skin and straightened hair still epitomized a "universal" black beauty in magazines and on television, while those with dark skin or African features remained stereotyped as hypersexual or primitive. Thus, while diversity-based advertising sought to promote products geared toward diverse populations, inclusion-based advertising aimed to normalize and neutralize all difference. Stated otherwise, where attempts at diversification would have rightfully singled out specific groups (e.g., black women) who had been historically ignored, the beauty culture industry instead took an inclusivity approach by promoting sameness—sameness of image/look and sameness in the marketing of products. Although the "before and after" images invoked by white-owned companies in the nineteenth century had long disappeared by the 1990s, there was still a sentiment that darker-skinned women, as compared to lighter-skinned women, were endowed with innate qualities that signified a wild, animalistic form of beauty. This chapter ultimately argues that when it comes to beauty culture, a move toward "sameness" has resulted in a whitewashing of difference that has done more harm than good to black women.

In 1993, CoverGirl focus groups concluded that black women did not want separate cosmetics lines, while Revlon's marketers found the contrary: black women wanted a line from a major company that specifically addressed who they were.[37] When Revlon launched its ColorStyle line in 1992, all ninety-eight of its products were given names that symbolically invoked "black culture" as *exotic*, such as Brazil Nut liquid makeup, West Indies Wine lipstick and Jungle Orchid nail enamel.[38] Under the guise of inclusion, the taxonomic language of these products not only made the *blackness* of blackness hypervisible but through the invocation of exotic landscapes (Latin America, the Caribbean, and Africa) each also perpetuated the historical association of blackness with the sexually primitive. Historically, as Petrine Archer-Straw observes, "the primitive represented the process through which Europeans suggested their own superiority by placing inferior status on others. This process was entirely one-sided: it was simply a way for Europeans to project their fear of difference onto other races."[39] While black women such as Veronica Webb joined the ranks of America's top models when she became a Revlon spokesmodel in 1992, cosmetics for the newly formed "ethnic market" tended to exaggerate, rather than celebrate, the difference of blackness either in the naming of the cosmetic product or in advertising campaigns featuring black models, like Webb. Since then, black women consumers have been inundated with advertising messages that increasingly ignore what a product can do (its use value) in favour of what the product is worth (its exchange value) in terms of status, success, image, and power.

When white women appear in skin care advertisements, for example, more often than not, the product's exchange value—enhancing their innate "natural" beauty—is emphasized. As Arjun Appadurai proposed, "the commodity situation in the social life of any "thing" [can] be defined as the situation in which its exchangeability (past, present, or future) for some other thing is its socially relevant feature."[40] In the 1990s, for example, Italian actress and model Isabella Rossellini was the face of L'Oréal's anti-aging brand Lancôme. In one representative advertisement in *Chatelaine* magazine in April 1994, a full-page close-up headshot of Rossellini appeared on one side of the page, while on the other side of the page the caption read, "A look that defies time. RÉNERGIE YEUX."[41] Her beauty was framed as an intrinsic part of her embodiment, which the product simply accentuated (and perpetuated). On the contrary, when actress and singer Vanessa Williams appeared in a Futur-e advertisement in August 1998, she was also captured in a headshot, but the benefit of the product (its use value) not her *innate* beauty (the exchange value) was emphasized. The advertising copy read, "L'Oréal invents the moisturizer of the future.... Skin looks smoother in just 1 day. Looks healthier in just 1 week."[42] It is important to note that, unlike black women, white women have had to deal with the burden of aging in an industry that values perpetual youth. In the documentary *About Face: Supermodels Then and Now* (2012), Rossellini commented, "Advertising is about dreams, not reality." This statement was in reference to having been replaced as Lancôme's spokeswoman by a younger model, even though market research showed that she was well liked. In the film, Rossellini opined that L'Oréal replaced her because the company's ideal was "youth, not reality."[43] Cosmetics, in addition to hair dyes, allowed black women to engage in the normalizing practice (in addition to hair straightening) that minimized the difference of blackness. This was especially true in the fashion world, where the markers of whiteness remained highly sought after by agents, casting directors, and magazine editors.

In the early 1990s, the world of high fashion initially sought black models who were dark skinned, such as Iman, Naomi Campbell, and Alek Wek, all of whom entered the ranks of the fashion runway and the pages of *Vogue, Harper's Bazaar, Mademoiselle,* and *Elle* magazines. In her autobiography, Sudanese model Alek Wek talked about her experiences as a model in Europe and America in the 1990s. In one example, Wek recounted her struggles convincing white executives that she was worthy enough to appear in a video shoot: "They wanted someone exotic who lived in a jungle," she recalls.[44] Similarly, in a 2006 interview, Iman spoke of not being "black enough" for some executives even though she is Somalian: "I hated being told that I look like a white girl only browner. I look very Somali, very Bantu. I didn't have to define myself as Black where I come from we are all Black."[45] When Naomi Campbell and singer-actress Grace Jones, both of whom were born in Jamaica, entered the fashion and modelling worlds, like Wek and Iman, they were highly sought after because of their dark skin. For example, Jones (who in the 1970s wore her hair in a shortly cropped Afro, a style known as the flat-top, which was an echo of Vidal Sassoon's wedge-cut of the 1960s) almost always appeared as the *exotic* black woman. At the same time these women entered the fashion world, however, they faced criticism from within black community because of their image.

Over the years, Campbell and Iman have been accused of "compromising" their heritage by wearing platinum and honey-blonde wigs, while Wek and Jones were criticized for not altering their hair at all. Despite the criticism, dark-skinned women may have ruled the runway and high fashion magazines in the 1990s, but when it came to beauty product advertising, light-skinned women such as Tyra Banks and Veronica Webb (who, in the 1990s, was not only a model and actress but also one of the first African

American women to secure major cosmetic contracts with global beauty firms) remained the rule. In general, black women still had not broken the colour barrier in the fashion and modelling worlds. A 1991 study found that out of more than 200 models associated with top New York agencies such as Elite Model Management, only 14 were black; of the 180 models with the Ford Modeling Agency, only 8 were black; and of the 124 models working at Wilhelmina, only 12 were black.[46] A 1991 report titled *Invisible People* tallied the number of black models appearing in over eleven thousand advertisements in twenty-seven different national magazines in the United States. The report, issued by the Department of Consumer Affairs of New York, noted the description of models' physical appearance and their positioning in each advertisement.[47] While approximately 11 percent of these magazines' readership was black, over 96 percent of the models were white. Additionally, most of the black women in advertisements appeared in group shots dominated by whites, and these women were usually light skinned and had long, wavy hair.[48]

When dark-skinned models appeared in *Chatelaine* throughout the 1990s, the magazine emphasized the difference of their blackness, categorizing it as "multicultural." In the September 1992 issue, for example, an article titled "Skin Color: Meet Your Match" featured a dark-skinned model alongside the subtitle "If your skin tone is ebony." The advertising copy read:

Beautiful skin comes in many shades. But for years, women of color have complained about foundations that are too pink, too ashy (caused by high levels of titanium dioxide, a white pigment commonly used in cosmetics) or simply the wrong shade. Now, the cosmetic industry is addressing the special needs of multicultural women by reducing the titanium dioxide and upping the pigment needed to keep cosmetic color true.... Try Maybelline's Shades of You collection: Mahogany Oil-Free Soufflé Makeup and Rich Mocha Oil-Free Pressed Powder.[49]

By invoking the word "multicultural," *Chatelaine* envisaged a colour-blind beauty and, by extension, a nation in which, as Augie Fleras argues, "the ethnicities of minority women ... are channelled ('de-politicized') into aesthetic pursuits in personal or private domains."[50] Susan Bordo similarly notes that it has become increasingly difficult in contemporary culture to sustain any significant political critique about beauty because "everything is the same in its unvalanced difference. ('I perm my hair. You're wearing makeup. What's the difference?') Particulars reign, and generality—which collects, organizes, and prioritizes, suspending attention to particularity in the interests of connection, emphasis, and criticism—is suspect."[51] Inclusion-based advertising, then, used multiculturalism as a tool to avoid the issue of race; stated otherwise, if we were all "multicultural," how could the beauty industry be accused of racism?

As black beauty culture has entered the mainstream, few African American-owned black beauty firms have managed to stay family-owned. Today, the list is few. There are Luster Products of Chicago (its most successful product is Pink Moisturizer), North Carolina–based Dudley Products Inc. (featured in Chris Rock's 2009 documentary, *Good Hair*), and Georgia-based Bronner Bros. Enterprise, which comprises Bronner Bros. Beauty Products (maker of BB, African Royale, and the Nu Expressions lines, and publisher of *Upscale* magazine). There are also smaller African American–owned companies such as Kizure Iron Works in Carson, California, a manufacturer of curling irons and pressing combs; Summit Laboratories in Illinois, a manufacturer of hair care and skin care products; and Lloneau Products in Los Angeles, which produces Liquid Gold Hair Bonding and Lace Front Adhesives (for wigs). As private, family-owned businesses, these African American–owned firms are up against global conglomerates—L'Oréal, P&G, Unilever, the Colomer Group, Shiseido (of Japan), Estée Lauder, Avon, and Johnson & Johnson. Combined, the aforementioned eight account for almost half of global revenues, competing with each other for market share in established and emerging markets.[52] L'Oréal and P&G also account for over one-fifth of total world sales of cosmetics.[53] Avon, the world's biggest beauty brand, was worth US$11.3 billion in 2008, and Unilever's Dove and P&G's Pantene, in second and third place, had sales of US$5.3 billion and US$4.5 billion, respectively.[54] With respect to black beauty, as of 2001, L'Oréal, Unilever, the Colomer Group, P&G, and Avon held over 50 percent market share. It is estimated that, as of 2013, L'Oréal controlled 61.9 percent of the hair-colouring market and 51.2 percent of the chemical-relaxer market.[55] That year, the black hair care market was also valued at US$684 million of the total US$7 billion US hair care market.[56] Black beauty culture is no longer a niche market; it is a global enterprise. Importantly, however, African American beauty entrepreneurs first began to worry about this takeover back in the early 1980s when several firms mobilized against what they believed was a forthcoming onslaught.

In 1981, ten African American hair care manufacturers joined forces and founded the AHBAI (American Health and Beauty Aids Institute).

The founding chairman, George E. Johnson, conceived the AHBAI to urge consumers to "buy black"; their logo, a profile of a black woman, produced by Chicago-based artist Richmond Jones, was meant to capture "the proud lady."[57] For a short time *Ebony*, *Essence*, and *Jet* magazines supported the AHBAI's efforts by refusing to feature advertisements from Revlon and other white-owned companies, but these efforts ultimately backfired as white firms simply solicited black celebrities to promote their products in advertisements in mainstream publications.[58] Today, the "Proud Lady" logo still appears on black-owned brands, but white-owned companies (such as L'Oréal, through its SoftSheen-Carson division) are also part of the AHBAI. The Luster family, the Dudley family, and the Bronner Brothers, to name a few, are all members of the AHBAI, and in recent years, at least one Korean businessperson sits on AHBAI's advisory board.[59] In chapter 5, I explore the growth of the hair weave and lace front wig markets, explaining the strategies Korean entrepreneurs used at the retail and distribution levels to gain control of the global hair trade.

Significantly, wherever black beauty products are sold at drugstores and department stores, they are strategically placed on separate store shelves. Back in 1977, the August edition of the *American Druggist*, a drug and pharmaceutical publication, noted that drugstores in the United States were given advice on how best to reach black women seeking more economical products, and product placement was one of the suggestions.[60] Where some retailers believed that black cosmetics should be given its own separate section, others felt that black cosmetics should be included in the regular cosmetic department. As one retailer explained:

> There's a dichotomy here and I don't know how to solve it. Blacks have a definite desire for ethnic cosmetics. But psychologically, no one wants to be singled out by announcing, in effect, "I'm black and I have to buy black cosmetics." With Revlon's Polished Ambers, she feels more comfortable because everyone buys Revlon. But if she buys Ultra Sheen, she's saying she's different. And in America, everybody wants to be the same.[61]

Robert E. Weems Jr. notes further that "although there existed a sizable market for high-priced black cosmetics during the 1970s, the beauty and personal care products industry did not ignore the needs of less-affluent African American women."[62] Despite the fact that the black population in the United States was, by the 1970s, diverse and one's racial identification was based on a myriad of factors including geographic location, language, and culture, white retailers still considered African American women a monolithic group, speaking for and about their conceptions of what it meant to be "American."

In comparison, Canada's black beauty market by the late 1980s was essentially an extension of the black beauty market in the United States. By the end of the decade, chemical relaxer advertisements for Johnson Products' Gentle-Treatment, Carson Product's Dark & Lovely, SoftSheen's Optimum and Wave Nouveau, Revlon's Realistic Permanent Creme Relaxer, and Alberto-Culver's TCB (Taking Care of Business) filled the pages of *Contrast* and *Share* magazine. Eaton's and Hudson's Bay continued to offer Fashion Fair, Flori Roberts, and Zuri Cosmetics; and drugstores became one of the prominent retailers of chemical relaxers, in addition to Walmart. Skin-bleaching creams from Ambi, Nadinola, and Dr. Fred Palmer were also widely available at these locations. There was, and remains, no manufacturer of black cosmetics or hair care products in Canada. The industry was (and remains an extension of African American–owned and white-owned conglomerates. Since the likes of Viola Desmond and Beverly Mascoll paved the road, however, only a few other African Canadian beauty entrepreneurs have tried to hold their own in product sales at the local retail level. In Toronto, Ragga Hair Studio and Beauty Store, on Dundas Street just east of Church Street, is one example of a black-owned hair salon that continues to thrive, despite the industry's challenges. "The ethnic market has never really been given a lot of respect and support from manufacturers in that they treat us all like we're in the US," Gordon Oliver, Ragga Hair Studio co-owner told me. "Because of the bilingualism requirements on Canadian packaging, it creates a big problem. With the market being very small and so diverse they say, 'Why should I spend the extra three cents on packaging just to accommodate that small market in Canada?'" Oliver, who opened Ragga Hair Studio in 1997, held a management position in Revlon's ethnic hair division for several years, so his perspective speaks directly to the conversations that are likely had within the walls of global conglomerates. While big-box stores such as Walmart do sell black beauty products, there is often very little in their business practices that could be construed as a celebration of black women's hair; the products are often placed in undesirable locations on the shelves (e.g., behind columns or in an out-of-the-way corner of the store), which also suggests that many of these efforts to accommodate black consumers are window dressing, at best. At black-owned hair shops, however, black hair products

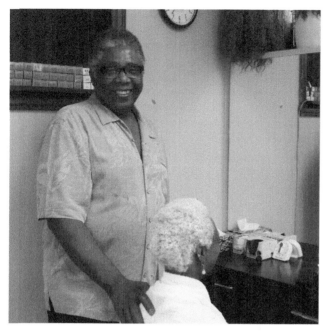

Figure 15a. Co-owner Gordon Oliver, Ragga Hair Studio and Beauty Store, Dundas Street East, Toronto, Ontario, 2018. Photograph by author.

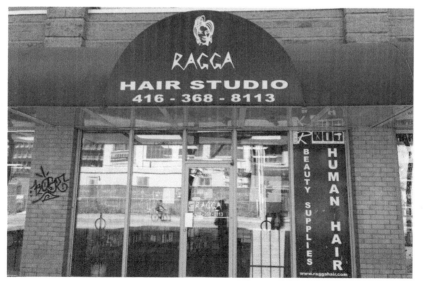

Figure 15b. Ragga Hair Studio and Beauty Store, Dundas Street East, Toronto, Ontario, 2018. Photograph by author.

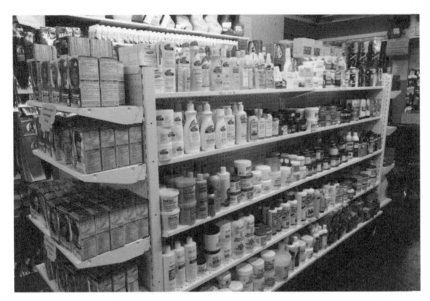

Figure 16a. Beauty products on store shelf, Ragga Hair Studio and Beauty Store, Dundas Street East, Toronto, Ontario, 2018. Photograph by author.

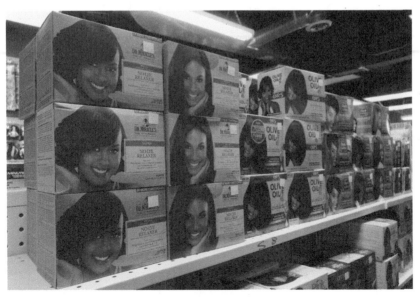

Figure 16b. Chemical relaxers on store shelf, Ragga Hair Studio and Beauty Store, Dundas Street East, Toronto, Ontario, 2018. Photograph by author.

are proudly on display throughout the store. Staff are also able to answer questions about the products and/or engage in hair care discussions that help black women learn about our hair. White-owned or Korean-owned hair product stores also are often ill equipped to offer any such services.

In comparison, a June 1988 article appearing in *Contrast*'s Western Canada edition reported, "There is a unique drug store situated two blocks south of Whyte Avenue, between the two Calgary Trails (North and South)....Maurice and Ann Walters own and operate the Plaza Drug Store. Plaza Drugs is the only black-owned drug store in Western Canada, and [operates] with the union of both Anne and Maurice's expertise."[63] The store carried a varied selection of merchandise catering to a "diverse population" including, cosmetics and black hair care products to "serve the needs of the black community (and other people of color)." The appearance of such editorials reveals that, by this time in Western Canada, there may have been a limited number of places where black women could find beauty products catering to their needs, but these places nonetheless did exist, and they understood their clientele. In 2014, Toronto's *CityNews* reported that Kemeel Azan's hair salon (first opened on Spadina Avenue just north of Queen Street in 1961, now with a location at Davenport and Avenue Road) was still in business after fifty-two years.[64] Back in 1978, in an interview with *Contrast*, Azan said, "Toronto is a haven for black professionals. Some of the finest black brains in the world are among us here, but we're too busy buying the house, the big car, the fur coats and living above our means."[65] While he did not specifically say this was one reason why the city lacked a black beauty company of its own, it does help to explain the mindset of black communities in Canada, which have generally been more apt to purchase imported black beauty products than to create and mass distribute products made right here in Canada. Overall, the wider distribution and sale of black hair care products at retail has been viewed by many as a sign of progress—that is, since the 1990s black beauty products have been more widely available—however, as I discuss in chapter 5, black women with natural hair were (and remain) entirely excluded from such developments.

At some point in the 1990s, black beauty was rebranded as "ethnic" beauty. It is unclear which firm (or firms) might have been responsible for this rebranding, but the term *ethnic* began to appear in the industry just as white-owned firms acquired black beauty firms. As an example, in 2012 while I was shopping in a Walmart in Brampton (a suburb northwest of Toronto), I came across a shipment order in the "black beauty" aisle in the store. Even though the products listed were chemical relaxers, and the faces on the boxes were all black, the order was labelled "ethnic hair and skin care." The appearance of this shipment order revealed that, in Canada, as in the United States, the term "ethnic" has become an industry-wide descriptor that depoliticizes black hair care and skin care products. If the faces on the boxes are black, and the target market for the products is black women, why are the products labelled "ethnic"? Why did the word "black" slowly disappear from products *for* black women between the 1970s and 1990s? The answer to these questions lies in the diversification of the hair-colouring market that took place during this period.

In the 1990s, industry marketers began to realize that black women changed their hairstyles more frequently than other women did, and that this fickleness extended to hair colour. At this point, companies formulated hair dyes specifically geared toward black women, and with this inclusion came the industry-accepted use of the terms "ethnic" and "diversity." In an advertisement appearing in *Share* in November 2003, for instance, SoftSheen-Carson's Hi Rez Hair Color was promoted in an advertisement for a local beauty-supply shop with the caption "Takes You from Dark to Rich Reds & Bold Browns the First Time & Every Time You Color!"[66] Revlon also launched HiLites, the first at-home semi-permanent highlighting kit created specifically for black women's hair texture, and Clairol launched its Beautiful Collection Gentle Creme Permanent Color, the first low-ammonia cream permanent hair colour designed for chemically relaxed hair.[67] All of these products ranged in shades from light ash blond to black. In 2004, the Chicago-based Hunter-Miller Group projected that African American spending power would grow from US$645.9 billion to US$852.8 billion by 2007, reporting that the African American spending share in the hair care sector was 30 percent of the overall market.[68] When most people think of black beauty advertising today, they probably think of Queen Latifah, Halle Berry, Beyoncé Knowles, Kerry Washington, or perhaps Lupita Nyong'o, who first appeared on the cover of *Vogue* in July 2014, or singer Janelle Monae, who has appeared in a series of advertisements for CoverGirl. Often, at the same time that these women have entered the beauty mainstream, their blackness has been minimized. Stated otherwise, while their racial difference is an empirical fact, in the multicultural contemporary such difference no longer carries political currency. To be "black" and beautiful is—ever since the 1990s—no longer about a "soul aesthetic" or a harkening back to the Motherland of Africa; it simply means that one's skin colour is a marker of ethnic difference, nothing more. The success of television screenwriter, producer, and author Shonda Rhimes has undoubtedly contributed to this industry-wide move toward a "post-racial" form of beauty.

In an editorial in *The New York Times* (*NYT*) in 2005 following the first season of *Grey's Anatomy*, for example, Matthew Fogel described the show as a "frenetic, multicultural hub where racial issues take a back seat to the more pressing problems of hospital life: surgery, competition, exhaustion and—no surprise—sex."[69] At that time, Rhimes told Fogel, "I'm in my early 30s, and my friends and I don't sit around and discuss race. We're post-civil rights, post-feminist babies, and we take it for granted we live in a diverse world." As Kristen Warner opines, the success of this series and of Rhimes "is tethered to the use of racialized bodies as signifiers of historical progress... as well as undermining the diversity of those bodies through a laundering, or whitewashing, of social and cultural specificity."[70] In addition to whitewashing black signifiers, since the 1990s, beauty advertising has also evoked the Caribbean and Latin America in a de-racialized, multicultural beauty. Most notably, in early 1994, a late-night television infomercial promoted a new method of hair care; the product, Rio, was said to have been used successfully for over forty years by Brazilians who wanted to straighten their hair without the use of chemicals. Despite the circulated image of a light-skinned Brazilian beauty with straight hair, as a site of transatlantic slavery, Brazil has the same skin and hair politics as other sites of black diaspora especially as it relates to the valorized difference in hair texture and skin colour. In her study of hair politics in Brazil, Kia Lilly Caldwell found that the concept of "bad hair" is associated with individuals who have black or African ancestry but Brazilian notions of *cabelo bom* (good hair) and *cabelo ruim* (bad hair) also permeate Brazilian society.[71] As a result, "it is not uncommon to hear white Brazilians describe someone as having 'bad' hair. Widespread familiarity with the significance of hair texture amongst all racial groups further underscores the significance of hair as a marker of racial and social identity in Brazil."[72]

Rio, produced by De Classe Cosmetics Ltd., a Rio de Janeiro–based company, but distributed by World Rio Corporation in Nevada, was advertised as an "all-natural, chemical-free relaxer" that was derived from "exotic flora" that grows in the rainforests of Brazil.[73] The product was also marketed specifically to black women. Rio infomercials told viewers that the product was "chemical free" and to prove it, a male spokesperson ate a portion of the product on the air. To sell the product, the infomercial also constructed a non–African American image of blackness by invoking the *exotic* Caribbean. As Noliwe Rooks explains,

The infomercial's set design evokes visions of a Caribbean resort, and audience members are seated in groups of three or four, at tables made of rattan and bamboo. Large palm trees and numerous "colorful" plants give the appearance of an exotic tropical locale, and a long, large structure in the middle of the set resembles a beach bar. The theme music sounds distinctly like steel drums and does indeed have a "rocking" calypso beat. The spokesman who joins Mary, the model and spokeswoman for Rio, is dressed in a tropical shirt. Mary is dressed in a red, skintight sundress. The set suggest informality. There is no pressure here. We are all relaxed and friendly.[74]

Other global brand conglomerates resurrected the tropical theme in the 1990s, as a strategy to reimagine the consumption of the "tropics" as *exotic*. As Krista Thompson writes, "The term *tropics*, from which *tropicalization* is derived, denotes the horizontal band on the earth's surface between the Tropics of Cancer and Capricorn in which many Caribbean islands are located," but it also characterizes how, "despite the geological diversity...even in a single Caribbean island, a very particular concept of what a tropical Caribbean island should look like developed in the visual economies of tourism."[75] In 1991, for instance, an American firm called Tommy Bahama started producing clothing and furnishing lines based on a tropical theme. Tommy Bahama was a contemporary testament to the power of the earliest tourism promoters to inspire travellers to seek out their tropical dreams by venturing to an island. "Now by simply attaching 'Bahama' to a brand, the company could persuade customers to go virtually native, to fulfill their tropical dreams without leaving home."[76] Rio similarly employed the tropical setting as a symbolic representation of taming the *naturally* untamed tropical black body into an *exotic* sexual body.

At one point in the Rio infomercial, André Desmond, a black man, spoke of his travels throughout Brazil: "Rio frees you. It doesn't put you in bondage. With Rio you are free." I have vivid memories of watching Rio infomercials at that time. While I did not purchase the product, I remember how the infomercial highlighted the product's Brazilian roots, and that the *exoticness* of South America made its women seem more beautiful than the blackness of people of African descent. Conveniently, the infomercial ignored the fact that the physical markers of blackness, namely hair and skin colour, are similarly politicized in Brazil. Using taped testimonials from black women, the infomercial disparaged natural hair, and by extension, reasserted the notion of light skin and straight hair as more beautiful than dark skin and natural black hair. In one testimonial, a dark-skinned black woman confided, "I hate my hair, it doesn't move at all. I just wake up in the morning and put on a hat." Not surprisingly, several other testimonials also applauded the product for working on their "bad hair" or for helping to fix their "kinky, fuzzy, and curly" hair problem. Historically, the terms "nappy," "kinky," and "fuzzy" have been hurled at black women as insults. In 2007, for example, Don Imus, a white American syndicated radio talk-show host referred to black women on the Rutgers University women's basketball team as "nappy-headed hos." In 2013, the term "nappy" also became fodder for controversy on the CBS television show *The Talk*. In a discussion about white model Heidi Klum saving the hair of her biracial children, Sheryl Underwood, the show's African American co-host, railed against what she called "nappy Afro hair."[77] "Why would you save Afro hair?" Underwood asked. When her white co-host, Sara Gilbert, responded that she, too, sometimes saves her children's hair, Underwood interjected, "[It's] probably some beautiful, long, silky stuff."

In black communities, the term "nappy" is synonymous with the phrase "bad hair" both of which are used to describe natural hair (i.e., hair that has not been altered). "Nappy," like "kinky," is also a descriptor for the supposedly "bad" texture of natural hair. The juxaposition between the supposed "bad" and "good" hair is so central to black women's beauty politics that there have even been films about the phrase. Most prominently, comedian Chris Rock's *Good Hair* (2009), which I discuss in more detail in chapter 5, sought to bring the "good hair" versus "bad hair" discussion into the spotlight. "Good hair" typically describes hair that is long and flowing and/or straight hair (altered or a hair weave) that is loosely textured. In both cases, "good hair" and "bad hair" are interconnected with skin colour. Girls/women with "good hair" are typically light skinned or of mixed race while "bad hair" is typically used to disparage girls/women who are dark skinned or have visible markers of an African ancestry, such as a wide nose. Whether good or bad, the American representation of, and public discourse about, black hair has brought black women's beauty politics into the mainstream lexicon.

Within a few months of Rio's debut, consumers began to report hair loss, baldness, and, in some cases, green hair colour. Instead of providing soft, flowing hair, as the infomercial had promised, Rio caused many users' scalps to itch and burn, while others said it took out their hair in clumps, leaving embarrassing bald spots.[78] By April 1995, more than fifteen hundred lawsuits had been filed and attorneys were considering consolidating them into one class action suit.[79] According to a Virginia newspaper, Arthur Rieman, general counsel for World Rio Corporation, argued that Rio was not to blame for any suffering that users might have experienced. In his opinion, the people who had problems with Rio probably did not follow the instructions properly.[80] In December 1994, the US Food and Drug Administration (FDA) warned consumers not to use Rio after the agency had received over fifteen hundred complaints. What Rio users did not know, and what many consumers in general do not know, is that cosmetics, unlike drugs, are not required to be tested by the FDA before they are sold to the general population.[81] Under the law, the FDA does not pre-approve cosmetic products and ingredients before they enter the consumer market-place, except for colour additives, and the FDA investigates a product after it is on the market only if consumers complain. Similarly, Health Canada investigates only after consumers complain about a cosmetic product, and there is very little information on its website about chemical relaxers or black beauty products in general. In June 2016, a report from the federal environmental commissioner found that Health Canada was not doing enough to protect Canadians from dangerous substances that may be found in some cosmetic products.

According to a *CTV News* report, since 2006, Health Canada has been part of the federal government's Chemical Management Plan, which aims to test about 4,300 chemicals found in consumer products for potential health risks by 2020.[82] The report claimed that chemicals considered "endocrine disruptors" are the most dangerous because they can cause a variety of neurological and immune disorders. Significantly, the environmental commissioner did not provide a list of the specific products, but made it clear that manufacturers and retailers are not legally required to inform Health Canada of any health-related incidents involving their products. It is unknown whether the study included a specific focus on black beauty products (e.g., chemical relaxers or skin-bleaching creams), but what we do know is that hair care products, like skin care products, also pose health risks. In April 2009, for example, Health Canada recalled two hair products—Wave Nouveau Revitalizing Mousse and Body & Shine (a conditioning enhancer), both sold under the SoftSheen brand name— for improper labelling.[83] There were, however, no reports of harm or injuries related to the use of these products.

After consumers complained to the FDA about Rio, the California Department of Health Services tested the product and determined that, despite claims to the contrary, it was not "all-natural and chemical-free" and that it contained harsh chemicals. The key ingredients in Rio—the cupric acid basic (the ingredients that turned the hair green), with the ascorbic acid acting as the stabilizer—were used at levels that were more acidic than is considered safe for use even in heavy industrial products.[84] While Rio was just an infomercial, the use of colloquial language around the *exotic* reveals how the depoliticization of difference permeated inclusive-based beauty advertising in the 1990s. At the same time that black women entered the ranks of mainstream beauty culture advertising, inclusion-based advertising continued to mask the realities of racial bias that have, since the nineteenth century, determined who is beautiful and who appears in beauty-product advertising in the first place.

In 1997, Halle Berry appeared as a spokesperson for Revlon lipstick; in 1998, Vanessa Williams appeared as spokeswoman for L'Oréal's Future moisturizer, and in 2000, singer-actress Brandy Norwood appeared in CoverGirl advertisements. With respect to Halle Barry, it is interesting to note that, in her early advertising campaigns for Revlon, she appeared alongside two white women or in a group shot with white and/or Hispanic women but that in 2000, she began to appear alone. This transition might have been because of her starring role as Storm in the box-office hit *X-Men* (2000), which catapulted her into Hollywood's mainstream. In 2001, Queen Latifah (Dana Owens) began her reign as CoverGirl's Queen Collection spokeswoman. In one representative advertisement, appearing in *Essence* in December 2007, a close-up shot of the rapper/actress/former talk-show host captured her with a flawless face, wearing the company's Natural Hue Foundation, below a caption that read, "Every woman is a queen, and deserves a makeup that celebrates her beauty."[85] In 2013 L'Oréal launched its True Match Foundation campaign; Yves Saint Laurent introduced its Le Teint Éclat foundation in twenty-two different shades, and Lancôme's Teint Idole Ultra 24H foundation was available in eighteen different shades. In 2014, when Lupita Nyong'o rose to fame after her Oscar-winning role in *12 Years a Slave* (2013) she became the first black spokeswoman for Lancôme. Of all these beauty brands, however, L'Oréal's True Match campaign stands as a contemporary example of how inclusion-based advertising raised other sets of concerns around the imaging of beauty in the "multicultural" era as far as black women are concerned. The True Match advertisement first appeared in 2013. In it, L'Oréal celebrated the fact that the new cosmetic product matched twenty-two skin shades, from warm to cool, and from light to dark. In a series of print advertisements, the company's slogan, "Whatever your skin's story, we have your match" also appeared.

In one representative advertisement, three skin types were shown: that of the Irish/Austrian/Italian woman (Aimee Mullins), the Ethiopian woman (Liya Kebede), and the Puerto Rican woman (Jennifer Lopez).[86] The accompanying "true match" makeup shades were named Nude Beige (for white women of mixed European heritage), Cocoa (for black women), and Sun Beige (for Hispanic women). The language of this ad turned the difference of blackness into an *exotic* difference, but it also equated black women with food. By naming cosmetic products for black woman after foods such as cocoa, which is indigenous to South America, the Caribbean, and Africa, such advertising evoked an association between the black female body and oral consumption, an association that harkens back to the nineteenth century. In her analysis of nineteenth-century portraits of black women subjects, Canadian art historian Charmaine Nelson found that still-life paintings of fruit are distinguished from those of flowers because "they presume the possibility of oral consumption that, for the most part, flowers do not. As such, they hold the potential of activating other senses beyond vision, like taste, smell and touch, in the imaginary anticipation of eating."[87] Meanwhile, in L'Oréal's conceptualization of a "true match," white and Hispanic women were constructed as different sides of the same coin—Nude Beige versus Sun Beige. The True Match ad also described Jennifer Lopez as "100% Puerto Rican"—she has straightened hair, and her body approximates the mainstream standard of beauty. Given Puerto Rico's Spanish colonial history (like that of Cuba, the Dominican Republic, and Brazil), there is no such thing as a "pure-blood" Puerto Rican. Thus, where we observe the ethnic difference of black women through the accentuation of their skin colour, Hispanic women, conversely, are often whitewashed and removed from histories of slavery and from a black ancestry. As Priscilla Peña Ovalle writes, "The 'Latina' body must change to simultaneously exhibit sameness and difference."[88] Stated otherwise, Hispanic women in beauty advertising, such as Jennifer Lopez and more recently Eva Longoria and Sofia Vergara, must conform to idealized beauty standards (i.e., straight hair, light skin) yet retain an *exotic* difference such as dark or curly-textured hair that positions them closer to black women, removing them from a European ancestry. At the same time, when black and Hispanic celebrities make disparaging comments about black and Hispanic women's bodies, it also reinforces a white standard of beauty.

On September 12, 2013, for instance, during an episode of *The View*, Barbara Walters asked her African American co-host Sherri Shepherd why she wears wigs. "Because if I didn't I'd look like a prisoner," Shepherd replied. Subsequently, on the short-lived return of the 1990s *Arsenio Hall Show*, Mexican-American comedian George Lopez appeared in an episode in which he said that black and Hispanics should have babies together because they would be so beautiful, but they would also have "some ugly hair." These comments reflect how members of black and Hispanic communities often ridicule black and Hispanic women because of skin that is "too dark" or hair that is "too coarse." Despite the mainstream beauty culture industry's move toward inclusive-based advertising, in 2017, dubbing itself "the number one global beauty brand in the world," L'Oréal launched a diversity-based advertising campaign for its True Match foundation, "Your Skin, Your Story." In a press release, the company stated that, with the thirty-three shades of True Match, "Your Skin, Your Story" champions the unique mosaic of American beauty and the L'Oréal Paris slogan "You're Worth It."[89] The "Your Skin, Your Story" campaign, which mounted integrated advertisements on social media, digital platforms, and television during the 74th Annual Golden Globe Awards, featured an artist and artisan native to Nepal; an American transgender model, actress and writer; a travel and food lifestyle blogger from Hawaii; and a millennial male model of Caribbean descent—each of whom "share[d] their unique heritage and skin story." While there are still aspects of this advertisement that miss the mark, such as the hyper focus on cosmetics as *being* the enabler of joy in a woman's life, this campaign stands as a positive sign that beauty firms, like L'Oréal, might be moving one step closer to achieving real diversity in their advertising, rather than whitewashed attempts to appear inclusive. In the fashion world, however, Elizabeth St. Philip's National Film Board (NFB) film *The Colour of Beauty* (2010), which followed black Canadian model Renee Thompson (no relation) as she tries to make it as a top fashion model in New York, exposed the fact that black (and Hispanic) models still struggle in an industry where white women continue to represent the standard of beauty.

The film observed that a 2008 survey of models during New York Fashion Week found that 6 percent were black, 6 percent were Asian, 1 percent were Hispanic, and 87 percent were white. To debunk allegations of exclusion, in July 2008 *Italian Vogue* released the "Black Issue," which exclusively featured black models. While the issue sold out in the United States and in the United Kingdom in just three days, as Thompson says in the film, "It was just an attempt to prove that [they're] not racist and unfortunately it worked." The unspoken truth about the beauty culture industry and by extension the fashion world is that whiteness continues to be the benchmark for beauty. Whether a model is black, Asian, or Hispanic, the "woman of colour" whose body and physical characteristics are more closely aligned with those of the white European is the one who appears most in fashion spreads and product advertising. As Margaret Hunter observes, "the lightest women get access to more resources because not only are they lighter-skinned and therefore racially privileged, but their light skin is interpreted in our culture as more beautiful and therefore they are privileged as beautiful women."[90] Thus, while dark-skinned women (usually celebrity actresses, not unknown models) do appear in beauty advertising today, they are more the exception than the rule. With respect to hair, Nyong'o stands as another exception to the industry standard of straight, flowing hair; in 2014, for instance, she was voted the Most Beautiful in the World according to *People* magazine's annual list, natural hair and all. Since the early 2000s, however, the ethnically ambiguous "woman of colour" has been most prominent in beauty advertising.

The idea of the ethnically ambiguous woman first arose as a topic of discussion in 2003 when the Fashion & Style section of *The New York Times* ran a feature titled "Generation E.A.: Ethnically Ambiguous."[91] Advertising executives and fashion magazine editors created the concept, which was essentially a marketing strategy. The *NYT* feature offered running commentaries on marketing trends for tweens, teens, and members of the hip-hop generation (defined as those blacks born between 1965 and 1984), in both the mainstream and high-end marketing. The feature explained, "Among art directors, magazine editors and casting agents, there is a growing sense that the demand is weakening for P&G, industry code for blond-haired, blue-eyed models." United States Census data for the year 2000 showed that nearly seven million Americans identified themselves as members of more than one race, giving advertisers "proof" of the marketability of ethnic otherness. A 2010 Statistics Canada report, "A Portrait of Couples in Mixed Unions," similarly claimed that more than 340,000 children in Canada were in mixed-race families, and that the number of mixed unions was growing much more quickly than that of other partnerships.[92] "Jennifer Lopez, Christina Aguilera, and Beyoncé Knowles have, from time to time, deliberately tweaked their looks, borrowing from diverse cultures and ethnic backgrounds," the *NYT* article noted.[93] "Beyoncé sometimes wears her hair blonde; Jennifer Lopez often takes on the identity of a Latina-Asian princess in Louis Vuitton ads, and Christina Aguilera, who is half Ecuadorean, poses as a Bollywood goddess on the cover of *Allure*," the article added. T. Denean Sharpley-Whiting observes that the collision between black celebrity culture and beauty culture has had visible impact on what black women consumers come to identify as desirable; in effect, what black women could once never *become*, they now believe they can buy.[94] Black women can now insert blue contact lenses, dye their hair blonde, and *become* more ethnically ambiguous. Rapper Lil' Kim (Kimberly Jones) is one noticeable example of the lengths to which some black women have gone to acquire this ethnically ambiguous look. On her 2003 album, *La Bella Mafia*, Kim presented herself as the "Queen Bee," a "gangsta-ass bitch" with a body other "bitches" envy and a Louis Vuitton lifestyle.[95] Today, Kim is almost unrecognizable. She has *become* more racially ambiguous not only by wearing coloured contacts and blonde wigs but also reportedly having bleached her skin and undergone rhinoplasty, breast implants, and liposuction. The desire for an ethnically ambiguous beauty has added new layers to the problem of racial inclusion in the mainstream beauty culture industry. While black and Hispanic women appear more frequently in beauty advertising today, to what lengths have women gone to appear *less* black?

In chapter 2, I referred to the "Brownskin" in *Ebony*'s postwar photojournalism as a figure who served to overturn the racist stereotyping of black women, who, prior to the war, were always depicted as dark-skinned, unattractive mammies and maids. By endowing the "Brownskin" with attributes historically denied black women—beauty, poise, and success— African American magazines also helped to position light-skinned black women as emblems of middle-class black progress. Since the 1990s, light-skinned and dark-skinned black spokeswomen have occupied somewhat similar space in beauty campaigns, which, for many, signals that the beauty industry is now "colour-blind." The appearance of "colour-blindness" has wide-reaching implications. In her writings about the television show *American Idol*, Janell Hobson has argued that reality shows have had the effect of reinforcing a new form of racism that ignores the "systemic racial hierarchies that continue to advance white supremacy or normalcy while non-white spectacle is always viewed as 'different.' ... [Such public representations] lull us into accepting the 'hyperreal' of what many like to call a 'postracial society.'"[96] This pretense of "transparency" has much in common with Jean Baudrillard's notion of the "hyperreal," which becomes "more real than the real, that is how the real is abolished."[97] In the context of beauty culture, the pretense of transparency and the illusion of inclusion have served to blind women to the realities of systemic racism, prejudice, and discrimination that continue to exist in the boardrooms and backrooms of the world's largest beauty companies.

In 2007, the Garnier division of L'Oréal and a recruitment agency it employed were each fined €30,000 (US$40,650) after they recruited women based on race, excluding non-white women from promoting Garnier's shampoo.[98] Back in 2000, a fax detailed the profile of hostesses sought by L'Oréal. It stipulated that women should be aged 18 to 22, size 38–42 (North American size 10–14) and "BBR"—the initials for bleu/blanc/rouge (blue/white/red), the colours of the French flag, which is a well-known code, used by right-wing conservatives in France, that means "white" French people and not those of north African, African, and Asian backgrounds.[99] In August 2008, L'Oréal was also accused of "whitewashing" Beyoncé in an advertisement in which the singer's skin appeared visibly lighter.[100] In December 2013, when Flora Coquerel, a nineteen-year-old biracial woman whose mother is from the West African country of Benin, was crowned Miss France, there were over 1.1 million tweets about it on Twitter that night, according to *TF1*, *Gala*, and *Le Télégramme*. A portion of those comments ranged from "I'm not a racist but shouldn't the Miss France contest only be open to white girls?" to "Fuck, a nigger" to "Death to foreigners." In an interview with *Elle.com*, Carol Mann, a professor of sociology and gender studies at the Paris Institute of Political Studies, said, "France has a deeply ingrained colonialist culture and still believes in a form of racial hierarchy and Gallic supremacy," adding that "the situation is especially touchy with women: 'la petite française,' 'la parisienne' are highly exportable and marketable myths that the French work hard at maintaining. And those expressions are usually synonymous with fair, European features such as Brigitte Bardot or Marion Cotillard."[101] As an editorial in the *New Yorker* explained in 2014, a study funded by the Open Society Institute showed that black and North African youths were much more likely to be stopped by police in France's equivalent of stop-and-frisk but, because researchers are forbidden from collecting official data, there are only general empirical studies on the subject (e.g., spending entire days hanging out at Paris subway stops where French police often conduct searches, noting the appearance of the people they saw stopped).[102] In a November 2013 advertising campaign for Chanel No. 5, the first perfume launched by Parisian couturier Gabrielle "Coco" Chanel, a series of vintage clips of the late Marilyn Monroe showed the "blonde bombshell" dazzling the paparazzi with her blonde curls and glamorous wardrobe, with a voiceover of Monroe recounting, "Marilyn, what do you wear to bed? So I said Chanel No. 5, because it's the truth." While fashion and women's magazines celebrated the thirty-second spot, it stands as another example of how blondeness (coded as whiteness) remains the pinnacle of beauty, especially in France.

In America, the politics of race still hover over beauty pageant winners. When Nina Davuluri became the first Indian woman to be crowned Miss America in September 2013, several racist comments appeared on Twitter, lambasting the pageant for its choice of winner.[103] In 2016, when Deshauna Barber (Miss District of Columbia—and a logistics commander in the US Army reserve) was crowned Miss USA, like Miss France, Barber was criticized. Naysayers took to Facebook and Twitter, insisting that the ethnically ambiguous Miss Hawaii, Chelsea Hardin, deserved the title; others suggested that one of the other white contestants should have won, and some even said they believed that the Miss USA Pageant should be segregated so that a black woman, especially a dark-skinned black woman, could not win the title again. The backlash against Barber hearkened back to previous black women who have won beauty pageants, most notably, Vanessa Williams. In 1983 when the green-eyed, light-skinned Williams became the first black woman to be crowned Miss America, it seemed like a positive step forward in that the colour barrier had finally been broken in America's most cherished pageant. When photographs of a nude Williams were made public shortly after the pageant, it played to the stereotype of the hypersexed black woman.[104] It also brought to the surface deep-seated issues related to skin colour that still permeated African American communities. The Congress of Racial Equality (CORE), for example, went so far as to issue a statement declaring that Williams was not "in essence black."[105] When *Chicago Tribune* columnist Leanita McClain wrote favourably about William's victory, she received calls and letters from angry African Americans.[106] The charge of "not black enough" reflects the extent to which black women in the public eye are held to both in-group and out-group standards of beauty. The charge of "not black enough" has even been levied against dark-skinned African American women, such as Kerry Washington. Despite her skin tone, Washington said in an interview in 2016 that she was once fired from two television dramas because (white) producers did not think she was "black enough."[107]

Thus, black inclusion into the mainstream via beauty advertising, beauty pageants, Hollywood films, and television has only made hypervisible the lack of real commitment on the part of executives (who continue to be predominantly white and male) to disrupt historical stereotypes and the standard of beauty. On the one hand, since the 1990s global conglomerates have increasingly relied on black women of all skin tones to cultivate black women consumers; on the other hand, these strategies have not coincided with dedicated efforts to shift who enters the beauty culture industry in the first place. The beauty culture industry has subtly persuaded us that the barriers that once prevented black women from entry are no more, but if beauty is now multicultural and *all* women are represented, why do black women still feel that they do not measure up to an unwavering standard of beauty? As Imani Perry observes, "the beauty ideal for black and Latina women [i.e., that of light skin and long, flowing hair] ... is as impossible to achieve as the waif-thin models in *Vogue* magazine are for white women."[108] If beauty firms now give the appearance of political and ideological gains but in reality only a specific "type" of black and Hispanic woman is permitted entry into advertising campaigns—those who approximate whiteness but are ethnically ambiguous at the same time—what impact has that had not only on African Americans but on black Canadian women, as well? With respect to Canada's mainstream beauty culture, *Chatelaine* provides us with an example of how the ethnically ambiguous woman, coupled with multicultural editorials, helped to depoliticize issues of race throughout the 1990s to celebrate Canada's national brand of "diversity."

In late 2004, Rona Maynard, who had been the editor of the stalwart women's magazine since 1997, retired; Kim Pittaway replaced her, but she would leave the magazine a few months later. Eventually Jane Francisco, *Chatelaine*'s fourth editor since 2004, took the helm and shifted the magazine's focus away from fashion and beauty to lifestyle features related to fitness and diet. In 2013, Francisco left the magazine to lead New York-based *Good Housekeeping*, a sign that *Chatelaine* was perhaps no longer the dependable voice for Canadian women that it had been for most of the twentieth century. Along with the new shift in content, models and/or celebrities no longer appear on *Chatelaine*'s cover. In the late 1990s, however, racially ambiguous women had made their first appearance on the magazine's cover. In June 1993, Hispanic model Serena Rojas appeared on the cover; in 1996, Filipino-Canadian model Joanna Bacalso made two cover appearances—in July and December; and in May 1998 a black woman finally appeared on the cover—alongside two white women—for a feature story on finding clothes that fit all sizes of women. As noted in chapter 3, Gloria Rueben and Deborah Cox were the first black Canadian women to appear solo on the cover of *Chatelaine* when both did so in 1999. If Rueben or Cox had not become famous in the United States, would they have even made a *Chatelaine* cover? Additionally, why did this accomplishment, and others like it, not catch the attention of Canadian media? Why is the inclusion of black models into Canada's mainstream often ignored as compared to when black women enter America's beauty mainstream?

For example, in the eight-two pages of the January/February 2014 issue of The Bay's *Beauty: The Guide*, a digital beauty magazine (launched in 2011) that mixes editorial content with e-commerce, there are three black models. A dark-skinned model on the runway appears on the cover, a light-skinned woman appears alongside two racially ambiguous women in an advertisement for Lancôme's Dream Tone, and R&B singer Alicia Keys appears in an advertisement for Kiehl's, the high-end skin care product line, alongside four black children in a campaign called "Keep a Child Alive."[109] There are no Asian or Hispanic women in this "guide to beauty." The July 2017 issue contains more of the same whitewashing: of its 106 pages (including the cover), white women occupy 43. There are so few black women (all of whom are light-skinned) that most readers likely do not even notice the absence when flipping through this digital magazine. And while there are numerous white men included, in advertisements from cologne to clothing, there are no black or Asian men in the entire guide.

The issue of inclusion, I argue, is not limited to Canadian print media. In the next chapter, I explore how novels, television, and film have tackled the issue of racial inclusion, and the ways in which natural hair has once again become a strategy to reconfigure the parameters of blackness. I also explore the short-lived Canadian sitcom *'Da Kink in My Hair*, and I examine why it has been so difficult for black women to wear natural hair in Canadian media, the workplace, and at school. While the beauty culture industry came a long way over the course of the twentieth century, there are new black beauty politics in the twenty-first century that require urgent attention.

CHAPTER FIVE

THE POLITICS OF BLACK HAIR IN THE TWENTY-FIRST CENTURY

In the second decade of the twenty-first century, a reoccurring image of black beauty began to circulate in advertising and women's magazines. This image was of the biracial woman and/or child with loosely curled, Afro hair. One notable example first appeared in a 2013 advertisement for Cheerios. The thirty-second advertisement opens with a cute biracial girl sporting a loosely curled Afro, who asks her white mother if it is true that Cheerios is good for the heart. After assurances from her mother, the girl exits the kitchen and approaches her black father, who is asleep on the couch; later, as he opens his eyes and awakes from his sleep, Cheerios spill down his chest (presumably because his daughter has put them there). This advertisement was widely criticized because of its depiction of an interracial union and offspring. Some critics noted that North American audiences are "so deeply wedded to antiquated racial ideals that the thought of a loving and devoted family created by people of different races is an anathema."[1] My concern with this representation had more to do with hair. A few years ago, I was in a mall in downtown Toronto and spied this image again—a biracial child with loosely curled, Afro hair, who appeared alongside a white child. This time, it was for the children's clothing store, OshKosh B'Gosh. The biracial woman and/or child with light skin and a loose, curly Afro has become a ubiquitous aesthetic in the twenty-first century, denoting a form of "multicultural" beauty that began in the 1990s. The case of Rachel Dolezal, however, reveals why this aesthetic is fraught with issues. In 2015, Dolezal, a civil rights activist, Africana studies instructor, and president of the Spokane, Washington, chapter of the National Association for the Advancement of Colored People

(NAACP), became fodder for media outlets when photographs circulated showing her childhood self (a white, blonde-haired girl) alongside her adult self (with darkened skin and a loosely curled Afro). These before-and-after portraits bring to mind Noliwe Rooks's discussion of nineteenth-century beauty advertisements geared toward African American women, in which such images were commonly used, and her assertion that "although no evidence suggests that any of these companies advertised widely or for extensive periods of time, the ads constituted a continuing discourse on the politics of constructing an African American female identity."[2]

Whether or not Dolezal was confused about her racial identity, her privilege as a white woman to "choose" to *become* phenotypically black—and her abuse of that privilege—is not my main concern in this chapter. What is significant is not only the hair politics that her case brought to light, but also the fact that, in years thereafter, she continued to receive a lot of attention from the Canadian media. For instance, in March 2017, both the *Toronto Star* and *CBC Radio* featured cover stories on the former "black" civil rights leader and her difficulties finding steady work since her racial identity became a matter of public interest. In a reprinted story from the Associated Press, the *Toronto Star* explained that in 2016, Dolezal legally changed her name to Nkechi Amare Diallo, a West African moniker that means "gift from the gods," to "give herself a better chance of landing work from employers who might not be interested in hiring Rachel Dolezal."[3] After the release of her memoire, *In Full Color*, also in March 2017, Dolezal appeared on the CBC Radio program *Out in the Open*, hosted by Piya Chattopadhyay. These two examples highlight the Canadian media's tendency to look southward to African American culture—even to a born-white woman—when it comes to race, often ignoring or downplaying the difficulties black women face here in Canada when it comes to racial identity, employment, and beauty politics. While Dolezal is unapologetic about her self-identified "blackness," her loose, curly Afro became a floating signifier for the crossing of racial boundaries. In the nineteenth century, scientific and popular literature became obsessed with the texture and stylization of black hair, so much so that some Europeans even went so far as to claim that hair served as a better indicator of racial identity than skin colour.[4] As Arthur Riss asserts further, "Hair has not stopped signifying racial identity. It may signify differently and have been thoroughly resignified, but hair nonetheless remains a crucial identity marker. Rather than having been emptied of social significance, it has become central to a liberatory politics, raising critical issues about standards of beauty and black self-definition."[5]

As for the loose, curly Afro, like tanning in the 1920s and the Black Is Beautiful Afro of the 1960s, it has become another aesthetic for white women to "put on" and "take off" when they so desire. One of the first examples of this trend appeared in the August 2015 issue of *Allure* magazine.

In the featured "how-to" piece, titled "You (Yes, You) Can Have an Afro" and modelled by white actress Marissa Neitling, readers were instructed on how to achieve a loose, curly Afro. The article made no mention of the hairstyle's black politics, most notably, its link to the Black Power movement, when the Afro became a symbolic aesthetic of socio-political change. After public outcry from African American hair bloggers, hairstylists, and cultural critics, Chris McMillan, the hairstylist responsible for Neitling's temporary Afro, told the *Huffington Post* that Barbra Streisand in *A Star Is Born* (1976) was the inspiration for his take on the Afro for white women.[6] "Yes We Can," the slogan attached to Barack Obama's 2008 presidential campaign, also became a single for Black Eyed Peas frontman will.i.am, "Yes We Can" (2008). The "we" in these two examples denoted a collective America, but on a connotative level it was a "knowing wink" to black America that unprecedented levels of political capital were now possible. *Allure* magazine's how-to guide was not just about hair; by removing the "we" (*blackness*) and replacing it with "you" (*whiteness*), editors signalled that the Afro, with all its latent blackness, was now available to white women as mere style. As noted in chapter 4, since the 1990s, the beauty culture industry has tried to present the illusion of inclusion. To signal that the barriers that once prevented black women from entry into its ranks are no more, beauty firms, advertisers, and women's magazines have tried to make us believe, as Susan Bordo has aptly argued, that "anything goes." She writes further, "all sense of history and all ability (or inclination) to sustain cultural criticism, to make the distinctions and discriminations that would permit such criticism, have disappeared."[7] *Allure* magazine could have hired a black woman to inform readers of how she styles her naturally curly hair. Instead, they chose a white woman to guide (presumably) other white women on how to recreate an artifice of blackness. Instead of acknowledging the corporeal politics of difference, borrowing from Bordo, we have endless differences, "an undifferentiated pastiche of differences, a grab bag in which no items are assigned any more importance or centrality than any others."[8]

This chapter is concerned with the contemporary politics of black beauty, specifically, black hair—its texture, styling, length, and colour. In many ways, the issues facing black women today are just as significant as they were a century ago. Black women have levels of agency today that women a century ago did not have, but many of the tensions with respect to hair and skin continue to circulate in the contemporary. One of the aspects of this book that cannot be overlooked is the fact of blackness and the marking of black bodies as Other. Stated otherwise, to speak of a black beauty culture requires that we acknowledge the debasement of not only the black body but also black aesthetic practices that occurred during transatlantic slavery, when black bodies were imbued with a visible, corporeal difference such that hair and skin became politicized aesthetics, irrespective of black women's intentions.

The moment Africans crossed the Atlantic Ocean through the Middle Passage to the "New World" (i.e., the Americas—North and South—and the Caribbean) in the fifteenth and sixteenth centuries, the black body formed part of a collective blackness. The meanings attached to enslaved black peoples' skin, facial characteristics, and especially hair (its length and texture) during slavery contributed to the classification of human types; this classification regarded black women and men (and children) as less morally, sexually, and intellectually developed than white, European colonialists, settlers, and wage labourers.[9] As Nadine Ehlers posits, "by conceptualizing blacks as inherently distinct due to differences in appearance, Europeans formulated a 'blackness,' and by implication a 'whiteness,' that conflated color with fictionized racial *identities*."[10] This "New World" was created on the basis of the slave-trade economy, and as such, the stigmatization of black people's bodies did not gain its historical intransigence by being a mere concept. Where race is a constitutive element of social structure and social division, hair and skin colour became powerfully charged with symbolic currency.[11] At the same time, enslaved Africans, those on plantations and those held in bondage in domestic slavery, as in Canada, would have lacked both the time for elaborate hairstyling practices and the implements with which such styles could most effectively be achieved— most notably, the African pick, or comb, whose long, smooth teeth did not snag or tear thick, tightly curled hair. As a result, black women's hair was sometimes unkempt, damaged, or covered under headwraps.[12]

Within colonial slave societies, black women (and men) were also separated along skin colour and spatial lines. This created a racialized and gendered hierarchy that functioned independent of, but because of, the dominant European culture. On the one hand, domestic slaves, who tended to be light skinned, generally lived in close proximity to their white masters (often living in the same house) and were forced to style their hair in imitation of the masters, including wearing wigs or shaping the hair to resemble a wig. On the other hand, field slaves, who tended to be dark skinned, lived in separate quarters and were often unable to properly care for their hair, which then went unkempt or covered by headwraps or bandanas (some enslaved men took to shaving their heads, wearing straw hats, or using animal shears to cut their hair short).[13] In terms of pitting "light-skinned" and "dark-skinned" black women against one another within black communities, Kathy Russell, Midge Wilson, and Ronald Hall pinpoint the social conditions under slavery as the starting point of this valorized juxtaposition. In some southern states, the authors write, "those with light-enough skin and European features commonly got around the law by simply passing as white."[14] To *pass* means to transgress the social boundary of race, to "cross" or thwart the "line" (both real and imagined) of racial distinction that has been a basis of racial oppression and exploitation since the seventeenth century. In *A Chosen Exile*, Allyson Hobbs posits that "white skin functioned as a cloak in antebellum America" in that, when attached to the "appropriate dress, measured cadences of speech, and proper comportment, racial ambiguity could mask one's slave status and provide an effectual strategy for escape."[15] As free black communities formed in mid-nineteenth-century North America, the resulting flood of manumitted and escaped blacks "darkened" many of these free black communities, and as a result, social distinctions within them were increasingly made based on skin colour (and hair texture), not to mention the length of time a person had been free.[16]

While many people are familiar with the transatlantic slave trade, fewer consider how Africans lived once they were shipped to the Americas and the Caribbean, especially how they engaged in self-care practices such as hair care. As Buckridge observes of Jamaican colonial society, "hairstyles consisted of plaits or braids or of combing the hair into 'lanes' or 'walks' like the 'parterre of a garden,' as is still done in West Africa. This display of African aesthetics in dress served as a marker to keep these women, the members of the slave community, separate from the world, and to identify those who did not belong."[17] Prior to the slave trade, African aesthetics were frequently changing, and by the sixteenth century, this adaptive and creative impulse permeated all aspects of Africans' wardrobe; from the combining of actual items of African and European dress to the reworking of cloth that composed that dress, Africans were as interested in dress and fine clothing as Europeans had become.[18] Once the slave trade commenced, the voyage through the Middle Passage on the slave ship was instrumental to the process of renaming and (re)identification.[19] This voyage had the effect, among other things, of homogenizing the African body—that is, of neutralizing ethnic and linguistic differences that had existed in Africa, as well as the varied hair care traditions among Africans. Hair also carried important cultural meaning in African societies.

Among the diverse societies along Africa's west coast (the Wolof, Mandingo, Mende, and Yoruba) and in distinct areas such as Upper Guinea (modern-day Sierra Leone), Guinea, Guinea Bissau, Senegal, Nigeria, the Gambia, the Gold Coast (present-day Ghana), and central and south-central Africa (present-day Congo and Angola), hair was used to indicate a person's marital status, age, religion, ethnicity, wealth, and social standing within the community. In the Wolof culture of Senegal, for example, young girls who were not of marrying age partially shaved their heads to emphasize their unavailability for courting, while a recently widowed woman would stop caring for her hair in order to look unattractive to men during her time of mourning.[20] Traditionally, the leaders of a community, both men and women, displayed the most ornate hairstyles, and only royalty or their equivalent was expected to wear a hat or headpiece, to signify their stature within the community.[21] Hair grooming in African societies included washing, combing, oiling, braiding, twisting, and decorating the hair with adornments including cloth, beads, and shells; the tools at their disposal were hand carved and specially designed to remove tangles and knots from the hair. Hairdressers were also prominent members of African society because a person's spirit was believed to be embedded in their hair.[22]

Any discussion of black beauty must always contend with the corporeal legacies of African enslavement. Whether we call ourselves Canadians, Americans, British, or even Continental Africans, black beauty is a contentious topic because it was first made so by eighteenth- and nineteenth-century Europeans. Some scientists, such as Peter A. Browne, a nineteenth-century "expert" of trichology (the study of hair), argued that the relationship between hair and race was more stable than the relation between skin colour and race, and that "the Negro's head was covered with wool rather than hair,"[23] thus serving as "proof" of the superiority of Europeans over Africans. During the eighteenth and nineteenth centuries, advances in print and visual media also helped to denigrate the black body. The public display and visual representation of an African woman named Saartjie Baartman (also known as Saat-Jee, Sara, or Sarah Bartmann) is the most enduring example of how Europeans naturalized supposed differences between black and white women.

Baartman, who was born in South Africa, was exhibited as a curiosity in Europe from 1810 to 1815—first in London, then in Paris—as the "Hottentot Venus" (early Dutch settlers of South Africa dubbed the South African natives "Hottentots" and "Bushmen").[24] Through her public display, Baartman's humanity was elided twice. "While alive, she was displayed; contained in various exhibitions and pressed to pose nude, she was positioned as popular and scientific entertainment for those who longed to stare at a woman thought to be their opposite," Lisa Gail Collins writes.[25] Then, after her death, her body was moved to a laboratory for further investigation and dissection and then to a museum shelf at the Musée de l'Homme, where her genitals were stored in a jar for over a hundred and fifty years until they were finally removed in 2002 and her remains repatriated to South Africa. Baartman's body became a symbol of black women's supposed inferiority to white women because, as Sander Gilman notes, "When the Victorians saw the female black [i.e., Baartman], they saw her in terms of her buttocks and saw represented by the buttocks all the anomalies of her genitalia."[26] In the nineteenth century, Western concepts of white feminine beauty were bound up with notions of purity, delicacy, modesty, and physical fragility; as such, black women like Baartman were seen to be physically amoral, exuding an "animal sensuality," which, to the European mind, was evidence of their inferiority.[27]

As discussed in chapter 1, at the beginning of the twentieth century, the "New Negro" sought to reimagine and re-image the black body as a site of emancipation, one that rebuked the centuries-long debasement of black hair and skin. One of the first attempts to announce the New Negro occurred in 1900 when Booker T. Washington, the African American civil rights activist and educator, helped edit a volume titled *A New Negro for a New Century*. Also in that year, at the Paris Exposition, one of the largest international exhibitions at that time, pan-Africanist W. E. B. Du Bois organized 363 photographs into three albums titled *Types of American Negroes*; *Georgia, U.S.A.*; and *Negro Life in Georgia, U.S.A.* As Shawn Michelle Smith observes, this exhibit challenged the photographic images of blackness that were made to uphold scientific discourses of "Negro inferiority" and "Negro criminality."[28] One of the reasons why Du Bois's exhibit was so significant is that, in the nineteenth century, advances in print and visual media helped to normalize the supposedly inherent differences between the races. Prints and photographs became symbolically interconnected with ideas, themes, and materials related to exchange, reproduction, and consumption. For the first time, printmakers and photographers were able to offer relatively inexpensive pictures of people and places, which could then be proudly displayed on living-room walls or stored privately in cases or folios.[29] At the same time, in the public sphere, photographs of black women and men were used as "proof" of their inferiority.

Most notably, in the 1850s, Robert W. Gibbes, a nationally recognized paleontologist, hired local daguerreotypist Joseph T. Zealy to make photographic records of first- and second-generation slaves on plantations near Columbia, South Carolina, for Swiss-born Louis Agassiz, the natural scientist and zoologist from Harvard University, who sought to use the images as "visual evidences" of photographic difference.[30] Using the frontal/profile combination that was first used in ethnographic photography, Zealy documented slave women and men in half- and full-length views, stripped to the waist or, in the case of some of the men, totally naked.[31] The result was a denial not only of black women's (and men's) humanity but also of control over the representation of their own bodies, removing all agency and power from their naked selves.[32] When the Eastman Kodak box camera hit the mass market in 1888, the proliferation of photographic "snapshot" images and postcards meant that by the end of the nineteenth century, the democratization of the image gave subjugated persons the ability to construct a new self-image that could stand as a counter-narrative to that which circulated within the dominant visual landscape. Whereas the white family posed as a photographic reproduction, and, as Smith opines further, "the photographic industry situated white middle-class women at the cornerstone of this technological process,"[33] the box camera made it possible to see the walls of photographs in black homes "as a critical intervention, a disruption of white control of black images."[34] In the world before racial integration, images empowered black subjects to express the human condition in new ways.[35] Thus, one of the best examples of this new form of black photographic freedom can be seen in the African American experience when they began to take photographs of themselves in the late nineteenth and early twentieth centuries; in so doing, they acquired levels of agency that they had previously been denied in the dominant cultural landscape.

Between 1895 and 1925, photography studios owned by and catering to African Americans in New York, Chicago, and Detroit were ubiquitous features of the urban landscape.[36] These studios offered African Americans the opportunity to cultivate an image of beauty that they were denied in fashion plates and women's magazines. The noted Harlem photographer James Van der Zee, for instance, made some of the best-known portraits of African Americans in the North during the period.[37] From images portraying well-groomed African Americans strolling around the streets of Harlem to numerous studio portraits of black women, Van der Zee imaged a distinctly urban people.[38] In her analysis of Van der Zee, Elizabeth M. Sheehan asserts that his images dramatized the process of transforming specific subjects into "types" through their composition, as his studio space and props transformed his sitters into the protagonists of recognizable bourgeois domestic scenes.[39] The combination of hair, cosmetics, and dress in Van der Zee's photographs positioned black women's bodies as modern. But at the same time, Sheehan notes further, "The prominence of and attention to dress in Van der Zee's images underscore[d] the malleable and fantastic nature of modern racial and gender identity and its reliance on external cues and props."[40]

This chapter argues that the issue of racial and gender identity is just as pertinent in contemporary culture as it was in the first decades of the twentieth century. The fact that *Allure* magazine saw no problem with its "how-to guide" for a black hairstyle that excluded black women altogether points to the historical denial of black women (even those black women who approximate the Western standard of beauty) from the purview of mainstream beauty culture. At the same time, when black women enter spaces where they hitherto have not been, such as sports, they often face criticism about their hair. At the London 2012 Olympics, for example, sixteen-year-old gymnast Gabby Douglas became the first African American woman to win gold in the women's artistic individual all-around competition; President Obama congratulated her, and she subsequently appeared on the cover of Kellogg's Corn Flakes. Despite all of that, the Internet exploded with criticisms about her hair. Most of the comments appeared on Twitter, where people commented that her hair looked "unkempt," and some even mocked her pulled-back bun. After her victory, instead of talking about her great achievement, Douglas had to face questions about her hair. "I don't know where this is coming from," she told the Associated Press. "What's wrong with my hair? I'm like, 'I just made history and people are focused on my hair?' It can be bald or short, it doesn't matter about [my] hair."[41]

In 2017, former Fox News host Bill O'Reilly was forced to apologize to California congresswoman Maxine Waters, who is also African American, when he made disparaging comments about her hair on the cable news program *Fox and Friends*. When asked his thoughts on Waters's criticism of President Donald Trump, O'Reilly said, "I didn't hear a word she said. I was looking at the James Brown wig."[42] "I didn't say she wasn't attractive," he said further, after Ainsley Earhardt, one of the hosts of *Fox and Friends* confronted him for talking about a woman's appearance. "I love James Brown. But it's the same hair James Brown, the 'Godfather of Soul,' had," he replied. From Don Imus's comments about members of the Rutgers University women's basketball team in 2007, to Gabby Douglas in 2012, to Maxine Walters in 2017, black hair—its styling, texture, and length—is still being judged, assessed, and criticized within and outside black communities, just as it was a century ago. In chapter 2, I discussed the "paper-bag" or "comb test" that was conducted at black churches in the late nineteenth and early twentieth centuries. While such tests are no longer practised today, the texture of black women's hair (along with skin colour) still holds tremendous social and cultural currency across sites of black diaspora.

In Jamaica, for example, Christopher Charles found that light skin is the cultural ideal for women and men who bleach their skin, while dark skin is anathema. "The negative images collectively create the hegemonic representation that light skin is superior to dark skin," he writes.[43] In the Dominican Republic, Ginetta Candelario notes that hair is the principal bodily signifier of race, followed by facial features, skin colour, and, last, ancestry. "*Pelo malo* [bad hair] is hair that is perceived to be tightly curled, coarse, and kinky. *Pelo bueno* [good hair] is hair that is soft and silky, straight, wavy, or loosely curled," she writes.[44] Candelario explains further that there are also colloquial expressions for women's hair texture. For Dominican women, "the notion of *pelo malo* implies an outright denigration of African-origin hair textures, while *pelo bueno* exalts European, Asian, and indigenous-origin hair textures. Moreover, those with *pelo bueno* by definition are 'not black,' skin color notwithstanding."[45] As noted in chapter 4, in Brazil the concept of "bad hair" is also associated with individuals who have black or African ancestry, but Brazilian notions of *cabelo bom* (good hair) and *cabelo ruim* (bad hair) also permeate Brazilian society as a whole.[46] As a result, it is not uncommon to hear white Brazilians describe someone as having 'bad' hair; widespread familiarity with the significance of hair texture among all racial groups further underscores the significance of hair as a marker of racial and social identity in Brazil.[47] Margaret Hunter also found that Mexican women shared painful experiences of being the "dark" one in the family, or of feeling less favoured than lighter-skinned family members were.[48] For his 2017 book, *Brown: What Being Brown in the World Today Means (To Everyone)*, Kamal Al-Solaylee travelled to Trinidad, Qatar, Hong Kong, the Philippines, Britain, France, and Canada to explore the question of skin colour. He also examined the intersections of visibility, the boundaries of space and the "crossing" of colour lines, and the impact of the sale of over-the-counter skin-lightening treatments, which have surpassed sales of tea and Coca-Cola in places like India, contributing to a ten-billion-dollar global industry.[49]

In 2007 when I interviewed black Canadian women about their hair, I asked them to describe what it means to have "good hair" and "bad hair." Their responses reflected a shared understanding of the power associated with adhering to the Western beauty standard of having hair that is straight, long, and flowing, in addition to having lighter skin.[50] In response to a question about natural hair, one of my interviewees said, "I used to go to the States and hang out with some of my cousins who were quite a bit older and they used to have their hair relaxed like everybody had their hair relaxed. Nobody had natural hair in New York; that was the style and that was what the cool kids were doing."[51] These comments point to the transnational exchange between black women in Canada and the United States as it relates to hair products, styles, and fashions.

In her 2006 study on the language of hair within the everyday lives of African Americans, anthropologist Lanita Jacobs-Huey found that humour was one of the prevailing forums where the phrases "nappy," "kinky" and "good hair" versus "bad hair" are continually used. Hair jokes, she writes, "often focus on...debates about 'good' versus 'bad' hair, Black women's hair rituals in beauty salons and kitchens, and common Black hairstyling dilemmas. Hair and head coverings...also emerge in some jokes as signifiers of 'authentic' racial and gendered consciousness."[52] The negative comments about black hairstyling also extend to dreadlocks. In 2001, New Orleans–based artist Kiini Ibura Salaam wrote about the different reactions she encountered in the Dominican Republic after she changed her hair to dreadlocks:

> More interesting than the multitude of hair transgressions I suffered, was the way I mutated from one race to another based on the way I wore my hair. When I arrived, the men on the street called me "morena" (brown girl/woman) and "india" (Indian) based on my skin colour and short curly afro. Halfway through my trip, I started locking [my hair], and suddenly I became "negra" (black girl/woman) and "prieta" (darky). Now I had experienced it all, hair had not only the power to make me unacceptable and uncool, but suddenly it had the ability to change my race! What power to place on the wiry strands growing from my scalp.[53]

While there are likely women with dreadlocks in the Dominican Republic who have not experienced such negative naming, there have been reports of people being punished for wearing dreadlocks in that country. In January 2013, the *Dominican Today* reported that San Pedro de Macoris prison authorities cut off rapper Vakero's dreadlocks.[54] Unlike the Afro, which is linked with a radical politics in North America, dreadlocks, which first appeared in the mid-1970s, did not originate in the United States. Thus, dreadlocks politics differed from those associated with the Afro, and the style's first adopters were different from those who sported the Afro hairstyle.

On August 12, 1976, Jamaican reggae artist Bob Marley appeared on the cover of *Rolling Stone* magazine.[55] The Annie Leibovitz photograph captured Marley with his arms raised and his dreadlocks flying. The iconic image marked the first time a reggae artist graced the cover of *Rolling Stone*, and it also introduced dreadlocks, Rastafari, and Jamaican culture to America. It is important to note that the reggae film *The Harder They Come* (1972) starring Jimmy Cliff was the first exported product from Jamaica to showcase dreadlocks and Rastafari culture; in fact, the film and its reggae soundtrack has been credited by music critics as the first film to "bring reggae to the world."[56] Outside of Jamaica, however, most people had never seen dreadlocks, and most knew very little about Rastafari or reggae.

Emerging in Jamaica's poorest black communities in the 1930s, the Rastafari movement openly defied British colonial rule by associating with Marcus Garvey's pan-Africanist movement. The name *Rastafari*, rooted in African spiritualism, is derived from Ras Tafari Makonnen, the black man who was crowned Haile Selassie I, Emperor of Ethiopia in 1930. Those who consider themselves "Rasta" believe that Haile Selassie I was the Second Advent of God; that is, Rastafari is a Rasta's religion. Stephen A. King asserts that as the movement challenged Jamaica's colonial society, Rastafari grew dreadlocks (an Ethiopian-inspired hairstyle), smoked marijuana, and proudly displayed the colours of the Ethiopian flag (red, gold, and green).[57] Dreadlocks are synonymous with Rastafari, but Rastafari did not invent the hairstyle. Bahatowie priests of the Ethiopian Coptic Church have locked their hair since at least the fifth century; in New Zealand, Maori communities wear dreadlocks for sartorial purposes; and in India, *sadhus* (and *sadhvis*, the female counterpart)—mendicant mystics of the Hindu faith—have also locked their hair for centuries.[58]

By the late 1970s, however, Rastafari was exported to sites of black diaspora through reggae music. Kobena Mercer asserts that dreadlocks embodied an interpretation of a religious, biblical injunction that forbade the cutting of hair (an act which paralleled the Sikh religion); however, "once 'locks were popularized on a mass social scale—via the increasing militancy of reggae, especially—their dread logic inscribed a beautification of blackness remarkably similar to the 'naturalistic' logic of the Afro."[59] Like Black Power and the Afro, Rastafari and dreadlocks were a symbolic reclaiming of Africa as an ancestral and cultural site of black culture. Whereas the Afro was linked to Africa through its name and its association with a radical politics, dreadlocks similarly signalled a symbolic link between the natural and Africa by way of a reinterpretation of biblical narrative, which identified Ethiopia as Zion or the Promised Land.[60] Dreadlocks ultimately negated the pervasiveness of the straight-haired aesthetic in black visual culture in the late 1970s by revalorizing Africa as a marker of blackness.

Initially, African Americans did not embrace dreadlocks or Rastafari. The hairstyle had come to America towards the end of Black Is Beautiful and the Afro, and while some African Americans dabbled with reggae and Rastafari, few adopted the hairstyle. In her introduction to Mastalia and Pagano's *Dreads* (1999), Alice Walker recalls:

> It wasn't until the filming of *The Color Purple* in 1985 that I got to explore someone's dreads. By then I had started "baby dreads" of my own, from tiny plaits, and had only blind faith that they'd grow eventually into proper locks. It was during a scene in which Sofia's sisters are packing up her things, as she prepares to leave her trying-to-be-abusive husband, Harpo. All Sofia's "sisters" were large, good-looking local women ("location" was Monroe, North Carolina), and one of them was explaining why she had to wear a cap in the scene instead of the more acceptable-to-the-period head-rag or straw hat. "I have too much hair," she said. Besides, back then (the 1920s) nobody would have been wearing dreads. Saying this, she swept off her roomy cap, and a cascade of vigorous locks fell way down her back. From a downtrodden, hardworking Southern Black woman she was transformed into a free, Amazonian goddess. I laughed in wonder at the transformation, my fingers instantly seeking her hair.[61]

When people think of dreadlocks today, many likely think of the *Color Purple*'s lead actress Whoopi Goldberg, who adopted the hairstyle in the early 1980s. Importantly, Goldberg was often criticized for wearing a style that many associated with a perceived "backwards island religion." As Russell, Wilson, and Hall note, Goldberg often had members of her own community tell her that her dreadlocks were disgusting and that she should "take those nappy braids out."[62] In 2010, I stumbled across a poster of "bad hair victims" in a window display in a hair salon in Toronto with the caption, "Oh My GAWD!!! I'm having a bad HAIR DAY." In addition to Marge Simpson, Whoopi Goldberg's dreadlocks were among the list of bad hair victims. Just like Cicely Tyson, who was told by members of the black community in the early 1970s that she might be a gifted actress but "her short natural hairstyle was detrimental to the image of black women,"[63] Goldberg's dark skin and dreadlocks have often positioned her as an aberrant figure as compared to other light-skinned, straight-haired black actresses.

Given the fact that black men were the first group to adopt dreadlocks, the hairstyle has often carried a masculine connotation for many people. Further, some African Americans also have felt that adopting dreadlocks, removed from Rastafari culture, is a co-optation that was inauthentic to the African American experience. As Kofi Taha explains, "the main problem [was] the absence of any of the original spiritual process that the decision to dred [one's hair] once implied, or any of the political action that gave the style that name."[64] In "Invisible Dread," Bert Ashe recalls why he hesitated to 'lock his hair in the early 1980s:

> My first real flirtation with dreadlocks happened while I was working as a radio disc jockey in Louisiana starting in 1983. Dreadlocks was standoffish, and did not respond to my flirtation at all. Actually, I'm not sure I could have gone through with it then, anyway. One reason was that I was dating a Caribbean woman who was adamant that dreadlocks were solely a sacred mode of expression for the Rastafari. She argued passionately that my wearing dreadlocks without "wearing" the religion would be a massive cultural insult.[65]

It was difficult for many African Americans who contemplated dreadlocks in the early 1980s to reconcile with the fact that the style could be more than just a symbolic gesture to Rastafari, that it might also present an alternative to Afros, cornrows, or chemical straightening. Over the course of the 1990s, dreadlocks became a lifestyle choice for many black women who viewed it as part of a natural way of life. As one woman in Chicago said of her dreadlocks in the early 1990s, "I love my hair like this. I wouldn't trade it for straight hair. There is something so spiritual and in-touch about my hair. I feel connected to my roots. My hair gives me a sense of oneness with nature."[66]

My own dreadlock journey started in October 2007. I had used a chemical relaxer from the age of fourteen until I was thirty, and during this period my hair went from long (straight) and healthy to short and damaged. For me, hair has always been a constant battle. Sure, it was long and healthy during my childhood, but after decades of using a chemical straightener, it grew increasingly damaged—a tale that rings true for millions of black women—and I became tired of repeating the "process" every six to eight weeks. Why am I doing this, I wondered? What does my thick, curly, frizzy hair look like? And, is there a way I can take care of my hair without using a chemical, a hot comb, or having to wear a wig? In January 2008, I shared my hair story for the first time publicly, and that is when my journey collided with Ruth Smith. One gloomy morning in February of that year, I walked into Strictly Roots (SR), a natural hair care studio—which means no measures are taken to alter the natural state of black hair—that was once located on Bathurst Street south of Richmond Street in Toronto. The studio opened in 2002, and at this point I had been a client of SR for months; however, this morning was different. As I entered the shop, Ruth was on the phone doing an interview about an article (titled "Why Do Black Women Fear the 'Fro?") that I had written a few weeks prior and which had recently been published in the *Toronto Star*. As I waited (and eavesdropped), I realized that that article had opened a Pandora's box on the black hair issue.

The decision to "go natural" today is just as politicized as it was a century ago, and as it relates to dreadlocks, misconceptions about cleaning and grooming in addition to misrepresentations in the media continue to play a role in demonizing the hairstyle. Just as the New Negro Woman refined blackness through a lens of racial uplift in response to a sociocultural milieu that debased black bodies, the remnants of this duality still exist in contemporary culture. Media culture is no longer infected with the rhetoric and ideology of eugenics and scientific racism that shaped the formation of the New Negro, but black women's bodies, and primarily their hair, continue to be debased and positioned as abhorrent.

Judy Davis observes that, because of the association between dreadlocks and Rastafari, people often believe that those who wear 'locks "do not wash or comb their hair, allowing it to become dirty and unkempt."[67] When *Essence* magazine began to run a series of how-to articles on dreadlocks in the 1990s, the magazine noted only marginally that the style was popularized in Jamaica, and, according to Ayana Byrd and Lori Tharps, a number of readers wrote in to lambaste the publication for having "crucified the dread!"[68] Following the Oscars in 2015, *E! Red Carpet* host Giuliana Rancic (who is of Italian descent) criticized eighteen-year-old actress Zendaya Coleman (who is biracial) on the television show *Fashion Police* because of her dreadlocks (which were not real but synthetic), saying, "I feel like she smells like patchouli oil and weed."[69] Despite such misconceptions, over the past thirty years, dreadlocks have become increasingly popular in urban cities across North America (and Europe), even among people not of African descent.

While there is some debate as to whether the choice of one's hairstyle automatically signifies one's alliance with, or opposition to, the European standard, what many often overlook, as Ashe aptly notes, are the specific male expectations about black women's hair that influence how women style their hair in the first place.[70] For some black women, heterosexual courtship dictates their hair choices and even the use of skin-bleaching products. In the United Kingdom, for example, Debbie Weekes observed that when black women talked about their identities, they were, like black Canadian women, highly gendered. The historical association of whiteness as a yardstick of beauty, she writes, "has become internalized not just by black women but by black men also. This process of negating the beauty of black textured hair and darker shades of skin has strong implications for black women in terms of appearing attractive to males."[71] Many straight black women believe that altering their hair will make them more attractive to men who equate straightened hair with femininity and natural hair with masculinity. Queer black women, on the other hand, have historically embraced their natural hair. It is hard to ignore the fact that Black Lives Matter Toronto, for example, is primarily made up of queer black women with natural hair. Without the pressure to adhere to the Western standard of beauty for which black men are also partially responsible, black queer women have "dared to go natural" in ways that many straight black women have not.

In addition to hair, the politics of black beauty still includes the struggle against the cultural imperative to remove dark skin and replace it with skin that is shades lighter or white. Dark skin is still connected to a "dark past" while lighter skin is positioned as a "brighter future."[72] The ubiquity of advertising imagery of bouncy, shiny, long, straight hair affects black women because this image is antithetical to what is naturally attainable for many women, especially those with darker skin. Amina Mama's research on black women demonstrates that there remains an ambiguous feeling among many black women with respect to a natural hair texture and darker shades of skin.[73] This straight-haired rule, as Paul C. Taylor posits, might be more precisely stated as "the principle that *long* straight hair is a necessary component of *female* beauty.... The straight hair rule dominates [black] culture to such an extent that one commentator can meaningfully [ask in 2000], 'Have we reached the point where the only acceptable option for [black] women is straight hair?"[74] In 2014 when I appeared on *Canada AM* alongside natural hairstylist Janet Campbell and comedian/playwright Trey Anthony to talk about why some black women are afraid of their own hair and of "going natural," I was surprised by the reaction I received from one of my white friends. Why was the segment so long? he wondered. He could not understand the issue. His response, however, spoke to the limited knowledge most Canadians have about black community, let alone black beauty politics. It is difficult to talk about varied aspects of black Canadian history; the conversation seems to be limited to Canada's role in the Underground Railroad and, well, that's about it.

In 1991, for instance, the Historica-Dominion Institute and the CBC co-produced a series of television commercials called *Canada: A People's History*. In one of these one-minute commercials, "The Underground Railroad," a black woman named Eliza stands worriedly in front of a window looking out for her (and her brother's) father to arrive in the "Promised Land" of Canada. She wears a brown dress, shawl, and headscarf, and a white woman, who wears a black dress and a bonnet, accompanies her. When Eliza's impatience forces her onto the street, we discover that their father has made it safely across the border by hiding in a wooden church pew. The voiceover then says, "Between 1840 and 1860 more than thirty thousand American slaves came secretly to Canada and freedom. They called it the Underground Railroad."[75] While a real Eliza might have lived in Canada during the mid-nineteenth century, her characterization in the *Heritage Minutes*, as they were also called, was fictional. The commercial represents a consistent institutional practice of positioning the mid-nineteenth century as the starting point of African Canadian history. It also represents the narrow depiction of black Canadian history, placing all people of African descent in a historical box as it relates to our contributions to the Canadian narrative. Vignettes like the *Heritage Minutes* forever frame the African Canadian narrative through the lens of immigration, as visitors to "our native land," not as contributors to the country's economic, political, and socio-cultural fabric.

As noted in chapter 2's discussion of Viola Desmond, rather than hearing about her entrepreneurial contributions, viewers of her *Heritage Minute* learn about her life only through the prism of black victimhood. The problem with this kind of nostalgia, as Lee Glazer and Susan Key aptly note, is that "[it] undermines the power of the present by bringing the past forward into the present, while simultaneously taking the present back to the past."[76] These two examples pinpoint how the dominant culture has viewed black Canadian history—as nostalgic fragments of our distant past. Such viewing acts as a form of hegemonic power that serves to keep black bodies and communities outside the dominant narrative, placing black Canadian stories on the periphery of *the* national story about Canada's becoming. The lack of diverse representation has had the effect of erasing blackness as being akin to Canadianness, and, as it relates to black beauty, it has helped to widen the gap between what the dominant culture does and does not know of black communities. When I was a graduate student at McGill University, for instance, I was invited to attend a media event. At the reception, I was the only black person in a room of approximately sixty people. This was not the first time this had happened, but it was the first time I was acutely aware of it. At one point, a white woman asked me and several other graduate students what our research interests were. When I told her about my dissertation on black Canadian beauty culture, she paused for a very long time, and then proceeded to ask someone else about his research. For her, black beauty culture was a frivolous topic of study. While there are black Canadian scholars who ardently believe that slavery is the most important aspect of black history and that it needs to be more central in Canadian historical studies, others believe that critiques of multiculturalism and the othering of blackness in Canada requires more attention in the annals of academic research. I believe that the study of black beauty culture and consumer culture, in general, are just as significant to the black Canadian narrative.

The cultural currency of African American beauty culture has also played a significant role in the cultivation of black beauty ideals in sites of black diaspora, so much so that black Americans have dominated the discourse on black hair. Althea Prince's *The Politics of Black Women's Hair* (2009) and Shirley Tate's *Black Beauty: Aesthetics, Stylization, Politics* (2009) are two of the first books to address the politics of black women's hair and beauty in Canada and the United Kingdom. Through interviews with black women, both authors explore how beauty ideals about skin and hair have been inscribed onto black women's bodies. Both texts locate

African American cultural production as having great impact on public perceptions of black beauty across sites of black diaspora. Americans novels and films, in particular, have helped to shape in-group and out-group attitudes about black beauty because these are the cultural products that have circulated transnationally and globally as representations of blackness.

Throughout the nineteenth and twentieth centuries, American novelists examined the politics of skin and the intersections of colorism (showing prejudice against darker-skinned blacks), hair texture, and the beauty of black women. The "literary mulatto" first emerged as a favourite theme of antislavery fiction in the mid-nineteenth century, embodying and dramatizing profound tensions and paradoxes of race and nation.[77] Eve Allegra Raimon asserts that the "literary mulatto" could be appropriated and exploited to "suit the sentimental conventions and readerly expectations of the day. In both lived experience and in fiction ... the mixed-race body was perpetually refigured, regulated, and neutralized all at once."[78] In 1854, for example, when English botanist, writer, and artist Amelia Matilda Murray visited Quebec and Ontario, on her first trip to Quebec City she noted, "Canadian ladies" are more like the French "in their enjoyment of passing moments, and are generally pretty natural, and well dressed, so that I have found their acquaintances agreeable."[79] On a visit to the Niagara region, on the other hand, in a letter dated October 28, 1854, she lamented, "One of the evils consequent upon Southern slavery is the ignorant and miserable set of coloured people who throw themselves in Canada."[80]

Harriet Beecher Stowe's "mulatto" and "quadroon" slave children (with strong Christian values) in *Uncle Tom's Cabin* (1852), arguably the most influential sentimental novel of the nineteenth century, had a great impact on British readers' conception of race. As an example of how *Uncle Tom's Cabin* resonated with the British, when Amelia Murray visited Charleston, South Carolina, in January 1855, she wrote:

> Mrs. Stowe's Topsy is a perfect illustration of Darkie's character, and many of the sad histories of which her book is made up may be true as isolated facts; but yet I feel sure that, as a whole, the story, however ingeniously worked up, is an unfair picture; a libel upon the slaveholder as a body. I very much doubt if a real Uncle Tom can be found in the whole Negro race; and if such a being is, or was, he is a great rarity as a Shakespeare among whites.[81]

When Stowe first introduces the character of Topsy, a stereotyped characterization of a black child, she is described by Stowe as "one of the blackest of her race; and her round shining eyes, glittering as glass beads, moved with quick and restless glances over everything in the room.... Her woolly hair was braided in sundry little tails, which stuck out in every direction."[82] When introducing Eva, the daughter of a Southern slave owner who befriends the enslaved Uncle Tom, Stowe describes her as "the perfection of childish beauty... the long golden-brown hair that floated like a cloud around it, the deep spiritual gravity of her violet blue eyes... all marked her out from other children."[83] Stowe uses hair to inscribe a black/white logic into the visioning of childhood which, as Robin Bernstein writes, "configured Topsy and Eva as a popularized dyad, the 'two extremes of society': the 'fair' child with a 'golden head,' and the 'cringing' black child who had been viciously beaten by her previous owners."[84] In the mid-nineteenth century, the "tragic mulatto" also emerged as the embodiment of a desire among whites to preclude mixed-raced women from full participation and acceptance in white society.

In order to draw an invisible line between the white body and the black body, laws against interracial unions began to appear in the United States as early as 1664.[85] In 1863 when the journalist David Goodman Croly published a pamphlet entitled "Miscegenation: The Theory and the Blending of the Races, Applied to the American White Man and Negro,"[86] the pamphlet coined the word *miscegenation*, combining the Latin *miscere*, "to mix," and *genus*, "race." Miscegenation was often the result of white males' exploitation of black slave women. In nineteenth-century America, a *mulatto* signified "one-half blood" or the child of a black and a white, a *quadroon* had "one-quarter blood" (or the child of a mulatto and a white), and an *octoroon* had "one-eighth blood" (or the child of a quadroon and a white). It is worth noting that, as Jennifer DeVere Brody points out, while octoroons might have had no trace of black blood in their *appearance*, they were still subject to the legal disabilities which attached them to the condition of blacks.[87]

The literary "tragic mulatto" was first introduced in two nineteenth-century short stories written by Lydia Maria Child: "The Quadroons" (1842) and "Slavery's Pleasant Homes" (1843). In both instances, Child portrayed light-skinned women, the offspring of white slaveholders and their black female slaves, as "tragic" by emphasizing their displacement in a society that needed to maintain boundaries between blacks and whites. The "tragic mulatto" was ignorant of both her mother's race and her own, and she believed herself to be white and free. Her heart was pure, her manners impeccable, her language polished, and she was beautiful. A similar portrayal of the *tragic mulatto* appears in *Clotel; or, The President's Daughter* (1853), a novel written by black abolitionist William Wells Brown. As one of the earliest published novels by an African American, *Clotel* perpetuated the doomed plight of the light-skinned woman. *Clotel* ends with a gang of white men chasing Clotel, a mulatto woman, who, unable to escape, drowns in the Potomac River within sight of the White House.[88] Harriet Wilson's *Our Nig* (1859), one of the earliest novels published by an African American woman, also drew from the "tragic mulatto" tradition to dramatize the theme of miscegenation.[89]

When African American writers penned narratives about "tragic mulatto" women, they emphasized the heroism of their light-skinned characters. In the novels of Charles Chesnutt, for instance, Claudia Tate found a "preponderance of light-skinned heroes and heroines, while the comic and local-color character roles are reserved for the folk who are literally black in hue."[90] Nella Larsen's *Quicksand* (1928) and *Passing* (1929) also depict beautiful mulatto heroines, although in both instances they struggle with their racial identity and their place in society.[91] By pitting light-skinned characters against dark-skinned characters, African American writers also contributed to black women's self-esteem issues with respect to skin colour, just as the stereotyped images circulating within the dominant culture had done, though it is unlikely this was their intention. Importantly, D. W. Griffith's 1915 film *The Birth of a Nation* (discussed in chapter 2), as the first feature-length film, entrenched the "tragic mulatto" character type that would dominate Hollywood films throughout the twentieth century. While there had been racially charged films before it, such as *The Debt* (1912), *The White Slave; or, The Octoroon* (1913), *In Humanity's Cause* (1913), and *In Slavery Days* (1913), which all relied heavily on "tragic mulatto" narratives and the fractioning of black blood, the significance of *The Birth of a Nation* can be seen in the wide-ranging influence it had on Hollywood. As Donald Bogle asserts, "one can detect in this single film the trends and sentiments that were to run through most every black film made for a long time afterward."[92] Bogle writes further that "the mulatto" was usually "made likable—even sympathetic (because of her white blood, no doubt)—and the audience believe[d] that the girl's life could have been productive and happy had she not been a 'victim of divided racial inheritance.'"[93] Her in-between status—as not black or white, living in a society divided by race—is what made light-skinned black women so tragic in the eyes of whites. The configuration of light-skinned black women as confused persons of a mixed progeny had a lasting impact on the visual image of black women through the 1950s and 1960s.

In the film adaptation of Fannie Hurst's novel *Imitation of Life* (1934), the story revolves around a young widow and mother, Bea Pullman (Claudette Colbert), who, as an aspiring entrepreneur, decides to appropriate the recipes and cooking skills of her African American housekeeper, Delilah Johnson (Louise Beavers), who becomes a waffle-making Aunt Jemima-type, working for Pullman. A subplot involves Delilah's light-skinned daughter, Peola (Fredi Washington), who is a "tragic mulatto" figure. In the film, Peola attempts to pass as white because she is embarrassed by her dark-skinned mother and by her own blackness. Twenty-five years later, Hollywood's fascination with the "tragic mulatto" narrative continued, as evidenced by the 1959 remake of *Imitation of Life*, this time featuring Lana Turner and Juanita Moore as the young widow and her housekeeper. As in the original, the housekeeper's light-skinned daughter rejects her mother and cuts off all communication with her so that she can pass as white. As Gayle Wald explains, passing entails not solely racial transcendence, "but rather struggles for control over racial representation in a context of the radical unreliability of embodied appearances."[94] In the March 1951 issue of *Ebony*, a first-person testimonial piece titled "I'm Through with Passing," appeared (without a byline) under the long descriptive subtitle "Negro girl tells of her 12 years of bitterness and frustration while posing as white to get decent job, finally decides to drop mask and return to her people." This feature affirmed that black-to-white racial passing was a common practice for many light-skinned blacks, as historically, transcending race has marked the boundaries of freedom (e.g., an enslaved person "passing as free") and the parameters of mobility (e.g., a black person "passing as white" to gain access to a higher level of employment). Because blackness carried negative connotations in the dominant culture, many people, if they could escape its grip, were willing to risk everything to do so.

In Wallace Thurman's novel *The Blacker the Berry* (1929), for example, the pain of being a dark-skinned woman in Harlem is reflected in the character of Emma Lou, who laments about her skin colour because "a black girl would never know anything but sorrow and disappointment."[95] In Toni Morrison's *The Bluest Eye* (1970), Pecola Breedlove is an eleven-year-old black girl who believes that she is ugly because of the way that people in her life treat her. Pecola comes to believe that if only she had blue eyes then she would become beautiful.[96] When Alice Walker introduces the light-skinned character of Shug Avery to the dark-skinned Miss Celie in *The Color Purple* (1982), Miss Celie recalls, "Under all that powder her face black as Harpo. She got a long-pointed nose and big fleshy mouth. Lips look like black plum. Eyes big, glossy.... She look me over from head to foot.... You sure *is* ugly, she say, like she ain't believed it."[97] In his reading of Toni Morrison's *Song of Solomon* (1977) and Zora Neale Hurston's *Their Eyes Were Watching God* (1937), Ashe found that both authors engaged how black women struggle between their own hairstyle preference and the hairstyle preference of black men. "These two authors offer dissimilar but compatible discussions of not only the black female's encounters with the white-female standard of beauty, but also the black female's difficulties negotiating her black-male partner's conception of that standard," he writes.[98]

In Chimamanda Ngozi Adichie's novel *Americanah* (2013), Ifemelu, a young black woman who comes to America from Nigeria, is faced with pressures to chemically straighten her hair to fit in with other African American women. After arriving, Ifemelu attends a West Philadelphia hair salon to get her hair chemically straightened:

> Since she came to America, she had always braided her hair with long extensions, always alarmed at how much it cost.... And so it was a new adventure, relaxing her hair. She removed her braids, careful to leave her scalp unscratched, to leave undisturbed the dirt that would protect it. Relaxers had grown in their range, boxes and boxes in the "ethnic hair" section of the drugstore, faces of smiling black women with impossibly straight and shiny hair, beside words like "botanical" and "aloe" that promised gentleness.... Ifemelu felt only a slight burning, at first, but as the hairdresser rinsed out the relaxer, Ifemelu's head bent backwards against a plastic sink, needles of stinging paint shot up from different parts of her scalp, down to different parts of her body, back up to her head.... Her hair was hanging down rather than standing up, straight and sleek, parted at the side and curving to a slight bob at her chin. The verve was gone. She did not recognize herself. She left the salon almost mournfully; while the hairdresser had flat-ironed the ends, the smell of burning, of something organic dying which should not have died, had made her feel a sense of loss.[99]

This passage captures the feelings of both excitement and loss that many black women experience after the application of their first chemical relaxer.

I, too, had mixed feelings when I chemically straightened my hair at the age of fourteen. On the one hand, I was excited to have hair that flowed and that I could style using a curling iron like white girls at school, but on the other hand, I missed the natural texture of my hair, its coarseness and its uniqueness. What I had gained was the ability to "fit in" with hair that flowed like everyone else, but what I had lost was the thing that made me unique—my tightly coiled natural hair. African American films rarely depict this sense of loss. Instead, on the big screen, black hair choices are often mocked and/or trivialized.

Spike Lee's *School Daze* (1988) for example, was one of the first films to provide a commentary on contemporary black beauty politics. The film, a satire about how colour and class continue to divide black communities, is set at a historically black college in the United States. Light-skinned blacks are caricatures of "wannabe" whites and the dark-skinned "jigaboos" are those who proudly affirm their love of blackness. This juxtaposition trivialized the issue of colour and the painful realities of colorism that have affected the lives of black women. In *Jungle Fever* (1991), however, Lee explored the issue of colour through the male lead character, Flipper Purify (Wesley Snipes), a dark-skinned man who is married to a light-skinned woman named Drew (Lonette McKee). The politics of skin are revealed in the film when Flipper has an extramarital affair with an Italian-American woman named Angie Tucci (Annabella Sciorra). Drew laments to her black girlfriends that she has been the victim of name-calling by African Americans throughout her life because of her light skin, but that, for Flipper, she must not have been "light" enough; but when Flipper discusses his affair with his black male friends, Angie's whiteness is framed as a site of curiosity. Flipper, like his friends, was attracted to her white skin because it was so different from their own much darker skin. *Jungle Fever* tried to present the complexity of race in America, but it failed to do so without reifying rigid, unchanging binaries of whiteness versus blackness, dark skin versus light skin, African American versus white. The film also reduced black beauty politics to matters of skin colour, ignoring altogether the complexities of hair.

Kathe Sandler's documentary *A Question of Color* (1993) explored the impact of colour consciousness within African American communities. Instead of focusing on other characters, however, Sandler used her own body (as a light-skinned, biracial woman) to examine constructions of blackness and colour relativity. As Janell Hobson points out, "Sandler seems anxious to 'prove' her blackness by donning Afrocentric attire and dwelling in a predominantly black urban neighbourhood. These actions imply that her very fairness, including her blonde hair and blue eyes, is not enough to establish her black identity."[100] In contrast to the filmic representation of black beauty as being in a constant binary position between light skin/dark skin, beautiful/ugly, an emulation of whiteness/a validation of blackness, many have lauded Julie Dash's *Daughters of the Dust* (1991) as one example that affirmed the beauty of all black women. The film tells the story of three generations of a black family in Georgia in 1902 as they prepare to migrate to the north, and it does so without privileging one body type, hair texture, or identity position over another.[101] Sadly, such representations have been rare.

Even Justin Simien's satirical comedy-drama *Dear White People* (2014), in its attempt to address the complexities of race, racial identification, and biracial beauty politics, failed to subvert the trope of having to "prove" one's blackness. Set on the campus of the fictional Winchester University, Sam White (Tessa Thompson) is a biracial student at the prestigious and predominantly white school. White is also the host of an edgy radio show that aims to politicize white racism on campus. Like Sandler, however, to authenticate herself as "black," White wears several Afrocentric hairstyles and surrounds herself with other like-minded black militants. In the end, however, when her *true* racial identity as a biracial woman (from a white father) with a white boyfriend is revealed, she is cast as "not black enough" to continue her political radio show, maintain her black-encoded hairdos, and associate with her militant (dark-skinned) black friends. This film is a contemporary example of how race, black beauty aesthetics, and in-group/out-group acceptance continues to bifurcate black communities in the twenty years since Sandler's and Lee's films. It explains why, in the first season of *How to Get Away with Murder*, for example, when Oscar nominee Viola Davis took off her wig—revealing her short Afro hair—and her makeup, many black women took to the blogosphere once again to comment on the act. Black hair, especially for dark-skinned women, remains a hot-button issue.

Back in 1925, sociologist Guy B. Johnson published a study titled "Newspaper Advertisements and Negro Culture" that examined advertising in six prominent African American newspapers. He discovered that most of the advertisements made their appeal to the desire for straight hair and light complexion.[102] In 1948, Vishnu V. Oak noted further that advertisements for hair and skin lotions remained the richest advertising contracts for the black press.[103] Just as products could deliver only a caricature of white standards of beauty, the images that accompanied skin-bleaching advertisements were also caricatures of a standard of beauty that was basically impossible for most black women to attain. The politics of skin colour and the prevalence of skin bleaching are still issues today.

In the documentary *Dark Girls* (2011), filmmakers Bill Duke and D. Channsin Berry document how colorism continues to divide many black communities. In interviews with black men, one said of dark-skinned women, "[They] have low self-esteem, while light-skinned women have more confidence because they're closer to white." A 2010 video project called *Shadeism*, created by undergraduate students at Ryerson University's School of Journalism in Toronto, similarly addressed the issue of light-skinned, long-haired black beauty ideals, the pressures to live up to such standards, and the ways in which family members treat young girls who are dark skinned as compared to those who are light skinned. Outside North America, the idea of whiteness as an enabler of confidence and blackness (or dark skin) as a disabling liability continues to circulate in contemporary advertising and media around the world. In India, for example, a 2009 television commercial for a skin-bleaching product featured two men— one with dark skin, the other with light skin—standing on a balcony overlooking a neighbourhood. The darker-skinned man turns to his friend and says, "I am unlucky because of my face." His lighter-skinned friend replies, "Not because of your face, because of the colour of your face." At the end of the ad, the darker-skinned man, now several shades lighter, appears with a woman by his side.[104] Such advertising circulates across Indian and Pakistan; in other versions, a young dark-skinned woman is not able to find a husband until she has lightened her skin.

Even though hydroquinone, the active ingredient in skin-bleaching creams, has been found to cause severe allergic reactions (rash; hives; difficulty breathing; tightness in the chest; swelling of the mouth, face, lips, or tongue), blistering, blue-black darkening of the skin, and excessive redness, stinging, and irritation,[105] it continues to gain in popularity. Black women (and men) in Canada—as in India, the United States, the Caribbean, and Africa (as well as Korea, Japan, and China)—use skin-bleaching creams because darker skin is still viewed as a liability, both socially and economically. Globally, the market for skin lighteners was expected to reach US$10 billion by 2015.[106] Hindustan Unilever, one of the largest consumer products companies in India, noted in a 2009 annual report that "skin lightening continues to be a major area of emphasis" for its skin care division.[107] Dancehall artist Vybz Kartel and Dominican baseball player

Sammy Sosa have publicly confirmed that they use bleaching creams. In 2011, Kartel also launched his own range of men's cosmetics, including a variety of skin-lightening creams called "cake soap." Cake soap was first introduced in the late 1970s in Jamaica as a dermatological wonder with the capacity to reduce the shine and "greasy" or "tarry" look on one's face, but by the 1990s, it was realized that the product had other qualities; it then took off as a skin whitener.[108] In a statement to Vibe.com, Kartel defended cake soap: "When black women stop straightening their hair and wearing wigs and weaves, when white women stop getting lip and butt injections and implants...then I'll stop using the cake soap and we'll all live naturally ever after."[109]

Significantly, such transformation, consumerist pursuits, and the alignment of skin-bleaching practices with the body-altering practices of black and white women point to how popular culture, as Bordo observes, applies no brakes to the fantasies of rearrangement and self-transformation, such that "we are constantly told that we can 'choose' our own bodies."[110] In her analysis of Tyra Banks, for example, Jessalynn Keller argues that the former model and talk-show host used her celebrity to position her hair-straightening ("relaxing") practices as a matter of personal choice, encouraging black women to make their own individualized hair choices, divorced from the broader political and social implications that these decisions may have.[111] Contemporary culture has also led many to believe that a person's bodily transformations and/or rearrangements are "undetermined by history, social location, or even individual biography."[112] In this regard, the continued practice of skin whitening points to the breadth and depth of the remnants of colonial domination.

In *Black Skin, White Masks* Frantz Fanon observed that if one is overwhelmed by a desire to be white, "it is because he lives in a society that makes his inferiority complex possible, in a society that derives its stability from the perpetuation of this complex, in a society that proclaims the superiority of one race."[113] While Fanon was writing in the 1950s, the convergence of beauty culture with popular culture has meant that the desire for whiteness shapes not only what is advertised and what is deemed beautiful, but also the sanctioned aesthetics of a black beauty. Karl Marx once described *commodity fetishism* as a theory that explains how the social relations represented in an object come to appear absolutely fixed or given, beyond human control, which in capitalist society helps to ensure that the social order is sustained in consumer culture and the reality of social inequality overlooked.[114] The convergence of popular culture and beauty culture has also neutralized the politics of race and class such that beauty firms have, since the 1990s, proudly claimed to be "hip" and "multicultural" despite engaging in systematic strategies that have removed the *blackness* of blackness from their advertising campaigns and product imagery. Black beauty has been *fetishized* into mere aesthetics, devoid of black-identified politics. Stated otherwise, as black women have entered mainstream beauty culture, a culture that claims to be "multicultural," issues surrounding hair texture and skin colour have appeared as non-issues. That we are surrounded by homogenizing and normalizing images, whose content, as Bordo has argued, is far from arbitrary "but instead suffused with the dominance of gendered, racial, class, and other cultural iconography"[115] seems on one level so obvious that it is hardly worth mentioning. On another level, however, the politics of hair and skin have typically been issues overlooked by mainstream beauty firms. Since white-owned companies, which for most of the twentieth century ignored black consumers, are now the leading manufacturers of black hair care and cosmetic products, we must ask renewed questions about the representation of black beauty in contemporary culture.

In the preface to *The Politics of Race in Canada* (2009), Maria Wallis observes, "Canadians continue to be widely applauded for promoting achievement over skin colour as a basis for recognition, rewards, and relationships. But like all powerful national dreams, this myth conceals more than it reveals, resulting in distortions that confuse or divide."[116] Racial bias does not dominate just by universalizing the values of hegemonic groups so that they become accepted as norm; as Mercer aptly writes, "their hegemony and historical persistence is underwritten at a subjective level by the way ideologies construct positions from which individuals recognize such values as a constituent element of their personal identity and lived experiences."[117] Mercer, writing in the 1990s, argued that hair functions as a key ethnic signifier because "compared with bodily shape or facial features, it can be changed more easily by cultural practices such as straightening."[118] I would argue that this reality has now changed. The composite nature of racial bias is both physiological and cultural, and it is intermixed with symbolic representations of racialized bodies.

In the twenty-first century, advancements in digital technology such as Photoshop have made it possible for phenotypical features such as dark skin, a wide nose, and coarse-textured hair to be malleable in photographic images. Further, improvements in plastic surgery have made the effects of scarring after surgery less significant for black women. Historically, keloid scarring has deterred many black women from getting plastic surgery, but this is less of an issue today. Where racial bias may dictate the colour of models in fashion spreads and advertising campaigns, hair texture still determines the coding of black beauty as either *exotic* (i.e., natural hair), ethnically ambiguous (loose, curly Afro), or both (long, flowing hair). Given this dichotomy, the pervasiveness of hair weaves and wigs among black models and actresses of all skin tones must be situated alongside the supposed "colour-blindness" of the contemporary mainstream beauty culture industry.

Hair weaves (which involve adding synthetic or real hair to one's own hair) became a popular hairstyling technique in the 1990s. The term "hair weave" was first patented in 1951 by an African American named Christina Jenkins, a housewife in Malvern, Ohio, who invented and then patented the style.[119] The widespread wearing of weaves did not occur until after 1990 when a reported 1.3 million pounds of human hair valued at US$28.6 million were imported to the United States from countries such as China, India, and Indonesia (where poor women sold their hair by the inch).[120] The "global hair trade," as it is now called, includes a supply-chain network where hair is sourced in Asia and South Asia, then sterilized, cut, and shipped to wholesalers in Europe and North America, who sell the hair to beauty supply shops, beauty parlours, and hair retailers. Since the 1990s, Korean immigrants have dominated the sale of human hair in the United States and increasingly in Canada, especially at the retail end-point. Whereas black celebrities such as Bob Marley and Whoopi Goldberg popularized dreadlocks in the 1970s and 1980s, by the 1990s it became virtually impossible to ignore the images of black women with coiffed, long, flowing, straight hair that circulated not only in mainstream beauty culture advertising but also in black media. In 1990, for instance, *Essence* magazine declared, "Sisters love the weave!"[121] From models (e.g., Naomi Campbell, Iman, Tyra Banks) to actresses and celebrities (e.g., Beyoncé, Janet Jackson, and Ciara), in order to attain long flowing tresses, black women in droves began to wear hair weaves. Many bloggers have questioned whether Oprah Winfrey wears a weave, a rumour she playfully refuted in 2009 when she allowed Chris Rock to rake his fingers through her scalp during a taping of her talk show. In the 1990s, she often used her talk show to out those black celebrities who wore hair weaves. Ironically, a series called *Houston Beauty*, which ran for one season on the Oprah Winfrey Network in 2013, chronicled the life of Glenda "Ms. J" Jemison, the owner and director of Franklin Beauty School, the oldest continuously operated licensed beauty school in Texas. The show predominantly featured hair weaves worn by the show's cast, and the preferred style taught at the school was hair weaving, in addition to chemical relaxing.

Even though women have been wearing weaves since the 1960s—and wigs and hair attachments since the nineteenth century—the weave of the late 1980s and early 1990s was a major improvement on prior weaves. The modern hair weave is less bulky than earlier versions, and it is available in a variety of colours and textures. Early hair-weaving techniques involved cornrowing the existing hair (i.e., braiding the hair in tight rows of braids); then hair extensions called "wefts" were sewn into "tracks" (strips of hair sewn into netting) directly onto the hair. This style eventually grew out of favour because it left a bump of hair at the crown of the head and gave rise to the joke "obvious weave" or "OW" for short. Current techniques involve a "bonding" method (where tracks are glued to chemically straightened hair at the roots) and "singeing" (using heat, synthetic hair is machine-pressed onto the wearer's natural hair). Another popular weave is the "lace front wig." With lace front wigs (given that name because they are often made with a French or Swiss lace cap base, a custom-fitted cap that is bonded to the head with tape or glue adhesive to create a hairline that looks more "natural" than a weave), the wig is placed overtop the lace cap and then attached to the adhesive. Like chemical relaxers, contemporary weaves and lace fronts also have ill health effects, primarily hair loss. As an example, a 2012 photograph on ABCnews.com of former supermodel Naomi Campbell revealed that the model's hairline had receded approximately two inches, likely a result of years of wearing weaves and lace front wigs.[122] In 2014, actress Countess Vaughn appeared on CBS's *The Doctors* to discuss the health issues she has suffered because of wearing lace fronts. After five years, her lace front wig, which requires the frequent reapplication of wig glue to stay in place, resulted in Vaughn developing a severe scalp infection, in addition to discharge from her scalp, hair loss, and skin discolouration on her scalp, the nape of her neck, and beneath her eyes.[123]

Hair salons in Toronto first began to advertise hair weaves in newspapers in the mid-1980s. Soul Cut, a black hair salon located on Bloor Street West, was one of the first hair salons to post an advertisement for its weave services. In October 1985, the salon told *Share* readers, "If your weave or braiding is unnatural, try the invisible look."[124] Sheer Advantage Hairstylists and Braiding Centre also advertised in *Contrast* in December 1986 that its stylists specialized in "all types of braids—curly braids and weave on."[125] In the 1980s, it was very common for beauticians to describe their weaving services as "weave on." The term described hair extensions (synthetic hair) that were sewn or glued to one's hair for length and texture. While a few hair salons in Toronto have specialized in dreadlocks and natural hair—such as Strictly Roots, once located on Bathurst Street south of Queen Street in the city's downtown; Nanni's Hair Studio, located in the city's north; and the Loc 'N Twists Natural Hair Studio in the northwest suburb of Brampton—black hair salons in Toronto have primarily specialized in hair weaves and/or chemical straightening. From 1987 onward, weaving and relaxing became the two main services provided at black hair salons in the city. At that time, however, few hairdressers worked with human hair on the weft; synthetic hair was more common.

In a rare article in September 1988, *Contrast*'s Montreal edition discussed the amount of care that a weave required. In an article titled "Caring Your Weaves," Doreen's Maison de Beauté on Victoria Avenue provided the following weave tips:

> Before washing weave, braid each weave section to avoid tangles. Cleanse hair and scalp between weave thoroughly as well as around weave base, run shampoo over braids. Do not massage or scrub weave. Always wash weave with lukewarm water. When shampoo and conditioning is complete, squeeze excess water out of braids then carefully remove braids and comb free tangles, remembering to hold weave at base so as not to loosen weave. Applying designing lotion to weave to help eliminate tangles and proceed with styling. Never apply spray or gel moisturizers to weave, they cause weave to mat. Use a lubricant daily such as designing lotion or oil sheen spray. Always hold weave at base while brushing or combing to avoid undo pressure on weave base. Do not sleep or set in pony tail when weave is wet for it will shrink up when drying.[126]

In April 1990, Armonie International, a hair-product distributor, announced in *Share* that it now offered "a new standard of quality in human hair weaves and braids."[127] The style ranged from straight to French refined, water weave, and deep wave. A "water weave" is wavy, not straight-haired like the "straight" or "French refined" hair. A "deep wave" is wavier than a "water weave" and more closely resembles loose, curly black hair, like that of some biracial women. Since synthetic weaves were very high maintenance, and by 1994, the label "100 percent human hair" began to appear on weaves and wigs, women increasingly sought "real human hair" weaves. In 1998, when Lisa Jones published "The Hair Trade," it was one of the first academic pieces to examine the growing global human hair trade. At the time, Jones explained that very few countries processed hair—that is, converted it, for example, from straight to curly/wavy textures. "Most 'raw hair,' as the trade calls it, is processed abroad, in Korea primarily, and sold prepackaged [in the US] at Asian retail shops," she noted.[128] The few American companies that traded human hair were based in New York and California. While African Americans were in the hair trade, the processing companies or "hair factories" were mostly family outfits operated by Jews and Italians.[129] Raw hair product was primarily sourced from China, Korea, and India, but in the early 1990s, Koreans began to buy from the same sources, processing the hair themselves and shipping it to their own retail networks in the United States. Jones also noted that to ask industry types where the raw hair came from and how the business was organized abroad was "to knock up against a covenant of silence."[130]

In May 2008, an *Ebony* feature titled "Guess Who Sells Your Weave?" by Adrienne Samuels noted that there were about nine thousand Korean-owned beauty supply stores in the United States.[131] Koreans first opened businesses in African American communities in the 1970s and 1980s by selling wigs, then weaves and extensions, and now they sell it all, including chemical relaxers, shampoos, hair dyes, and moisturizing products. The impetus for the article was to put a spotlight on what some feel are the "wrong owners" of black hair care product distribution and sales. The *Ebony* article also revealed that popular media portrayals of Korean merchants (since the 1992 L.A. Riots) as so hardworking, driven, and self-sacrificing as to seem "barely human" continues to add fuel to the hair battle. In the 2006 documentary *Black Hair: The Korean Takeover of the Black Hair Care Industry*, Aron Ranen explored how Korean interests gained control of the human hair trade. The film, which is viewable on YouTube, explains that distributors in Korea began to sell products to Korean stores strategically located in African American communities, thereby cancelling out opportunities for local distributors to sell their products to black consumers. In the 2009 documentary *Good Hair*, comedian Chris Rock attempted to turn a spotlight on this human hair trade. In the film, Rock investigates the global hair trade and the relationship black women have with hair weaves and chemical relaxers (said relaxers being euphemistically called "creamy crack" throughout the film). Most notably, Rock exposes the fact that many black women spend upwards of a thousand dollars (US) on hair weaves, sometimes deferring payment through a layaway plan, to maintain the facade of long flowing hair. Rock also goes on a voyage to India; he interviews black hairstylists and celebrities such as Nia Long and Raven-Symoné; and he visits Dudley Products' North Carolina facility, one of the few surviving African American–owned hair-product firms, where he learns how chemical relaxers are made. *Good Hair* then follows competitors through a season of the annual Bonner Bros. Hair Battle in Atlanta, which attracts upwards of 120,000 hair care professionals and showcases almost exclusively hairstyles that involve weaves and chemically relaxed hair.[132]

While *Good Hair* sought to explore the question of whether black women spend countless hours and hundreds of dollars in hair salons to make their hair straighter and silkier because they want to "look white,"[133] it simplified the complexity of the global hair trade. Hair weaving is not singularly a black woman's practice; today, hair weaves, hair extensions, and wigs catering to all ethnicities are offered for sale at beauty-product shops. In fact, walk through any mall in North America and you will likely stumble upon a hair-extension business, selling 100 percent human hair. Numerous celebrated white and Hispanic women have admitted to wearing hair weaves and/or extensions, most notably Céline Dion, Angelina Jolie, and Cameron Diaz. Human hair is so highly sought after that it is now the target of criminals. In metropolitan Atlanta in 2011, for instance, in a series of smash-and-grabs at beauty-supply stores, at least US$100,000 worth of hair was stolen, and similar thefts have occurred in Chicago, Houston, and San Diego, where the take—per heist—has ranged in value from US$10,000 to US$150,000.[134]

Today, the largest black hair-care trade magazine, *OTC Beauty Magazine*, is published in Korean as well as English. According to its website, *OTC Beauty Magazine* serves retailers, store employees, manufacturers, and distributors; the magazine, published for the United States beauty-supply industry has international distribution through outlets in South Korea, China, and the Caribbean. The magazine also uses the tagline "multicultural" even though black hair is its primary focus. In the November 2011 issue, an article (written in English and Korean) titled "Hair, Hair, Hair: Human, Synthetic, Animal" explained the variations in human hair currently on the market.[135] The article describes eight types of human hair imported to the United States and Europe:

> "French, European or Italian hair" is considered the highest quality hair because it is less coarse than Asian or Indian hair but is essentially hair from a "Caucasian" person. "Cuticle hair" is human hair

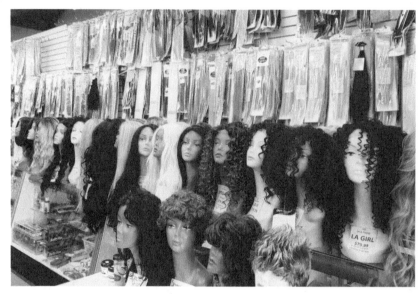

Figure 17. Synthetic wigs and 100% human hair on display, Ragga Hair Studio and Beauty Store, Dundas Street East, Toronto, Ontario, 2018. Photograph by author.

that has been scrutinized to insure that the cuticles are in the same direction on each strand, a procedure that prevents tangles, snarls and matting when the hair is combed. "Synthetic hair" is made from nylon and polyester fibers. "Yak hair" is culled from a yak, an animal native to Thailand; it most resembles human hair and grows long enough to be harvested. "Virgin hair" is human hair or sometimes animal hair that has not been chemically treated. "Yaky, Yaki or Yakie hair" most closely resembles natural black hair that has been chemically relaxed and is also referred to as Afro Yaky, Perm Yaki, Curly or Geri Curl Yaky. "Remi hair" is high quality human hair that is usually silky, straight and smooth, it is also considered to be Virgin hair because it is not processed with chemicals. "Indian hair" describes the source of the hair and it is obtained as a result of a religious ceremony called Tonsure, whereby the hair is shaved from the heads of women.[136]

Thus, while *Good Hair* gave the impression that human hair is culled exclusively from women in India, human hair is traded in Asia, as well. But whereas African Americans are about 13 percent of the United States population, they are responsible for over 80 percent of hair sales, which explains why Korean-owned beauty-supply stores are located predominantly in black neighbourhoods. Koreans also import approximately 85 percent of all commercial hair in the United States.[137] Approximately 60 percent of sales in most Korean-owned beauty-supply stores involve commercial hair and related grooming products. In Britain, according to the UK *Guardian*, the hair-extensions industry is estimated to be worth between £45 million and £60 million (according to London-based industry research firm IBISWorld, revenue from hair and beauty salons was £3.64 billion in 2012–13).[138] The US government has mandated that hair labelled as "100 percent human hair" can legally contain up to 10 percent of fibres other than human hair, such as synthetic or animal hair.[139]

While the Canada Border Services Agency has a customs tariffs schedule that includes "Human hair, unworked, whether or not washed or scoured; waste of human hair," the importation of human hair is not governed by specific regulations from any government agency. Since there are no known mandates in Canada, labelled warnings on these products are purely superficial. Weave wearers (and women who wear braids in which synthetic or real hair is attached to one's real hair) know very little about the hair on their heads or where it comes from, and one is hard pressed to find any labels that identify in detail how the hair is treated or its supply chain. In 2000, Eric Choi, a Korean businessman and CEO of a hair care company based in the United States told *Share* in an interview that he had plans to expand into Canada, most notably Toronto.[140] Eric Choi's firm, headquartered in Syracuse, New York, was the parent company of YTT Canada, with six outlets throughout the northeastern United States; it was, at that time, the largest mass merchandiser in the region. Three months before the *Share* interview, the first of five superstores opened in Toronto; one store in the city's east end had 3,100 square feet of retail space. There has been a virtual silence in Canada about the increased Korean ownership of black hair care, in addition to the health concerns related to hair weaves. Korean-owned and black-owned beauty-supply shops and big-box retailers in Toronto sell hair weaves, as is the case in Montreal, Edmonton, Calgary, and Ottawa. In recent years, salons and supply stores have also started to offer synthetic dreadlocks.

Since the late 1990s, wig and weave advertisements in *Share* have included Beverly Johnson's Black Is Beautiful human-hair wig collection, which has been available for sale in Canada since 1998, and the Calypso Silky Straight human-hair brand. Since 2008, SoftSheen-Carson has also offered for sale a weave care product specifically geared toward synthetic and human-hair extensions. In 2011, advertisements from the Beauty Supply Warehouse began to appear in *Share*; these advertisements included images and accompanying names for the human-hair weaves available for purchase at retail in the Greater Toronto Area. Hair weaves and wigs at retail are typically sold under celebrity brand names, such as the Beyoncé or Rhianna, or with the descriptors "Brazilian" or "Malaysian." In some cases, celebrities are unaware that their name is being used to sell hair. In 2013, Tyra Banks filed a lawsuit in a Los Angeles County Court claiming that ten wig companies had been wrongfully using her name to sell wigs.[141] Further, hair labelled "Brazilian" and "Malaysian" does not really originate in either country; the labels are typically used to frame "virgin Remy" hair as *exotic*. Thus, the question of black beauty today is essentially the same question of a century ago: Why is long, straight hair so important to black women that many are willing to spend exorbitant amounts of money that they do not have, wear animal hair that has been chemically processed (which may result in irrevocable hair loss), and endure health problems, such as uterine fibroids, all so that their hair "swings from side to side"? As Jones poignantly notes, "If hair is the key racial signifier after skin, then the trade makes a fine mockery of it. Processed Asian hair passes as black hair. Italian stock is allegedly blended with hair from the Third World and this passes as European. The hair of yaks...passes as nappy hair."[142] While hair weaves remain popular, natural hair has re-entered the mainstream, not necessarily as a political act but simply as an alternative to relaxers, hair weaves, and lace front wigs.

In 2009, Solange Knowles, Beyoncé's sister, took off her weave and cut her hair into a short pixie cut. At the 2012 Academy Awards, Oscar winner Viola Davis appeared not in her usual weave but in a short, auburn-coloured Afro. Singer Jill Scott also flaunted a natural in 2012, and that same year actress Nicole Ari Parker revealed a short natural curly hairstyle, after years of wearing hair weaves. In June 2012, Parker, along with University of Pennsylvania professor Anthea Butler, cultural critic Joan Morgan, and CurlyNikki.com founder Nikki Walton, also appeared on Melissa Harris-Perry's talk show on MSNBC. The show reported that as of 2011, 36 percent of African American women no longer chemically straighten their hair.[143] In 2013, songstress Goapele appeared at the premiere for the film *Baggage Claim* with a short Afro, and author and spiritual advisor Iyanla Vanzant graced the February 2013 cover of *Essence* with a short, auburn-brown Afro hairdo. In addition to the return of the natural among black celebrities, there are now several natural hair websites in the United States and Canada, and hair care companies catering to women with natural hairstyles are giving black women the opportunity not only to purchase natural products but also talk to other black women about hair. One example of a natural hair care company is Carol's Daughter.

Founded by Lisa Price in 1993, the African American–owned Carol's Daughter was initially a mail-order business, but after the first retail store opened in Brooklyn in 1999, it expanded. Black celebrities such as Jada Pinkett Smith, Mary J. Blige, and Solange Knowles have all endorsed the company's products. Inevitably however, L'Oréal, eager to get in on the "neo-natural" movement, seized an opportunity to purchase Carol's Daughter in 2014 after its retail locations filed for bankruptcy.[144] With that acquisition, Carol's Daughter products joined other brands such as Urban Decay and Kiehls as part of L'Oréal's US lineup. Rumours that Carol's Daughter was up for sale first began to circulate as far back as the spring of 2013. L'Oréal was then believed to be a prospective buyer, as were other white-owned conglomerates that had already made inroads into the black beauty products market, such as Estée Lauder, Shiseido, and Procter & Gamble. In response to L'Oréal's purchase of Carol's Daughter, CosmeticsDesign.com USA, one of the most-read North American news websites for the cosmetic industry, described the move as a signal that L'Oréal was looking to launch a "multicultural division."[145] "This acquisition [of Carol's Daughter] will enable L'Oréal USA to build a new dedicated multicultural beauty division as part of our Consumer Products business, and strengthen the company's position in this dynamic market," said Frédéric Rozé, president and CEO of L'Oréal USA.[146] This is exactly what L'Oréal has done. In recent years, it also launched a natural hair care line, known as the Dark & Lovely Au Naturale.

While mainstream beauty companies laud the "multicultural beauty" as the future of the beauty market, and industry market research has shown that the "naturals" market is outpacing the overall cosmetics market, one must wonder what the larger impact of this recent shift will be. In 2013, for instance, the naturals market saw 7 percent growth, in contrast with 2 percent for the larger beauty market, and in 2014, market-research firm Kline & Company reported that the naturals market at the manufacturing level was approaching US$30 billion in global sales, including double-digit growth in the previous twelve months.[147] Just as the Afro was commodified and depoliticized as a mere fashion aesthetic in the late 1970s, natural hair today runs the risk of becoming just another "look" with no political currency. In 2013, Jill Scott and Nicole Ari Parker once again appeared with hair weaves in television and film roles, and Viola Davis and Iyanla Vanzant have also returned to straightened hairdos, indicating that natural hair remains a difficult commitment for many black women in a culture that continues to place a premium on long, flowing, straight hair. As Judy Davis argues, hair-product advertising's "emphasis on relaxer products and on straight-textured 'fake' (manufactured) hair teaches [black] women to continue to embrace a non-black standard of beauty, often at great monetary expense...and frequently to the detriment of the health of their own hair and scalp."[148] Despite the fact that hair weaves, skin bleaches, chemical relaxers, and tight braids cause irrevocable damage, the capitalist machine behind the straight-haired rule in advertising remains so powerful that for all those women who resist it, the battle is still an uphill one. Significantly, the politicization of black hair, and in some cases its near-criminalization, especially in the workplace and at schools, is one overarching reason why many black women find it difficult to fully embrace a natural hairstyle and keep one for years. Like those who wore braids in the 1980s, black women and men since the 1990s have continued to be punished for wearing dreadlocks, braids, and/or any variation on a natural hairstyle.

In 1996, education officials in the Cayman Islands refused to allow a five-year-old boy back into any government-funded primary school until he "complie[d] with the dress code" and cut his long dreadlocks.[149] That same year, school policies at several Chicago-area junior high and high schools designated that hairstyles such as braids and dreadlocks violated school dress-code policies. School officials argued that the codes had nothing to do with race and culture but instead had to do with "keeping kids safe and preventing distractions in the classrooms." Thomas Ryan, superintendent of District 168, said further, "We have never had a gun in the school or a kid stabbed. I don't ever want to call to a home and say to a parent, 'Your kid was stabbed in school.'"[150] In 1998, seventeen-year-old Michele Barskile of North Carolina was told by her black sorority, Alpha Kappa Alpha, that because she wore her hair in dreadlocks, she would not be allowed to attend the debutante ball.[151] In April 2006, Susan Taylor, then executive editor of *Essence* magazine, cancelled a speaking engagement at the historical black college Hampton University in Virginia, when she learned that a department had a strict "no-braids, no-dreadlocks policy" for its students. After cancelling the engagement, Taylor issued a statement, which read in part, "The freedom to wear our hair in ways that cel-

THE POLITICS OF BLACK HAIR IN THE TWENTY-FIRST CENTURY   235

ebrate our heritage is one of our 'rites of passage.' Students would benefit from learning how to care for and groom locks and braids and wear them in ways that are appropriate in a business setting."[152] Hair—its texture, length, and colour—continues to function as a battleground where issues related to the politics of personal appearance and beauty are fought.

In the United States, lawsuits involving black hair have included claims against police departments, prison authorities, schools, and retailers, all of which have "rules against knotted 'locks [that] unfairly single out [Rastafari] in particular and [blacks] in general."[153] As Deborah Grayson aptly notes, "because of the hierarchical structure of beauty culture, the choices black women make about their personal appearance are political choices whether we intend them to be or not."[154] In November 2002, for instance, two years after Patricia Pitts began working for a theme park in Valdosta, Georgia, she decided to wear her hair in a cornrow style. Wendy Greene recounts that Pitts's manager informed her that she did not approve of her cornrow hairstyle and suggested that "she should get her hair done in a 'pretty' hairstyle." Attempting to satisfy her supervisor's request, Pitts revamped her hairstyle by placing extensions on her hair and styling it in two-strand twists; however, because Pitt's hair had the appearance of dreadlocks, her supervisor again disapproved of her hairstyle. Shortly thereafter, the company issued a memo barring "dreadlocks, cornrows, beads, and shells" unless they were "covered by a hat [or] visor."[155] The US military also had a longstanding anti-braid policy. In the 1980s, several women were fired or threatened with dismissal for wearing braids or cornrows. These occurrences, however, led to lawsuits that eventually outlawed discrimination in the workplace based on hairstyle. Ironically, it transpired that the US Navy abolished its anti-braid policy in 1994 after Navy Board of Dress Regulators became convinced that braided hair was actually more practical for ship-bound black women.[156]

In November 2013, the *New York Daily News* reported that a white woman, Katherine Lemire, who served as special counsel for NYPD Commissioner Raymond Kelly, claimed she was terminated from the position at a leading security firm for standing up for a black colleague, Chanissa Green, who wore a braided hairstyle.[157] In the filed lawsuit it is alleged that Green's supervisor told her that "when someone like me...sees someone with a style like that, we think ghetto—not professional," and further, the supervisor is alleged to have said, "I'll tell you what's beautiful: my daughter, with blond hair and blue eyes." A few weeks later, twelve-year-old Vanessa VanDyke, who wore an Afro, was allegedly told that she would have to leave her school, the Faith Christian Academy in Orlando, unless she cut her hair.[158] In May 2017, after admonishment from the Massachusetts attorney general's office, a Boston-area charter school that punished black girls for wearing braided hair extensions had to suspend its dress-code policy that many felt was discriminatory toward black children. A *Toronto Star* reprint of a *Washington Post* article reported that, after the school banned hair extensions, fifteen-year-old twins Mya and Deanna Cook had been kicked off school sports teams and banished from prom and had received hours of detention for refusing to change their professionally braided hair.[159] After the American Civil Liberties Union filed a discrimination complaint with the state Education Department, and school officials met with the state Attorney General Maura Healey, the school suspended its hair ban. Importantly, not only hair style but hair colour has also resulted in punitive reprimand for black women.

In *Santee v. Windsor Court Hotel* (2000), a black woman lost an employment opportunity and her job not because she wore dreadlocks, cornrows, or braided extensions but because she dyed her hair blonde.[160] In April 1999, Andrea Santee applied for a housekeeping position at the Windsor Court Hotel in New Orleans; when she interviewed for the position, she had dyed blonde hair.[161] In the Executive Housekeeper's opinion, Santee's hair colour was "extreme under the parameters of the [h]otel's grooming policy [and therefore] she inquired into whether [Santee] would be willing to change her hair color for the job."[162] Other cases involving black women and blonde hair include *Burchette v. Abercrombie & Fitch* (2009) and *Bryant v. BEGIN Manage Program* (2003).[163] Dulazia Burchette, who worked for the clothing retailer Abercrombie & Fitch, decided to wear blonde highlights to work one day. A supervisor allegedly told her that she could not continue to work at the store with blonde highlights because they were "not natural." Shirley Bryant, who worked as an Orientation and Assessment Facilitator for a work-study program for BEGIN (a US federally mandated assistance program that helped welfare recipients return to the workforce), wore her short, curly hair in a shade of blonde. In Bryant's case, the issue was the fact that the other black women at BEGIN wrapped their hair in African-inspired headdress and wore "Afrocentric" clothing while Bryant, who was light-skinned, did not. As such, Bryant's supervisor, a black woman, allegedly terminated her not because she was black but because she was light-skinned, wore business attire (i.e., "white" clothing), and dyed her hair blonde; Bryant claimed that the supervisor also called her a "wannabe" for such aesthetics. Considering that blonde hair is a rare colour for *all* women, and is much more common in children than in adults,[164] the fact that black women who dye their hair blonde are reprimanded for a supposed artifice speaks to the pervasiveness of racial bias. In Canada, several "hair cases" have also made national news in recent years.

In March 2015, an alleged hair discrimination case made headlines when a hostess at Madison's New York Bar and Grill in downtown Montreal said she was a victim of discrimination because of her hair. Nineteen-year-old Lettia McNickle told Global News she was told to go home when she showed up for work with braids in her hair.[165] After investigating the incident, the Centre for Research Action on Race Relations (CRARR) filed a complaint with Quebec's Human Rights Commission on behalf of McNickle. On November 27, 2018, the Commission ruled that McNickle was a victim of workplace discrimination and the owner of Madison's was ordered to pay over $14,500 to the young woman.[166] In December 2015, school officials allegedly sent home a black Grade 8 student at Amesbury Middle School in North Toronto because of her crochet braid hairstyle. In an interview with the *Toronto Star*, the child's mother, Terressa Sutherland, said that the principal of the school, who is also a black woman, approached her daughter several times about her hair and had brought her daughter to her office.[167] And in March 2016, Akua Agyemfra, a black waitress at Jack Astor's Bar and Grill in Toronto, was also sent home during her shift because of her hair, which was not styled like that of her white counterparts and therefore a "problem" for her supervisors.[168]

If we go back to *Rogers v. American Airlines* (1981), the groundbreaking hair case discussed in chapter 3, we see that its outcome continues to speak to how black women's hairstyling choices, coupled with external pressures, still create a series of conflicting juxtapositions: wear it chemically straightened or natural, cut it low or wear it long, braid it or wear it "out." In her analysis of the *Rogers* case, Paulette Caldwell opined that the court chose to base its decision principally on distinctions between biological and cultural conceptions of race, and it treated the plaintiff's claims of race and gender discrimination as independent of each other, thereby denying any relationship between the two.[169] The way the court distinguished between phenotype and cultural aspects of race were twofold. First, the court rejected Rogers's claim that braids were akin to Afros. The court argued that the two were not the same because braids were not the product of natural hair growth but were in fact "artifice."[170] Second, in response to Rogers' argument that, like the Afro, the wearing of braids reflected her ethnic and cultural identification, the court distinguished between the unchangeable aspects of race and those characteristics that are socially and/or culturally associated with a particular race.[171] Stated otherwise, the court positioned braids as a matter of personal choice, and not reflective of one's cultural heritage or race. The *Rogers* case ultimately helped to position braids as a style separate from black culture, and by implication, a style derived from white women; and because mainstream (white) beauty culture determines what is popular, braided hair has been trivialized as mere style or treated as a fashion trend throughout the decades since Renee Rogers' case, an attitude that continues to the present day.

As these numerous contemporary hair cases reveal, the lasting impact of hair cases is that black women across North America still must "prove" or justify their hair choices to the dominant culture at large. Some black women, however, refuse to allow hair discrimination to go unchecked. As noted in the introduction to this book, in 2016, the 11th US Circuit Court of Appeals ruled against a lawsuit filed by the Equal Employment Opportunity Commission (EEOC) against Catastrophe Management Solutions (CMS) for firing a black woman, Chastity Jones, because she wore her hair in dreadlocks.[172] In 2018, the NAACP Legal Defense and Educational Fund (LDF) filed a petition to add *EEOC v. Catastrophe Management Solutions* to the US Supreme Court's docket so that the case can be heard by the highest court in the country. As reported by the news and opinion website VOX, Jones, who lives in Alabama, was offered a job as a customer service representative at a call centre in Mobile in 2010.[173] During the interview, Jones's dreadlocks were worn short, and she was dressed in a business suit and pumps. A human resources manager later told Jones that dreadlocks violated the company's grooming policy because they "tend to get messy." She told Jones that she could not wear her hair that way at work, and when Jones refused to cut her hair, the job offer was rescinded. "Black women who wish to succeed in the workplace feel compelled to undertake costly, time-consuming, and harsh measures to conform their natural hair to a stereotyped look of professionalism that mimics the appearance of white women's hair," lawyers for the LDF wrote in their petition to the Supreme Court.[174]

I have also been affected by societal pressures to wear my hair in a "presentable" (read: white) manner in the workplace. After graduating from the University of Windsor in 2001, I landed a job as an insurance claims adjuster in downtown Toronto. In this position, I had to wear "business casual" attire to work. Every day I went to work with my hair up in a ponytail. At the time, I used a chemical relaxer, so my hair was straightened and always neat. One day, one of my white colleagues asked me why I did not wear my hair down. In his opinion, I would look more attractive if I did so. The next day, I woke up two hours earlier to curl my hair and wear it as suggested. When I arrived at work, and over the next ten minutes, I was surrounded by several white colleagues who "had to see what I looked like with my hair down." My hair had not only interrupted my morning, it had transformed me from colleague into spectacle. Thus, the choices black women must make regarding our hair are not mere juxtapositions; in some instances, they mean the difference between social acceptance and ostracization, employment and unemployment. While black women may be more visible in the mainstream culture via advertising, film, and television, this ascendency has only made hypervisible the ways in which Western standards of beauty continue to impose limits on black women's choices. Instead of mainstream beauty culture, and Western culture in general, expanding to include different hairstyles and aesthetics, it has simply narrowed the parameters of beauty by demanding that the visible markers of racial difference are muted. We can attribute some of the ignorance regarding black hairstyling in Canada to a lack of public awareness about black hair. For one thing, there have been very few representations of black hair in Canadian media.

In 1999, the CBC program *Rough Cuts* aired the Canadian film *Black, Bold and Beautiful*, which explored the issue of black women's hair. Directed by Nadine Valcin and produced by Jennifer Kawaja, Julia Sereny of Sienna Films, Karen King of the NFB, and Jerry McIntosh of CBC Newsworld, the film explored the "dilemmas" black women face in terms of hairstyling choices, but also celebrated the bonds that women form while tending to each other's hair. An article in *Share* titled "CBC Explores Black Hair" described the film as allowing the viewer into debates not only on black hair but also on the position of black people in Canada.[175] In the years that followed, however, no other Canadian-produced programming focusing on black women's hair aired on a national network until Trey Anthony's *'Da Kink in My Hair* (*'Da Kink*) appeared—over fifteen years later.

In 2007, Global TV brought *'Da Kink* to Canadian television. Set in a Jamaican beauty parlour in Toronto's Little Jamaica neighbourhood on Eglinton Avenue West, *'Da Kink*, prior to its television incarnation, appeared as a stage play, first in 2001 at New York's Fringe Festival, then in 2003 at Toronto's Theatre Passe-Muraille, and in 2005, it became the first black Canadian production to appear at the Princess of Wales Theatre. *'Da Kink* also appeared at the San Diego Repertory Theatre in San Diego and at the Hackney Empire in London, England. In the initial Passe-Muraille production, the narrative centred on monologues by black women about their hair, their experience of abuse in black communities, and self-esteem issues. The play was set on a small, black-curtained stage, and each of the women wore natural hair—either a short Afro or dreadlocks. By the time of the Princess of Wales adaptation, the show had had a Mirvish Productions makeover—the dramatic monologues disappeared into comedic scenes that focused on Anthony as a dark-skinned, overweight woman with brightly coloured wigs, hair weaves, and extensions. Before its appearance on Global, the play was again transformed, this time into an hour-long television pilot that aired on Vision TV in 2004. When 'Da Kink was revamped for Vision TV, African American actress Sheryl Lee Ralph joined the cast. In this version, the story centred on Novelette "Letty" Campbell (Ralph), her hair salon, and her sister Joy (Trey Anthony), who also worked as a hairstylist. While the show returned to its dramatic Passe-Muraille roots, with Anthony playing a supporting role, the station did not pick it up for further episodes.

When 'Da Kink premiered on Global on October 14, 2007, Anthony (who by then had lost a significant amount of weight) was still a supporting character but her "ghetto fabulous" outfits, intermittent use of Jamaican patois, multi-coloured wigs, and off-the-cuff humour once again returned. Instead of Sheryl Lee Ralph as the lead character of Letty, theatre actress Ordena Stephens-Thompson assumed the role. Letty, who now spoke a Standard English and dressed conservatively, was a single mother raising a young boy while dating a professional black man, unlike her sister Joy, who was perpetually single or dating "Mr. Wrong." The nuances of the stage play, especially those related to hair and beauty, were largely expunged from the black hair salon, which was represented as a space where chemical relaxers, weaves, and wigs—along with the backlog of appointments that frustrates many women who frequent black hair salons—take place. The show touched on other issues such as interracial dating, immigration, and dancehall music, but 'Da Kink had lost much of the cultural currency that had made the stage play so successful. It was as though 'Da Kink, in a space of Canadian hegemony—whether a large theatre house or a national broadcaster—had to be whitened; the narrative had to appeal to a mainstream audience that presumably knew very little about black women's beauty politics and/or were not interested in learning about such topics. In 2009 after two seasons, 'Da Kink was cancelled. As the first black-focused television show in Canadian history, with a predominantly black female cast, were there constraints placed upon the show by the network to downplay its racial and gendered difference? Was the show's target audience black women, the patrons of black hair salons, or white Canadians, who have never set foot in one nor mingled with the black Canadians they would find there? 'Da Kink ultimately stands as a compelling example of how difficult it is for black women to find a place in mainstream (that is, white) Canadian media, as well as in the country's mainstream beauty-culture industry. Despite the illusion of inclusion in contemporary beauty advertising, beauty pageants, and the fashion and modelling worlds, the question of black beauty remains as political and contentious as ever.

Since Black Is Beautiful no longer exists, can or should black beauty culture once again embrace a natural hair movement? Is it possible to have a black hair revolution without co-optation from mainstream beauty culture? These questions remain unanswerable, but one thing is undeniable—black beauty politics are as salient in the lives of black women today as they were two centuries ago. Black women may be more socio-politically empowered and financially able to make decisions about their hair and skin today than those in prior generations, and in this sense, we *have* overcome, but there is still a very long way to go before we can truly proclaim that black beauty is *free* from its historical politics. Is a new black beauty revolution, a new Black Is Beautiful, possible? This question cannot be answered in this book, but hopefully its contents have provided a depth of understanding about where black beauty politics come from, what the issues are today, and how we might resolve them in the future.

CONCLUSION

It was difficult to write a conclusion for this book. How do you conclude something that is still in a process of becoming? There were and remain so many areas that I simply could not attend to in writing this book, most notably, the innumerable undocumented oral histories from black women and men who have laboured for decades as hair stylists, barbers, and natural hair care practitioners. Bringing these stories to light will do more to broaden the scope of the black Canadian narrative as it relates not only to beauty culture but also black community. Further, I was not able to delve into the politics of barbering in Canada. Since 1998, Ontario's Ministry of Training, Colleges, and Universities, for instance, has grouped all trades related to hairstyling, including barbers, under the trade name of hairstylist. Given the great number of barbershops on Eglinton West in Toronto and in other black communities across the city, such as in Scarborough and North Etobicoke, there is a dire need to start documenting and telling the stories of black barbers and the barbershop, not only those in Ontario but across Canada. After spending eight years researching this topic, what I can say for sure is that Canada's black culture is too often ignored, minimized, or framed solely as an extension of African American culture.

For example, several years ago I attended a concert in Toronto that featured an African American soul singer who, at some point during the show, started talking about "soul food." As a Jamaican Canadian, my "soul food" is ackee and saltfish, a traditional Jamaican dish (also the Jamaican National Dish), and beef patties. This artist mentioned African American staples such as collard greens and cornbread, as if these foods were also the "soul food" of the mostly black Canadian audience. In her defence, there is simply so little known of black Canadian culture that even black Canadians often have a hard time pinpointing foods and/or experiences that speak to a collective sense of identity. In this regard, one of the aspects of the black Canadian experience that I have tried to elucidate in this book is the fragmentation of black communities across the country. How can we connect the experiences of black people in Vancouver with those in Halifax, or those in Calgary and Edmonton with those in Toronto and Montreal, and all of those voices with the voices of historical African Canadian communities in rural towns across the country when we still lack the infrastructure for a national black media? Thus, one of the questions that remains unanswered in *Beauty in a Box* is how black communities can become more connected. One possible obstacle preventing more connectivity is the geographic distance between, and even within, communities.

York University geography professor Joseph Mensah writes that "unlike the situation in the United States, where Blacks live in extreme segregated inner-city neighbourhoods...Canadian Blacks are less spatially concentrated, with many of them living in suburban areas of our gateway cities." Furthermore, whereas there are "recognizable spatial concentrations of Blacks...in some neighbourhoods in Toronto, Montreal, and Halifax," generally speaking, the extent of "segregation among Canadian Blacks certainly pales in comparison with what persists in US cities,"[1] he writes. Because African Americans are more geographically concentrated, there exist more opportunities to speak to and among each other, to continually define and redefine what it means to be African American. Comparatively, black communities in Canada might not be spatially segregated from the dominant population, but culturally, these communities remain at a distance, both symbolic and literal, from one another. Therefore, any discussion of the black Canadian experience across time and space is a difficult one to engage in.

That said, *Beauty in a Box* has accomplished three goals. First, it provides a material and discursive account for the extent to which black media has recorded and documented the lives and experiences of African Canadians and Caribbean Canadians. For too long, the experiences of black Canadians have been removed from Canadian history, except for discussions of slavery and anti-black racism, and in turn, many of these experiences have been expunged from the collective memory. This book has accounted for that absence in terms of not only Canadian history but also media studies. The field of media and communication studies has ignored black Canadian media as an area of inquiry. This book makes it difficult to continue to do so. Second, this book provides a historiography of the development and expansion of black cultural practices such as hair care and product distribution but also the role of promotional culture, consumer culture and advertising, and entrepreneurship in black communities. By exploring the lives of black women such as Viola Desmond, Beverly Mascoll, and the many others who are accounted for in the pages of black community newspapers such as *Contrast* and *Share*, *The Clarion*, and the *Dawn of Tomorrow*, there is now a record of how black Canadians have contributed to the cultural and economic landscape, not only through the discourse on transnational migration but through transnational media networks and economic and cultural exchanges as well.

Third, and perhaps this book's biggest contribution, is to twentieth-century Canadian history. The gap in historical knowledge about black Canadians between World War I and 1967 is staggering. I was, in fact, shocked to discover, when I began researching this book, how little work had been done to recuperate the varied and numerous stories, lived experiences, triumphs, and struggles of black Canadians during this period. Dionne Brand's oral history accounts of black women in the 1920s through 1940s, David Austin's writings about the Sir George Williams Affair in 1960s Montreal, and Barrington Walker's numerous works on twentieth-century legal history stand out as a few of the contributions that have recuperated this gap in the historical knowledge about black Canadians. As a black cultural project, however, *Beauty in a Box* has not only expanded the scope of information about black beauty culture (beyond the African American narrative), but it has also filled a gap in the literature regarding twentieth-century black life.

Additionally, one of the most profound realizations I had after completing this book was just how little the tensions, politics, and issues that defined black beauty culture in the twentieth century have changed in the twenty-first. In many ways, there has been progress, especially as it relates to inclusion in global advertising campaigns, and there is now a broader range of products geared toward black women consumers for sale at retail, but in other ways, there has been little or no change whatsoever. For example, in the 1940s and 1950s, two African American scientists, Dr. Kenneth Clark and Dr. Mamie Clark, first published studies about the effect of whiteness as the measure of beauty on young black children. The Clarks conducted a series of experiments in an effort to assess the psychological effects of segregation on African American children. They asked black children to choose between a black doll and a white doll whose features were exactly the same; the only difference was the dolls' skin colour.

In the experiment (which became known as "the Clark doll test"), the Clarks showed black children between the ages of six and nine two dolls, one white and one black, and then asked a series of questions: "Show me the doll that you like best or that you'd like to play with," "Show me the doll that is the 'nice' doll," "Show me the doll that looks 'bad.'" Most of the black children attributed the positive characteristics to the white doll and the negative characteristics to the black doll.

In 2006, filmmaker Kiri Davis recreated the Clarks' experiment.[2] In *A Girl Like Me*, Davis asked four- and five-year-old children at a Harlem primary school the same set of questions the Clarks had asked fifty years before, and she found that the children's answers remained the same. In Davis's test, fifteen of the twenty-one children said that the white doll was good and pretty, and that the black doll was bad. In 2010, CNN hired child psychologist Margaret Beale Spencer to recreate another Clark experiment at eight schools in the New York area, and the results were the same.[3] These tests confirmed the fact that there is a multi-generational pathology that continues to influence how black children see themselves, and in turn who they become as adults. Since whiteness continues to determine what is sold in beauty culture (and in Western culture, in general), hair straightening and, for some, skin bleaching are still practices that are used to approximate this ideal. In the 2006 single "I Am Not My Hair," India Arie sang, defiantly, that her identity is not to be tied to her hair or her skin or to anyone's expectations but to "the soul that lives within."[4] While these lyrics are inspirational for many black women, the beauty-culture industry has continually reinforced the fact that we *are* our hair and our skin.

From our earliest childhood experiences through to our adult lives, there are constant reminders in the media and advertising positioning black women's bodies as Other and the visible markers of blackness—dark skin or "kinky" hair—as aberrant. In her experiences with her biracial child Cassie, Susan Bordo once described how the straight-haired aesthetic *as* beauty sends a conflicting message to black children, especially those who are of a mixed ancestry:

> It pains me when Cassie tells me she hates her curls (as she calls them). But how could she not, when even [Queen] Latifah—one of her idols—has hair like satin? In the doll world, there's been an explosion of "ethnic" or "urban" production and marketing, as dolls like the saucy and style-conscious Bratz have started to give Barbie a real run for her money (or rather, ours). But although some of these

dolls have hair done in cornrows and braids, undo those dos and it's
still the same old white-girl hair.... These dolls are clearly an illus-
tration of the principle that this culture mostly lets "difference" in
by exoticizing it.[5]

The exoticization of difference is not just limited to North America. In 2012,
the *Guardian* posted the following editorial on its Facebook page regarding
white models wearing Aunt Jemima earrings on a catwalk at a Dolce and
Gabbana show during Milan fashion week:

> Some might argue that they're harmless, even cute, but there's noth-
> ing cute about two white men selling minstrel earrings to a majority
> non-black audience. There wasn't a single black model in Dolce and
> Gabbana's show, and it's hard not to be appalled by the transparent
> exoticism in sending the only black faces down the runway in the
> form of earrings [of stereotypes of black women].[6]

The editorial continued, "When you're explicitly pandering to such a
shameful era of western racism and colonialism, it's time to move on to
the future."

In January 2014, the *Huffington Post* reported on an editorial released on
the Martin Luther King, Jr. holiday in the United States, which appeared on
the Russian website Buro 247.[7] In it, Dasha Zhukova, the Russian editor-in-
chief of *Garage* magazine is photographed perched atop a chair designed to
look like a half-naked black woman. The piece, created by Norwegian artist
Bjarne Melgaard, was part of a series that "reinterpreted" artworks from
historical artists such as Allen Jones. Both Zhukova and Melgaard apologized for the photograph after the fact, claiming it was not their intent to
be "racist," but it simply reaffirmed the problem of the contemporary in
which bodies are depoliticized as neutral canvases without histories and/or
politics. The photograph also hearkened back to the historical categoriza-
tion of black women as furniture; under slavery, black slave women were
frequently documented as "chattel." Since black women remain marginally
represented in the beauty and fashion worlds, and when they are, there is
a heightened exoticism attached to and projected onto their bodies, these
images are never neutral.

Even when consumer brands try to be inclusive and appear to embrace
a diversity of women's bodies, hair textures, and skin tones, a racial bias
remains. In 2010, the Dove Movement for Self-Esteem was launched at

the G(irls) 20 Summit. Modelled after the G20 Economic Summit, this convention brought together young women from Argentina, Brazil, Canada, China, India, Indonesia, Japan, Mexico, Russia, Saudi Arabia, South Africa, South Korea, Turkey, and the United States, as well as the United Kingdom, France, Germany, Italy, and other countries in the European Union to discuss education, health, and economic initiatives that could stimulate girls' activism and advancement in their communities. Dove, the personal care products division of Unilever in operation since 1957, emerged as an agent of female empowerment via beauty consumption in the global marketplace through the Movement and, by extension, its brand Campaign for Real Beauty (CFRB).[8] The construction of CFRB was based on Dove's 2003 global research study, "The Real Truth about Beauty." This research involved the participation of thirty-two thousand women, ages eighteen through sixty-four, in ten countries, in a twenty- to twenty-five-minute-long telephone interview. The study found that less than 2 percent of women feel beautiful; 75 percent want representations of women to reflect diversity through age, shape, and size; and 76 percent want the media to portray beauty as more than physical.[9] Based on these findings, Dove announced its challenge to the dominant beauty industry, and by doing so, it affirmed a commitment to feature "real" women and girls of "various ages, shapes, and sizes" in its television and print advertising, billboards, new media, and national and grassroots outreach campaigns.[10] The Dove Movement for Self-Esteem launched in Canada and the United States in the fall of 2010. On the surface, the campaign appeared to challenge the dominant standard of beauty, but it has not gone far enough, as far as black women are concerned. In 2017, another Dove campaign proved that the global consumer brand is not as attuned as it might claim to issues of race and the privileging of white women's bodies over black women's bodies that have been a mainstay in the beauty culture industry for centuries.

The campaign, which was posted on social media in October of that year, featured a static compilation of four images. The first frame showed a dark-skinned black woman in what appeared to be a bathroom removing her brown shirt; a bottle of Dove body wash sits in the lower right-hand corner. In subsequent frames, the woman slowly lifts up her shirt, and by the last frame, not only is she wearing a white undershirt, but in the process the dark-skinned black woman has transformed into a red-haired white woman. In a *Toronto Star* reprint of a *Washington Post* article, the author penned a series of questions: "Was Dove saying that inside every black woman is a smiling red-headed white woman? Was Dove invoking the centuries-old stereotype that black is dirty and white is pure? Or that black skin can or should be cleansed away?"[11] Dove is not the only beauty brand that attempted to bring back these centuries-old tropes about the purity of whiteness and the dirtiness of blackness. Earlier that year, Nivea, the German-based global skin care brand, produced an advertisement that declared "White Is Purity."

Anne McClintock has argued that one of the consequences of centuries of colonial domination is that whiteness functions as a form of both spectacle and desire in capitalist production. The manufacture of soap had burgeoned into an imperial commerce at the beginning of the nineteenth century, and as a consequence, "Victorian cleaning rituals were peddled globally as the God-given sign of Britain's evolutionary superiority, and soap was invested with magical, fetish powers."[12] The cult of domesticity positioned white women's bodies within the domestic space, but the imperialist production of soap advertising equated monogamy ("clean" sex) with industrial capital ("clean" money), Christianity ("being washed clean"), and class control ("washing and clothing the savage").[13] Soap companies even went so far as to use caricatures of black children to sell whiteness as "clean" and conversely, blackness as "degenerate." In 1844, for instance, the New York–based N. K. Fairbanks Company introduced the cartoon images of two black children, the Gold Dust Twins (Goldy and Dusty), to promote its brand of soap. Meanwhile in Canada an advertising print produced by John Henry Walker (1831–99), which depicted the stereotype of Sambo covered in buttermilk, a symbolic representation of a black child subsumed in whiteness, circulated between the 1850s and 1880s. As Thomas Hine aptly notes, these racist images that "reflected ethnic stereotypes, provided products with personalities that were apparently unthreatening. They were a kind of servant just about anyone could afford, with the frequent exception of people who belonged to the groups shown on the package."[14] The connection between empire and cleanliness was also promoted in hair care. By the 1870s, Britain began exporting shampoo to Europe and soon thereafter, to the colonies.[15]

Thus, the issues that profoundly affect black women such as hair (i.e., the historical valorization of straight, long, flowing hair) and skin colour (i.e., the preference for light skin over dark skin) are still as widely circulated today as they were centuries ago. The difference today, however, is that these are global campaigns that claim to be for *all* women and young girls. The beauty-culture industry in the twenty-first century is still far from "multicultural." In a 2014 Jergens lotion commercial, for example, a black model with light skin appeared in a "before" shot with dry skin and "frizzy" hair, but in the "after" shot she appeared with soft, moistened skin and straightened hair. This juxtaposition, when placed in historical context, is a reminder of how the same tropes related to skin colour grada- tion from the nineteenth century continue to appear in the contemporary. A campaign for *real* beauty that does not confront the politics of skin and hair is mere window dressing and does little to shift ideologies that deeply affect black women's lives. Many young black girls (and boys) continue to believe that dark skin is anathema. Thus, the question remains whether the legacies of racism and colonialism, interwoven into the fabric of West- ern culture, can be undone. Is it possible to produce counter-hegemonic beauty ideologies and images in the twenty-first century?

In April 2013, Procter & Gamble released the film *Imagine a Future* in conjunction with its consumer campaign "My Black is Beautiful" (MBIB). With the participation of the United Negro College Fund (UNCF) and BLACK GIRLS ROCK! (an organization founded by DJ Beverly Bond in 2006 to promote positive images of women of colour in the media), the documentary examined the topic of beauty among black women and the self-esteem issues that challenge black women and girls. The film aired in the United States and Canada on Black Entertainment Television (BET) in July 2013. MBIB's mission is stated on their website:

> Imagine a Future. Imagine a future where every black girl believes her black is beautiful. You know your black is beautiful...but what about young black girls? Together, we can empower the next generation of black women to confidently be their best, most beautiful selves. Three years. One million black girls. A beautiful future starts with you.[16]

If the problem with the beauty-culture industry was simply a matter of its unrealistic depiction of thin, youthful (increasingly sexualized) bodies, MBIB campaigns would not need to exist. MBIB is a contemporary example of a counter-hegemonic response to CFRB-type campaigns; it also points to two possibilities. First, that the consumer marketplace can be a site where the diversity of black womanhood is represented, and second, that white- owned conglomerates can work alongside black women to not only celebrate our beauty but also raise questions about the images of beauty that are absent in the dominant media. Significantly, however, not all black-focused media aim to challenge the beauty ideal of straightened hair and light skin.

A quick glance at black hair care magazines such as *Today's Black*

Woman, Upscale, Sophisticate's Black Hair, Essence, Ebony, and even *Black Hair: Fashion, Beauty, Style* reveals that there is a clear preference for straight hair, especially hair that is chemically relaxed or hidden under a weave and/or lace front wig. In the twenty-first century, hair alteration remains a valorized ideal. In these black periodicals, advertisements from white-owned black beauty brands like SoftSheen-Carson (L'Oréal), Creme of Nature (Colomer), Motions (Unilever), Clairol (Bristol-Myers Squibb), Ambi (L'Oréal), and Pantene (P&G) continue to dominate their pages. When natural hairstyles appear in these magazines, it is typically under the theme of "how to care for your troublesome hair." Constructed as burdensome, natural hair is not celebrated by these magazines the way chemically relaxed hair and weaves are. At the same time, a 2013 report from the consumer trends firm Mintel revealed that chemical-relaxer sales had declined 26 percent since 2008 (when sales were at US$206 million) and 15 percent since 2011 (when sales were US$179 million).[17] "In 2013, nearly three-fourths (70 percent) of black women said they currently wear or have worn their hair natural (no relaxer or weave), more than half (53 percent) have worn braids, and four out of ten (41 percent) have worn dreadlocks," the report continued.[18] Between 2013 and 2015, sales of chemical relaxers dropped by 18.6 percent.[19]

Despite this, advertisements for chemical relaxers and hair weaves have not declined in the pages of African American magazines. The contemporary beauty milieu is thus marked by a paradox as far as black women are concerned. On the one hand, African American celebrities increasingly throw their support behind natural hair—for instance, in 2017, Gabrielle Union launched the brand Flawless, with a range of shampoos, conditioners, styling products, and oil treatments for naturally textured black hair. In an interview with *Harper's Bazaar*, Union said, "I didn't love my skin colour, I didn't love my lips. I didn't love my nose, I didn't love my hair. I didn't love anything."[20] "More and more black women have set their own beauty standards and begun to embrace their God-given tresses," she added. This realization compelled her to develop a natural hair care brand specifically for women with "textured hair." On the other hand, such celebrities are not fully committed to embracing the natural texture of their own hair. Union, for example, has never appeared in a television show or film with natural hair; she has always had long, flowing, straight hair (on occasion, she wears synthetic braids).

In 2012, *Ebony* magazine also ran a feature titled "Loc'd Out: Has the Style Lost Its Luster?"[21] in which the longest-running African American

252 BEAUTY IN A BOX

magazine essentially made the argument that, while the natural hair market is booming, the style just does not provide black women with the versatility that other hairstyles do. (In 2015, Mintel reported that black consumers in the United States continue to embrace the natural hair movement; sales of styling products for naturally textured hair increased 26.8 percent from 2013 to 2015, reaching US$946 million, comprising 35 percent of black hair care sales. This negatively affected sales of relaxers, which dropped 18.6 percent during the same period.)[22] The *Ebony* writer said further, "The thought of trading in my ten years of curldom for a fixed look is out of the question.... Locs are gorgeous and I highly doubt they'd ever get dumped in a retro category like thick 90's braids but are they simply not versatile for today's new natural?" These comments affirmed what marketers have known for nearly twenty-five years: as noted in chapter 4, black women get bored with their hair and change it more frequently than other women do, a fickleness that also extends to hair colour. What such editorials ignore, however, is the fact that chemical relaxers and hair dyes have health risks that are finally receiving long overdue medical attention.

As discussed in chapter 3, since the early 2000s, researchers have found that the damage caused by chemical relaxers and hair weaves includes shaft dryness, increased fragility of the hair cuticle, and baldness. An increased risk of uterine leiomyomata (known as uterine fibroids) has also been linked to the use of chemical relaxers. In 2017, a study found that African American women and white women who regularly chemically straighten their hair or dye it dark brown or black have an elevated risk of breast cancer. According to *The Globe and Mail*, the study of 4,285 African American and white women was the first to find a significant increase in breast cancer risk among black women who used dark shades of hair dye and white women who used chemical relaxers.[23] Why would researchers study the effects of chemical relaxers on white women when, according to their own findings (adult women from New York and New Jersey, surveyed from 2002 through 2008, who had been diagnosed with breast cancer), "the vast majority—88 percent—of blacks had used chemicals to relax their hair, [and] only 5 percent of whites reported using relaxers."[24] By linking their findings about hair dyes (58 percent of the white participants said they regularly dyed their hair dark shades, while only 30 percent of the black participants did) with black women, and conversely, chemical relaxers with white women, this study gave a skewed perception of who actually uses chemical relaxers (and hair dyes) in the first place. Since José Baraquiel Calva's invention in the 1950s (discussed in chapter 2) black women have *always* been the predominant users of chemical relaxers. Thus, even regarding health, black women remain linked to white women; we cannot exist in our own right. At the same time that there might be a neo-natural hair movement going on, black hair is still politicized, and often turned into mere spectacle.

In 2013 in New York City's Union Square for example, Antonia Opiah, founder of the website Un'ruly.com, extended an open invitation to all curious passersby for an exhibition she called "You Can Touch My Hair." According to a feature in the *Huffington Post*, Opiah sought to explore the "tactile fascination" with black women's hair by gathering women with different hair textures and styles (dreadlocks, chemically straightened, weaves, naturally curly, and Afro) and allowing strangers the opportunity to fondle the women's hair without fear.[25] The accompanying short video and twenty-two-page photographic slide show of the event revealed that each of the black women who participated wore a sign that read "You can touch my hair," and while a few black men were curious, it was overwhelmingly white men and women who touched each black woman's hair and posed for photographs.

On the surface, this type of spectacle appears to depoliticize black hair (because black women are inviting the touch and gaze of whites), but on a deeper level, it points to the disturbing contemporary trend of trivializing a personal and collective issue. It is also a reflection of how intertwined black women now are in the mainstream media culture where, as Rosalind Gill observes, there is the almost total evacuation of notions of politics or cultural influence, and "notions of choice, of 'being oneself' and 'pleasing oneself,' are central to the postfeminist sensibility that suffuses contemporary western media culture."[26] There is a desperate need for scholars to begin to deconstruct how postfeminism and the socio-political milieu that increasingly constructs people as rational, calculating, self-regulating individuals who bear full responsibility for their life biographies affect black women and their conceptions of beauty and their bodies. The September 2013 issue of *O, the Oprah Magazine* is yet another example of the urgent need to probe the intersections of race, consumption, and beauty.

The issue, dedicated to women's hair, featured Winfrey on the cover wearing an Afro wig so large that it engulfed nearly the entire top half of the page. The sixteen-page feature, titled "Hair Extravaganza!" began with general statistics on the hair care market: "Every year American women fork over more than $22 billion for haircuts, $30 billion for hair color, and most of the $7 billion spent on shampoo, conditioner, and styling products.

(That's nearly $59 billion—more than three times the annual budget of NASA.)"[27] From there on, women—mostly white women—shared their hair stories: the longing for the "right" hairdo, the big hair 1980s, difficulties finding the right hair colouring, what to do when you lose all your hair, and what to do about greying hair. The only depiction of black hair was through the story of Bridgett Davis, a woman for whom "going natural meant losing a lifelong hairstyle—and finding her true self."[28] Black hair in the context of O was removed from any politics (that would be associated with a neo-natural hair movement) and was framed in the context of (postfeminist) choice and self-exploration. On one page, titled "The Natural," a light-skinned woman with straight hair gazed into a mirror of her reflection with a curly, Afro hairdo. On the facing page, photographs of Davis (who is dark skinned) captured her in "transition" from relaxed to natural hair.

The mirror imagery paralleled artist Carrie Mae Weems's 1987 satirical photo-text "Mirror, Mirror" from her *Ain't Jokin'* series (1987–88). In Weems's piece, a white spectral female appears in a mirror, returning the gaze of a black woman. In the caption, the spectre responds to the woman's question, "Who's the finest of them all?" with "Snow White, you black bitch, and don't you forget it!"[29] As Janell Hobson posits, "the irony, of course, is that this 'joke' of seeking one's image in the mirror, only to find it un-mirrored by the dominant Other, 'ain't no joke.'"[30] The irony of a light-skinned woman with straight hair seeing an image of herself with a loose, curly hairdo speaks to how hair-texture and skin-colour issues, though made to appear as natural, everyday (universal) struggles, are, in reality, "no joke" when it comes to black women. Despite the scarcity of positive images of black beauty in the dominant media culture, however, the Internet has become a new vanguard in producing positive images of black womanhood and beauty.

Many black women have started to view the Internet as a place (and a resource) where they can celebrate not only their natural hair but black beauty, in general. As Moya Bailey asserts, "the creation of digital networks and images that are primarily intended for communities of origin are two ways I see Black people asserting their significance outside of commoditized survival-oriented citizenship. I see the representations being created by marginalized communities directly challenging depictions in mainstream and medical media."[31] Millennial black women, in particular, have started to create how-to videos on YouTube; they use Pinterest and Instagram to share photographs that act as catalogues of natural hairstyles; and various other websites now provide black women (and girls) with instructions on how to transition from hair weaves, chemical relaxers, and wigs to dreadlocks, Afros, and naturally textured twists. The Internet has created a counter-hegemonic space for a new standard of black beauty, a space in which it can exist, flourish, and expand. There are dozens of websites, vlogs, and blogs in United States, Canada, and globally today that are dedicated to natural hair.[32]

In 2015, natural hair advocate Amber Starks gave a TEDxPortland talk titled "A New Standard of Beauty," in which she talked about the struggles that black women who "go natural" continue to face. At the same time, Starks loudly proclaimed, "It's not a fad, it's a movement." There is evidence to support her claims. As Tonya Roberts, Multicultural Analyst at Mintel observes, "As more and more Black women consumers are embracing their natural self and walking away from relaxers, it is presenting opportunities for natural brands to enter the market.... Research indicates that wearing their natural hair makes Black women feel liberated, confident and different from others, giving them a tremendous sense of pride in being Black while displaying their natural beauty."[33] In 2017, *The New York Times* even dedicated multiple pages of its newsletter "Race/Related" to the work of Tasha Dougé, a New York–based artist whose exhibit "This Land is OUR Land" directly tackled the intersection between history, art, hair, and identity.[34] In response to the question of what hair means in the African American community, Dougé said, "Either we subscribe to the European aesthetic and spend all our money there, or we try to buy African hair and products from shops in our communities, but owned by people outside of our race. Either way, the money never funnels back into the black community." These comments point to the historical tension in African American communities about the encroachment upon the black hair care market by Korean Americans, discussed in chapter 5. They also speak to the problem of equating black hair with the consumer marketplace, rather than with knowledge of self and with a self-love that comes with embracing your natural hair texture.

In November 2017 Atlanta-based artists Regis and Kahran Bethencourt, the husband-and-wife duo behind the photography studio Creative-Soul Photography, brought an artistic vision to life that highlighted the beauty of black girls and their natural hair. The series *Afro Art* appeared online at MyModernMet.com, and it featured portraits of black girls with Afro-textured hair, as well as visual stories. "We feel that it is so important for kids of color to be able to see positive images that look like them in the media," Kahran told My Modern Met.[35] "Unfortunately the lack of diversity often plays into the stereotypes that they are not 'good enough' and often forces kids to have low self-esteem." In the first decades of the twenty-first century, such examples point to the existence of a new natural hair movement that is not just happening on the big and small screens or in the world of black celebrity; it is happening on Main Streets across North America, Europe, and Africa, and globally, thanks to the Internet.

In the state of Oregon, as an example, black women have also begun to challenge laws that have unfairly punished natural hair salons. In June 2013, thanks in part to Oregon State Representative Alissa Keny-Guyer and Senator Jackie Dingfelder, the House and the Senate passed the Natural Hair Act, signed by the Governor of Oregon, which joined California and Washington State in acknowledging the training and legitimacy of natural stylists without requiring them to attend cosmetology school. Formerly, in Oregon, it was illegal to provide natural hair styling (i.e., braiding, twisting, combing, or brushing) without a cosmetology licence. The natural hair website Conscious Coils, founded by Amber Starks in Portland, Oregon, was instrumental in changing the law by lobbying for a separate licence (a natural styling license) that would allow natural stylists to perform their trade upon the completion and passage of a licence test; her actions point to the contemporary milieu where black women have the agency and global reach (via the Internet) to affect real shifts in the culture and ideology of black beauty. In recent years, even tennis player Venus Williams has worn a natural hairstyle, both on and off the court, proving that natural hair is just as versatile and manageable as straightened hair. The natural hair movement is not political in the historical sense of collective black pride, but it is political in that it aims to challenge the hegemony of Western beauty culture that still positions straight hair and lighter skin as the ultimate symbols of beauty. With respect to the latter, the ever-expanding global skin-lightening market tells us that whiteness is still sold around the world as the ultimate state of being as far as beauty is concerned.

In October 2017 the Guardian published a feature titled "Nivea's Latest 'White Is Right' Advert Is the Tip of a Reprehensible Iceberg."[36] "Now I have visibly fairer skin, making me feel younger," declared Nigerian actress Omowunmi Akinnifesi (who is dark skinned) in the advertisement for a new face cream that was intended to reach only a West African audience but—thanks to the Internet—was watched and shared millions of times around the world, according to the Guardian's reporting. While Nivea, like Dove, apologized, stating that the ad "was not intended to offend," as writer Afua Hirsch lamented in the article, "offence is not the point. The global market for skin lightening products, of which west Africa is a significant part, is worth $10bn (£7.6bn)," adding that "ads speak of 'toning' as code for whitening."[37] A few years ago, the article continued, Paris-based Lancôme (owned by L'Oréal) also got into trouble when it used British actress Emma Watson's image to market its Blanc Expert line in Asia, which emphasized that it does not lighten, but rather "evens skin tone, and provides a healthy-looking complexion...an essential part of Asian women's beauty routines." In countries such as Ghana and Nigeria, the *Guardian* noted, an estimated 77 percent of women currently use skin-lightening products, and while the brands focus on "health," as noted throughout this book, skin-lightening products are highly toxic and include ingredients such as hydroquinone, mercury, and corticosteroid. It is also not uncommon for these to be mixed with caustic agents such as automotive battery acid, bleaching agents, and detergent, all of which can have serious adverse health effects. The images of black beauty that still circulate in the global marketplace—Lupita Nyong'o and Sudanese model Nyakim Gatwech being the exceptions to the rule—are light-skinned with long, flowing hair and/or straightened hair, such as Beyoncé or Rhianna.

In 2017, for instance, *Teen Vogue* published an article on its website that harshly criticized Hollywood for its continued colour bias. Author Tiffany Onyejiaka lamented, "Over the past few years, the 'Black Girl Magic' movement has exploded into the movie and television screens across the country. And while it's a *huge* step for on-screen representation, there's just one problem: This representation tends to be limited by Hollywood's colorism problem."[38] While Hollywood has openly embraced dark-skinned male actors, such as Idris Elba, John Boyega, and Daniel Oyelowo, conversely it has consistently preferred light-skinned black women, even in roles where they are portraying dark-skinned women. Infamously, in 2016 for instance, Afro-Latina actress Zoe Saldana was harshly criticized when she was cast to portray Nina Simone in the biopic *Nina*, for which she wore a prosthetic nose and had her skin darkened to mimic Nina's appearance. In *X-Men* comics, the character Storm is of Kenyan descent and has dark skin, yet she has been portrayed by lighter-skinned biracial actresses such as Halle Barry and Alexandra Shipp in film adaptations. In the summer of 2017, the release of the film *Wonder Woman* marked a significant milestone in the representation of women onscreen. It premiered more than seventy-five years after the character's creation, and while Wonder Woman is one of the most recognizable superheroes and an integral part of the DC Comics legacy, she had never before been featured as the lead character in a film.

In an article for *Harper's Bazaar*, Cameron Glover lamented that the film's narrative connected black people to brute strength, a trope that dates back to slave-selling auctions, where a black person's value was directly linked to how physically fit they were; she also pointed out the legacy of that trope, wherein "today, Black women athletes like Serena Williams are still endlessly ridiculed, their physical strength mocked in anti-Black insults which demean their womanhood."[39] While I have, admittedly, not seen the film, her observations point to the continued problem of misrepresenting black women in the visual landscape as somehow less beautiful and less "woman" than white women.

In India, women have started to fight back against this bias toward lighter skin. Kavitha Emmanuel, for example, founded a non-governmental organization called Women of Worth and in 2009 launched the "Dark is Beautiful" campaign, which runs media literacy workshops and advocacy programs in schools across the country to counteract colour bias.[40] If you consider that global spending on skin lightening is projected to triple to $31.2 billion by 2024, according to a report released in June 2017 by the research firm Global Industry Analysts,[41] it is clear that the task of combating colour bias will be a decades-long battle.

Ultimately, when *all* women acknowledge that the same companies that market to American women are the companies that market to Canadian women and to the rest of the world, we can begin to have a conversation about "real beauty." Until women of varied racial and ethnic backgrounds collectively challenge the dominant beauty ideal that casts darker skin against lighter skin or excludes women on phenotypical differences—such as nose shape, eyelid size, or lip size—the beauty-culture industry will only continue to divide, not unite the very women whom companies like L'Oréal insist are "worth it." In 2016, for example, CoverGirl named Denver-based beauty vlogger Nura Afia, who is Muslim and wears a hijab, its new brand ambassador, joining Colombian-born Sofia Vergara and Katy Perry in the "diversity-focused #LashEquality campaign."[42] Time will tell if this kind of inclusion is *really* about diversifying the beauty standard or whether it is just another whitewashing of ethnic difference, folding such women into the unwavering beauty standard for which European ideals still determine what and who is beautiful. At the same time, there are women such as Rachel Dolezal who have claimed a lived "blackness," and other white women such as Martina Big, a German model and actress known for her body modifications, who made headlines in late 2017 for "transitioning" into a black woman, including taking supplements to darken her skin, lip implants, a nose job, various liposuction procedures, and hair weaves. Martina Big, like Dolezal, captured the global media's attention. The mere fact that a born-white woman's physical metamorphosis into blackness was given the wide-reaching platform it was given points to the continued erasure of real black women and our stories.

While there is a plethora of options available to black Canadian women today in terms of buying hair care products at mainstream retail stores, finding a black hair salon, and purchasing products for natural hair, there are few media outlets promoting such activities. The short-lived lifestyle magazine *Sway*, aimed primarily at African and Caribbean Canadians, attempted to show the diversity of black women's beauty; however, it was unsuccessful. Launched in 2005 (its last issue was July 2012), at one point the Star Media Group publication had a circulation of fifty thousand across the Greater Toronto Area.[43] Advertisements from natural hair studios along with features on black women with dreadlocks and other natural hairstyles appeared throughout the magazine, but in the end, its inability to garner enough advertising from mainstream beauty firms contributed to the publication's demise. The failure of a glossy black Canadian magazine served as more proof that it is very difficult for black beauty culture to attract the interest of American advertisers who, a generation ago, relied on Canada's black press to promote their products. Even in the pages of *Share*, there are fewer and fewer advertisements from companies such as Revlon, SoftSheen-Carson, and Pro-Line. Why have American beauty firms stopped advertising in black Canadian newspapers? What has changed? And what role are retailers now playing in the sale and promotion of black beauty products?

Beauty in a Box did not answer every question, but it has shone a light on the history of Canada's black beauty culture, laying a foundation for deeper understanding of the interconnectedness of the beauty-culture industry's ideologies and practices with slavery and colonialism, race and racism, and the iconographic legacies of advertising, photography, film, and television. If there is one overarching statement that could be said to sum up Canada's black beauty culture, it would simply be that there is no black beauty culture entirely removed from American black beauty culture; the industry has been, and continues to be, mostly a proxy for American products, services, and beauty imagery. There are, however, glimpses of change in the twenty-first century that are worth mentioning. For instance, in recent years, Bulk Barn, the largest bulk-food retailer in Canada, has offered for sale black Canadian-owned natural skin care and hair care products that are formulated with black women's skin and hair texture in mind. Most notably, the retailer sells handmade, all-natural products from Toronto-based Maiga Shea Butter, which has collation and processing operations in Burkina Faso, West Africa. This is a step in the right direction in terms of being more open to black Canadian beauty-product manufacturers while also acknowledging the growing natural product movement.

Ultimately, if this book has given black Canadian women a deeper understanding of our identities, our histories, and our connectedness with other black women across the country and transnationally across multiple sites of diaspora such as the United States, Europe, Africa, and the Global South, *Beauty in a Box* has served its ultimate purpose. I wrote this book out of sheer curiosity to know the roots of my own hair care practices and beauty-product choices. From that curiosity came something that can be used to further the goal of widening the scope of knowledge about black Canadian history. In the end, I hope that *Beauty in a Box* has started a conversation that will continue for decades to come and that it will also be the spark that changes historical patterns of exclusion, misrepresentation, and misinformation in black beauty advertising, product labelling, and promotional campaigns. Black beauty, in other words, can no longer be placed in a box.

NOTES

Introduction

1 Brand, *No Burden to Carry*, 31.

2 Burman, *Transnational Yearnings*, 9.

3 Trotz, "Rethinking Caribbean Transnational Connections," 43.

4 Grewal, *Transnational America*, 8.

5 Ibid., 11.

6 Winks, *Blacks in Canada*, 411.

7 Ibid.

8 Thomas, "Cultural Tourism," 434.

9 Berger, "Race, Visuality, and History," 95–96.

10 Ibid., 96.

11 Belisle, *Retail Nation*, 7.

12 Ibid., 10.

13 Ibid., 25, 23.

14 See Matthews, "Working for Family."

15 "Dupuis Frères Dept. Store, St. Catherine Street East," McCord Museum, http://www.mccord-museum.qc.ca/en/collection/artifacts/MP-0000.813.13.

16 Henry, *Black Politics in Toronto*, 12.

17 James, *Beauty Imagined*, 98.

18 Walker, *Style and Status*, 15.

19 Winks, *Blacks in Canada*, 334.

20 Toney, "Locating Diaspora," 76.

21 Henry, *Black Politics in Toronto*, 12.

22 Williams, *Road to Now*, 90.

23 Toney, "Locating Diaspora," 76.

24 Ibid.

25 Belisle, *Retail Nation*, 47.

26 Hine, *Total Package*, 109.

27 Wolf, *Beauty Myth*, 62.

28 Belisle, *Retail Nation*, 81.

29 Smith, *American Archives*, 22.

30 Nelson, "'Hottentot Venus,'" 118–19.

31 Archer-Straw, *Negrophilia*, 12.

32 Ibid., 6.

33 Conor, *Spectacular Modern Woman*, 14.

34 Ibid., 7.

35 Mathieu, *North of the Color Line*, 4.

36 Ibid.

37 Belisle, *Retail Nation*, 69.

38 Ibid., 67.

39 Bernstein, *Racial Innocence*, 34.

40 Sutherland, *Monthly Epic*, 156–57.

41 Rymell, "Images of Women," 97.

42 Grove, "Castle of One's Own," 166.

43 Spencer, *Lipstick and High Heels*, 38.

44 Topsy doll advertisement, *Chatelaine*, September 1937, 57.

45 Stowe, *Uncle Tom's Cabin*, 351.

46 Rooks, *Ladies' Pages*, 17–18.

47 Wallace-Sanders, *Mammy*, 2.

48 Mammy Pad advertisement, *Chatelaine*, December 1936, 84.

49 McLaren, *Our Own Master Race*, 47.

50 Korinek, *Roughing It*, 284.

51 Belisle, *Retail Nation*, 69.

52 Korinek, *Roughing It*, 125.

53 Rooks, *Ladies' Pages*, 4.

54 Shaw, "'Most Anxious to Serve,'" 545–46.

55 Joseph Whitney, "An Open Letter to the Colored Race in Canada," *Canadian Observer*, July 31, 1915, 1.

56 Young Women's Christian Association advertisement, *Canadian Observer*, April 15, 1916.

57 Hair advertisement, *Canadian Observer*, June 17, 2016, 6.

58 Toney, "Locating Diaspora," 80.

59 "History of the *Toronto Star*," *Toronto Star* website, http://www.thestar.com/about/history.html.

60 "Mrs. C. E. Jenkins," *Dawn of Tomorrow*, November 6, 1926, 1.

61 Willis and Williams, *Black Female Body*, 148.

62 Sheehan, "The Face of Fashion," 181.

63 Mathieu, *North of the Color Line*, 6.

64 Ibid.

65 Reynolds, *Viola Desmond's Canada*, 1.

66 Ibid., 2.

67 Walker, *West Indians in Canada*, 12.

68 Ibid.

69 Aronczyk, *Branding the Nation*, 112.
70 Walker, "Introduction," 11.
71 Maynard, *Policing Black Lives*, 53–54.
72 Russell, Wilson, and Hall, *Color Complex*, 1.
73 Cordelia Tai, "Report: The Spring 2017 Runways Were the Most Diverse in History—Sort Of," Fashion Spot, October 14, 2016, http://www.thefashion spot.com/runway-news/717823-diversity-report-spring-2017-runways/.
74 Nathalie Atkinson, "The Bay Launches Digital Beauty Magazine with E-Commerce," *National Post*, September 6, 2011, http://news.nationalpost .com/life/the-bay-launches-digital-beauty-magazine-with-e-commerce.
75 Cordelia Tai, "This Black Model Is Calling Out the Industry by Recreating Whitewashed Campaigns," Fashion Spot, December 8, 2016, http://www .thefashionspot.com/runway-news/726613-black-mirror-project/#/slide/1.
76 Ibid.
77 Noel Gutierrez-Morfin, "US Court Rules Dreadlock Ban during Hiring Process Is Legal," NBC News, September 21, 2016, http://www.nbcnews .com/news/nbcblk/u-s-court-rules-dreadlock-ban-during-hiring-process -legal-n652211.
78 Verity Stevenson, "Demonstrators Declare: Black Hair Is Beautiful," *Toronto Star*, December 4, 2015, https://www.thestar.com/yourtoronto/ education/2015/12/04/demonstrators-declare-black-hair-is-beautiful.html.
79 Makda Ghebreslassie, "Jack Astor's Waitress Claims She Was Sent Home Because Hair Was in a Bun," CBC.ca, March 9, 2016, http://www.cbc.ca/ news/canada/toronto/jack-astors-hair-1.3484037.
80 Phillip Lee-Shanok, "Zara Employee Accuses Store of Discrimination Over Her Hairstyle," CBC.ca, April 9, 2016, http://www.cbc.ca/news/canada/ toronto/ballah-zara-discrimination-hairstyle-1.3527977.
81 Rooks, *Hair Raising*, 26.
82 Gill, "I Had My Own Business," 169.
83 Blackwelder, *Styling Jim Crow*, 3.
84 Jacobs-Huey, *From the Kitchen*, 5.
85 Collins, *Black Feminist Thought*, 79.
86 hooks, *Black Looks*, 62.
87 Bailey, "Redefining Representation," 73.
88 Tate, *Black Beauty*, 1.
89 Ibid.
90 Rooks, *Ladies' Pages*, 19.
91 Winks, *Blacks in Canada*, 407.

Chapter 1

1 Shaw, "'Most Anxious to Serve,'" 549.
2 Hastings, "Territorial Spoils," 457.
3 Bennett, *Shaping of Black America*, 269.

4 Walker, *Style and Status*, 15.
5 Williams, *Road to Now*, 40.
6 Ibid.
7 Carby, *Reconstructing Womanhood*, 164.
8 Cited in Rooks, *Ladies' Pages*, 17.
9 Rooks, *Ladies' Pages*, 18–19.
10 Walker, *Style and Status*, 28.
11 White and White, *Stylin'*, 184.
12 Ibid.
13 Sheehan, "Face of Fashion," 181.
14 Willis and Williams, *Black Female Body*, 4.
15 Mathieu, *North of the Color Line*, 152.
16 Toney, "Locating Diaspora," 80.
17 "Toronto Jamaica Folk Attend Smart Wedding," *Toronto Daily Star*, July 29, 1926, 25.
18 "Church Bulletins," *Canadian Observer*, December 12, 1914, 3.
19 Toney, "Locating Diaspora," 80.
20 Reynolds, *Viola Desmond's Canada*, 45.
21 Mathieu, *North of the Color Line*, 32.
22 Ibid.
23 Ibid., 51.
24 Ibid.
25 Library and Archives Canada, "Orders in Council—Décrets-du-Conseil," RG2-A-1-a, vol. 1021, PC 1911-1324, August 12, 1911.
26 Dowbiggin, *Keeping America Sane*, vii.
27 Young, *Fear of the Dark*, 50.
28 Dowbiggin, *Keeping America Sane*, vii–viii.
29 Henry, *Black Politics in Toronto*, 12.
30 White and White, *Stylin'*, 124.
31 Ruck, *Canada's Black Battalion*, 27.
32 Goldberg, *Racial State*, 79.
33 Walker, *Style and Status*, 85.
34 Maynard, introduction, 7.
35 Ibid.
36 Rooks, *Ladies' Pages*, 107.
37 Spencer, *Lipstick and High Heels*, 6.
38 Thanks a Million, *Sunday Star*, February 2, 1986.
39 Conor, *Spectacular Modern Woman*, 8.
40 Ibid., 9.
41 Berlant, *Female Complaint*, 122.
42 Young, *Fear of the Dark*, 53.
43 Peiss, *Hope in a Jar*, 231.
44 Toney, "Locating Diaspora," 78.

45   Williams, *Road to Now*, 13.

46   Ibid., 14.

47   Bristol, *Knights of the Razor*, 2–3.

48   Gill, "I Had My Own Business," 170.

49   Cooper, "Search for Mary Bibb," 180.

50   Adams, "Making a Living," 33.

51   McFarquhar, "Black Occupational Structure," 55.

52   Shadd, *Journey from Tollgate to Parkway*, 167.

53   Williams, *Road to Now*, 31.

54   Spray, *Blacks in New Brunswick*, 65–66.

55   Blackwelder, *Styling Jim Crow*, 47.

56   Henry, *Black Politics in Toronto*, 2–3.

57   Ibid., 4.

58   Mathieu, *North of the Color Line*, 152.

59   Marano, "'Rising Strongly and Rapidly,'" 253.

60   Mathieu, *North of the Color Line*, 105.

61   Marano, "'Rising Strongly and Rapidly,'" 236–37.

62   Brand, *No Burden to Carry*, 16.

63   Toney, "Locating Diaspora," 82.

64   Reynolds, *Viola Desmond's Canada*, 141.

65   Ibid.

66   Alexander and Glaze, *Towards Freedom*, 169.

67   Nicholas, "Gendering the Jubilee," 261.

68   Mathieu, *North of the Color Line*, 6.

69   Winks, *Blacks in Canada*, 411.

70   Rooks, *Ladies' Pages*, 4.

71   Conor, *Spectacular Modern Woman*, 14.

72   Rooks, *Hair Raising*, 47.

73   Toney, "Locating Diaspora," 80.

74   Hill Collins, *Black Feminist Thought*, 60.

75   Alexander and Glaze, *Towards Freedom*, 144.

76   Pierre Bourdieu, *Distinction: A Social Critique of the Judgment of Taste* (Cambridge, MA: Harvard University Press, 1984), quoted in Brand, *No Burden to Carry*, 9.

77   Willis, *Reflections in Black*, 35.

78   Rooks, *Ladies' Pages*, 18–19.

79   Spray, *Blacks in New Brunswick*, 66.

80   Winks, *Blacks in Canada*, 400–401.

81   Pachai and Bishop, *Historic Black Nova Scotia*, 42.

82   Ibid.

83   Ibid.

84   High Class Pocket Billiards and Barber Shop advertisement, *Canadian Observer*, January 2, 1915, 1.

85 Lorinc, introduction, 12.

86 Toney, "Locating Diaspora," 80.

87 Hair Dressing Parlor advertisement, *Canadian Observer*, June 12, 1915, 1.

88 Scalp Specialist advertisement, *Canadian Observer*, June 26, 1915, 1.

89 Plitt, *Martha Matilda Harper*, 120.

90 Peiss, *Hope in a Jar*, 73.

91 Ibid., 80.

92 Gill, "I Had My Own," 169.

93 Peiss, *Hope in a Jar*, 109.

94 Blackwelder, *Styling Jim Crow*, 20.

95 Rooks, *Ladies' Pages*, 64.

96 Russell, Wilson, and Hall, *Color Complex*, 50.

97 Ibid., 142.

98 "Music in the Home," *Globe*, August 25, 1923, 25; "*Shuffle Along* Scores Again," *Dawn of Tomorrow*, January 19, 1924, 6.

99 Peiss, *Hope in a Jar*, 150.

100 Detweiler, *Negro Press*, 113–14.

101 Scott's White Lily Toilet Wash advertisement, *Christian Recorder*, September 30, 1886.

102 Weems, "Consumerism," 166.

103 Rooks, *Hair Raising*, 26.

104 Russell, Wilson, and Hall, *Color Complex*, 50.

105 Ibid.

106 Beautiwhite Company advertisement, *Chicago Defender*, March 17, 1923, 2.

107 Horne, *Rise & Fall*, 16.

108 No-Mor-Kink advertisement, *Chicago Defender*, November 30, 1929, 2.

109 Pachai and Bishop, *Historic Black Nova Scotia*, 45–46.

110 Thompson, "Cultivating Narratives," 32.

111 Winks, *Blacks in Canada*, 402.

112 See *London Free Press*, 1950.

113 Peiss, *Hope in a Jar*, 213.

114 "Miss Ethel Shreve," *Dawn of Tomorrow*, July 28, 1923, 2.

115 "Madame Berry-Hunter," *Dawn of Tomorrow*, August 25, 1923, 1.

116 Ozonized Ox Marrow hair straightener advertisement, *Dawn of Tomorrow*, April 12, 1924, 6. The company also posted similar advertisements in August and September 1924.

117 Peiss, *Hope in a Jar*, 67.

118 Ibid.

119 Horne, *Rise & Fall*, 27.

120 Rooks, *Hair Raising*, 49.

121 Mitchell C. Brown, "The Faces of Science: African Americans in the Sciences," November 25, 2007, https://webfiles.uci.edu/mcbrown/display/walker.html.

122 Blackwelder, *Styling Jim Crow*, 25.

123 Sherrow, *Encyclopedia of Hair*, 186.

124 Peiss, *Hope in a Jar*, 113.

125 Blackwelder, *Styling Jim Crow*, 17.

126 Cited in Horne, *Rise & Fall*, 28.

127 Real Hair Grower advertisement, *Canadian Observer*, September 16, 1916, 3.

128 Real Handmade Human Hair advertisement, *Canadian Observer*, July 21, 1917, 6.

129 Mesdames Wells and Hunter advertisement, *Dawn of Tomorrow*, February 2, 1924, 3.

130 "Madame Lillian D. Wells," *Dawn of Tomorrow*, December 29, 1923, 1.

131 J. M. Jefferson Hair Dressing and Shaving Parlor advertisement, *Dawn of Tomorrow*, March 1, 1924, 6.

132 Yale Tonsorial and Beauty Parlors advertisement, *Dawn of Tomorrow*, November 5, 1927, 6.

133 Barber Business for Sale advertisement, *Dawn of Tomorrow*, April 25, 1925, 6; Wolverine Barber Shop advertisement, *Dawn of Tomorrow*, November 5, 1927, 6.

134 Wavine advertisement, *Dawn of Tomorrow*, June 20, 1930, 6.

135 Alex Marks advertisements, *Dawn of Tomorrow*, October 11, 1924, 4, and October 24, 1925, 4.

136 Harriet Hubbard Ayer Face Cream advertisement, *Dawn of Tomorrow*, May 1937, n.p.

137 Du Barry advertisements, *Dawn of Tomorrow*, April 1942, 3, and September 1944, 4.

138 Walker, *Style and Status*, 20.

139 Eaton's advertisement, *Dawn of Tomorrow*, August 1946, n.p.

140 "Ebony," *Dawn of Tomorrow*, September 1946, n.p.

141 Winks, *Blacks in Canada*, 394.

142 Rooks, *Ladies' Pages*, 131.

143 Haidarali, "Polishing Brown Diamonds," 13.

144 Higginbotham, *Righteous Discontent*, 192.

145 Ibid., 193.

146 Haidarali, "Polishing Brown Diamonds," 13.

147 Ibid., 15.

148 Ibid.

Chapter 2

1 *Canada: The Story of Us*, "Expansion (1858–1899)" and "A New Identity (1946–1970)," directed by Renny Bartlett, P.J. Naworynski, and Tim Wolo-chatiuk, written by Michael Allcock, Greg Beer, and Carl Knutson, aired March 26–May 14, 2017 on CBC.

2 Francis, *National Dreams*, 11.

3 Grewal, *Transnational America*, 8.
4 Ibid., 9.
5 Peiss, *Hope in a Jar*, 238.
6 Haidarali, "Polishing Brown Diamonds," 12.
7 Ibid.
8 Russell, Wilson, and Hall, *Color Complex*, 28.
9 Ibid., 25.
10 Ibid., 27.
11 Higginbotham, *Righteous Discontent*, 195.
12 Ibid., 194.
13 Ibid.
14 Bernstein, *Racial Innocence*, 230.
15 Blackwelder, *Styling Jim Crow*, 146.
16 Russell, Wilson, and Hall, *Color Complex*, 27–28.
17 Blackwelder, *Styling Jim Crow*, 154.
18 Rooks, *Hair Raising*, 127.
19 Ross D. Perry, "Have We a Color Line?" *Globe and Mail*, February 26, 1947, 15.
20 Brand, "We Weren't Allowed," 174.
21 Ibid., 174–75.
22 Reynolds, *Viola Desmond's Canada*, 3.
23 Ibid., 55.
24 Thomas, "Cultural Tourism," 435.
25 Winks, "Canadian Negro," 288.
26 Ibid., 297.
27 Winks, *Blacks in Canada*, 420.
28 Ibid.
29 Ibid., 449.
30 Ibid.
31 *Montreal Daily Star*, October 4, 1921, 1.
32 *Hamilton Spectator*, March 24, 1923, 1.
33 "Claim Women's Canadian Ku Klux Klan Has 1000 Members Here," *Hamilton Herald*, March 20, 1925.
34 Shadd, *Journey from Tollgate*, 213.
35 *Globe*, March 1, 1930, 1.
36 Silva, Introduction, 5.
37 Ibid.
38 Christine Sismondo, "The KKK Has a History in Canada. And It Can Return," *Maclean's*, August 18, 2017, https://www.macleans.ca/news/canada/the-kkk-has-a-history-in-canada-and-it-can-return/.
39 Mathieu, *North of the Color Line*, 25.
40 Cited in Mathieu, *North of the Color Line*, 168. See also *Winnipeg Free Press*, November 20, 1920.

41 "Fight Is Ours Birth of a Nation Play Cancelled," *Canadian Observer*, December 4, 1915, 1.

42 "Amherstburg Racial Trouble," *Globe and Mail*, August 12, 1965, 5.

43 Cited in Winks, *Blacks in Canada*, 435.

44 Mensah, *Black Canadians*, 71.

45 Walker, *West Indians*, 12.

46 Ibid.

47 Kibler, *Rank Ladies*, 119.

48 Gold Dust Washing Powder advertisement, *Daily Mail and Empire*, December 3, 1897.

49 Alexander and Glaze, *Towards Freedom*, 172.

50 Winks, *Blacks in Canada*, 406.

51 Oak, *Negro Newspaper*, 67.

52 Haidarali, "Polishing Brown Diamonds," 16.

53 Backhouse, *Colour-Coded*, 232.

54 Ibid.

55 Robson, *Sister to Courage*, 35.

56 Higginbotham, *Righteous Discontent*, 196.

57 Robson, *Sister to Courage*, 38.

58 Backhouse, *Colour-Coded*, 234.

59 McAndrew, "Twentieth-Century Triangle Trade," 795.

60 Ibid.

61 Spencer, *Lipstick and High Heels*, 7.

62 Rita Cummings, "My Daughter Married a Negro," *Chatelaine*, May 1959, 25.

63 Ibid., 76.

64 Korinek, *Roughing It*, 186.

65 Mensah, *Black Canadians*, 152.

66 Walker, *West Indians*, 10.

67 Williams, *Road to Now*, 105.

68 Ibid., 107.

69 Mensah, *Black Canadians*, 151.

70 Williams, *Road to Now*, 108.

71 Locke, "Are Canadians Really Tolerant?" *Chatelaine*, September 1959, 27.

72 Belisle, *Retail Nation*, 81.

73 Robson, *Sister to Courage*, 40–41.

74 Backhouse, *Colour-Coded*, 240.

75 Harrison, "'Shining in the Sun,'" 43.

76 Higginbotham, *Righteous Discontent*, 196.

77 Backhouse, *Colour-Coded*, 243.

78 Ibid., 245.

79 Higginbotham, *Righteous Discontent*, 186.

80 Ibid., 188.

81 Ibid., 193.
82 Backhouse, *Colour-Coded*, 246.
83 Reynolds, *Viola Desmond's Canada*, 59.
84 Pachai and Bishop, *Historic Black Nova Scotia*, 46–47.
85 "Women's Hair Styles That Men Prefer," *Ebony*, November 1956, 50–57.
86 McCracken, *Big Hair*, 151–52.
87 Meyerowitz, "Women, Cheesecake," 18–21.
88 Haidarali, "Polishing Brown Diamonds," 25.
89 "Hair Attachment," *Ebony*, June 1947, 36.
90 Ibid., 38–39.
91 "Canada's Crimeless Colored Community," *Ebony*, December 1946, 24.
92 Ibid., 25.
93 Ibid., 27.
94 Ferrell, *Let's Talk Hair*, 16.
95 Lustrasilk advertisement, *Ebony*, December 1948, 58–59.
96 Lustrasilk advertisement, *Ebony*, September 1948, 54–55.
97 "New Hair Culture Discovery," *Ebony*, June 1948, 58–59.
98 Rooks, *Hair Raising*, 128.
99 Winks, *Blacks in Canada*, 404.
100 Pachai and Bishop, *Historic Black Nova Scotia*, 47.
101 Robson, *Sister to Courage*, 112.
102 Mirror Tone advertisement, *The Clarion*, February 16, 1949, 5.
103 Peiss, "Making Up, Making Over," 322.
104 Peiss, *Hope in a Jar*, 128.
105 Ibid.
106 Korinek, *Roughing It*, 33.
107 Peiss, *Hope in a Jar*, 239.
108 Ibid., 101.
109 Ibid.
110 Max Factor True Color Lipstick advertisement, *Chatelaine*, August 1940, 27.
111 Tobias, *Fire and Ice*, 47.
112 Basten, *Max Factor*, 69, 71.
113 Peiss, *Hope in a Jar*, 87.
114 Ibid., 105.
115 Helena Rubinstein advertisement, *Chatelaine*, May 1944, 28; Elizabeth Arden advertisement, *Chatelaine*, February 1945, 32.
116 Helena Rubinstein advertisement, *Chatelaine*, September 1945, 41.
117 Elizabeth Arden advertisement, *Chatelaine*, September 1953, 49.
118 Avon advertisement, *Chatelaine*, November 1945, 37.
119 Avon advertisement, *Chatelaine*, June 1946, 48.
120 Walker, *Style and Status*, 270.
121 Koehn, "Estée Lauder," 222.

122 Eaton's advertisement for Estée Lauder, *Toronto Telegram*, March 19, 1968, 19.

123 Haidarali, "Polishing Brown Diamonds," 32–33.

124 Peiss, *Hope in a Jar*, 259.

125 Nadinola advertisement, *Ebony*, November 1946, 16.

126 Nadinola advertisement, *Ebony*, January 1957, 145.

127 "Ten Types of Colors of Beauties Emphasize Racial Harmony of West Indian Island," *Ebony*, February 1956, 30–34.

128 Rowe, "'Glorifying the Jamaican Girl,'" 51.

129 Barnes, "Face of the Nation," 474.

130 Ulysee, "Uptown Ladies and Downtown Women," 153.

131 Shaw, *Embodiment of Disobedience*, 5.

132 "Miss West Indies in Miss Universe," *Ebony*, November 1954, 79–83.

133 Buckridge, *Language of Dress*, 9.

134 Barnes, "Face of the Nation," 477.

135 Rowe, "'Glorifying the Jamaican Girl,'" 44.

136 Kristina Rodulfo, "Miss Jamaica Wore an Afro at Miss Universe 2017, and We Are SO Here for It," PopSugar, December 25, 2017, https://www.popsugar.com/beauty/Miss-Jamaica-Davina-Bennett-Afro-Miss-Universe-2017-44301922.

137 Nancy J. Dawson, "George E. Johnson." *The African American Experience: The American Mosaic*, http://africanamerican.abc-clio.com/.

138 Byrd and Tharps, *Hair Story*, 85.

139 Ibid., 17.

140 Ibid., 86.

141 "How the Male Entered Beauty Culture Field," *Chicago Daily Defender*, January 2, 1963, 9.

142 "Beautician Answers Questions about Chemical Hair Relaxers," *Chicago Daily Defender*, October 17–23, 1964, n.p.

143 Archer-Straw, *Negrophilia*, 97.

144 Walker, "Black Is Profitable," 255.

145 Kelley, *Yo' Mama's Disfunktional*, 27.

146 Austin, "All Roads Led to Montreal," 206–35.

147 Walker, "Black Is Profitable," 274.

148 "Why Use Chemicals for Modern Day Hair Care?" *Chicago Daily Defender*, August 2, 1966, 18.

149 Peiss, *Hope in a Jar*, 263.

150 Walker, "Black Is Profitable," 269.

151 Raveen Au Naturelle advertisement, *Ebony*, November 1968, 22.

152 Clairol advertisement, *Ebony*, December 1970, 167.

153 Sherrow, *Encyclopedia of Hair*, 10.

154 Brody, *Impossible Purities*, 88.

155 Ibid.

156 Etcoff, *Survival of the Prettiest*, 118.
157 Taylor Orci, "The Original 'Blonde Bombshell' Used Actual Bleach on Her Head," *Atlantic*, February 22, 2013, http://www.theatlantic.com/health/archive/2013/02/the-original-blonde-bombshell-used-actual-bleach-on-her-head/273333/.
158 Etcoff, *Survival of the Prettiest*, 118.
159 Polykoff, *Does She... or Doesn't She*, 31.
160 Craig, *Ain't I a Beauty Queen?*, 3.
161 Barnes, *Cultural Conundrums*, 62.
162 Farrington, *Creating Their Own Image*, 150–51.
163 Witt, *Black Hunger*, 44.
164 Clairol's Born Blonde Lotion Toner advertisement, *Chatelaine*, April 1966, n.p.
165 These Clairol ads appeared in *Chatelaine* in April and May 1966, and January and February 1967.
166 Revlon advertisement, *Chatelaine*, October 1971, 7.
167 Freeman, "From No Go to No Logo," 831.
168 Harry Bruce, "Women of Halifax Pattern Breakers," *Chatelaine*, December 1974, 38.
169 "Black Canadian Culture Workshop Set for Saturday," *London Free Press*, April 25, 1975.
170 Prince, *Politics of Black Women's Hair*, 107.
171 Johnson Products Afro Sheen advertisement, *Ebony*, November 1968, 207.
172 Byrd and Tharps, *Hair Story*, 67.
173 *Essence*, December 1972, 92.
174 Kelley, *Yo' Mama's Disfunktional*, 27.
175 "The Natural Look—Is It Here to Stay?" *Ebony*, January 1969, 104.
176 Ibid.
177 Ibid., 108.
178 "For Women Who Wear It Like It Is," *West Indian News Observer*, November 1968, 7.
179 "Black Is In," *West Indian News Observer*, November 1968, 7.
180 "Azan's Beauty World," *West Indian News Observer*, December 1968, 9.
181 Patrick Martin, "Reflections on the Black Press," *Ryerson Review of Journalism*, April 1, 1993, http://rrj.ca/reflections-on-the-black-press.
182 "Today's Look—The Natural You," *Contrast*, April 1969, 8.
183 Ken and Tony of Jamaica Beauty Salon advertisement, *Contrast*, April 1969, 10.
184 "Hair Relaxing Clinic," *Contrast*, April 1969, 8.
185 Weems, "Consumerism," 171.
186 Tessa Judi Been, "Keep Your Natural Looking Great," *Contrast*, May 1969, 9.

Chapter 3

1 Aronczyk, *Branding the Nation*, 107.
2 Ibid., 112.
3 "Caribana '68," *West Indian News Observer*, July 1968, 3.
4 Trotman, "Transforming Caribbean," 187.
5 Ibid., 188.
6 Alexander and Glaze, *Towards Freedom*, 223.
7 Lyndon Watkins, "Antigonish," *Globe and Mail*, May 2, 1972.
8 Walker, *Racial Discrimination*, 19.
9 Alexander and Glaze, *Towards Freedom*, 221.
10 Neal, "Sold Out on Soul," 120.
11 Alexander and Glaze, *Towards Freedom*, 223.
12 Hill, *Women of Vision*, 21.
13 Ibid., 7.
14 Ibid., 14.
15 Ibid.
16 Cecil Foster, "How Toronto's Black Press Taught Me to Find Hope Despite the Despair of Exclusion," CBC.ca, February 3, 2017, http://www.cbc.ca/2017/how-toronto-s-black-press-taught-me-to-find-hope-despite-the-despair-of-exclusion-1.3963493.
17 "Black Business Directory," *Contrast*, September 16, 1970, 15.
18 "Black Business Ownership on the Rise in Toronto," *Contrast*, March 20, 1970, 5.
19 "15 Minutes of Manipulation," *Contrast*, April 4, 1970, 2.
20 King, "'Who's That Lady?'" 94.
21 Ibid.
22 Austin Clarke, "This Is Canada, Not the United States," *Contrast*, October 1, 1970, 4.
23 Liz Cromwell, "Shopping for a Black Doll in Toronto," *Contrast*, December 21, 1973, 19.
24 Ducille, "Dyes and Dolls."
25 Roberts, *Barbie*, 44.
26 Ducille, "Dyes and Dolls."
27 Azan's Beauty World and Nouveau Femme advertisement, *Contrast*, May 1, 1970, 12.
28 Ken Johnson, "Glamorous Models!" *Contrast*, June 1, 1970, 11.
29 Third World Books advertisement, *Contrast*, August 1–15, 1970, 10.
30 Mr. Stephen advertisement, *Contrast*, August 1–15, 1970, 10.
31 Townecraft Industries advertisement, *Contrast*, August 1–15, 1970, 13.
32 "Dashiki Party," *Contrast*, February 16, 1970, 10.
33 Van Deburg, *New Day in Babylon*, 195.
34 Eveleen Dollery, "Sparkle in Your Own Holiday Life-Style," *Chatelaine*, December 1970, 36–39.

35 Willis and Williams, *Black Female Body*, 133.
36 Ibid.
37 Wallace-Sanders, *Mammy*, 1.
38 Charlotte Gray, "Yes, 11 Ministers," *Chatelaine*, January 1991, 21–23, 86–88.
39 Elspeth Cameron, "Who Is Marlene Nourbese Philip, and Why Is She Saying All Those Terrible Things about PEN?" *Chatelaine*, November 1990, 87, 123–25, 127–28.
40 Cecil Foster, "Can Jean Augustine Deliver?" *Chatelaine*, November 1994, 52–56. Also see "Why Blacks Get Mad," *Chatelaine*, November 1992, 70–75, 118.
41 CoverGirl advertisement, *Chatelaine*, December 1994, 11.
42 Rob Colapinto, "Gloria!" *Chatelaine*, March 1999, 82–86, 88, 90.
43 Beth Hitchcock, "Soul Survivor," *Chatelaine*, December 1999, 56–58, 60–62, 64–66.
44 O'Donnell, "Visualizing the History," 352.
45 Cachet advertisement, *Chatelaine*, April 1979, 37.
46 Clairol advertisement, *Chatelaine*, February 1982, 2.
47 "Black and White...Always Right," *Chatelaine*, June 1986, 68–71.
48 Weems, "Consumerism," 172.
49 Walker, *Style and Status*, 175.
50 Joan Young, "Now Black Can Be More Beautiful," *Contrast*, April 19, 1971, 7.
51 Flori Roberts advertisement, *Contrast*, July 19, 1971, 13.
52 Eaton's Wig Shop advertisement, *Toronto Star*, September 17, 1968, 58.
53 Eaton's Wig Shop advertisement, *Telegram*, October 21, 1968, 16.
54 Posner advertisement, *Contrast*, July 19, 1971, 11.
55 Eaton's Estée Lauder advertisement, *Toronto Star*, March 18, 1968, 57.
56 Flori Roberts advertisement, *Contrast*, September 18, 1971, 13.
57 "Black-Oriented Afro Sheen Being Introduced in Canada," *Contrast*, August 1, 1971, 21.
58 Beverly Mascoll advertisement, *Contrast*, September 18, 1971, 11.
59 Beverly Mascoll advertisement, *Contrast*, December 22, 1972, 16.
60 Monette Cosmetics advertisement, *Contrast*, February 21, 1975, 10.
61 Weems, "Consumerism," 172.
62 Koehn, "Estée Lauder," 227.
63 Walker, *Style and Status*, 176.
64 Fashion Fair advertisement, *Contrast*, December 20, 1975, 12.
65 Clark, "Commodity Lesbianism," 494.
66 Arvidsson, "Brands," 244.
67 Sandy Newton, "Enhancing the Beauty of the Black Woman," *Contrast*, April 11, 1975, 3.
68 Barbara Walden Cosmetics advertisement, *Contrast*, April 4, 1975, 5.
69 Fashion Fair advertisement, *Contrast*, May 27, 1976, 17.
70 Walden Cosmetics advertisement, *Contrast*, May 20, 1976, 5.

71 Nadinola advertisement, *Contrast*, February 1, 1972, 9.

72 Nadinola advertisement, *Essence*, November 1972, 29.

73 Dr. Fred Palmer advertisement, *Share*, May 31, 1980, 2.

74 Ambi advertisement, *Ebony*, October 1975, 6.

75 Ambi advertisement, *Share*, June 26, 1983, 2.

76 Russell, Wilson and Hall, *Color Complex*, 51.

77 Nadinola advertisement, *Share*, February 7, 1985, n.p.

78 Azan's Beauty World advertisement, *Contrast*, November 16, 1973, 3.

79 "Beauty Bar's First Anniversary," *Contrast*, April 4, 1970, 14.

80 Peiss, *Hope in a Jar*, 257.

81 *Globe*, February 24, 1928, 16, and *Globe and Mail*, June 26, 1947, 29.

82 Marvel Beauty School advertisement, *Contrast*, September 29, 1972, 9.

83 French Perm advertisement, *Contrast*, April 12, 1974, 13.

84 Ibid.

85 French Perm advertisement, *Contrast*, June 28, 1974, 2.

86 Royal Crown advertisement, *Contrast*, May 10, 1974, 13.

87 Anupa Mistry, "Inside Toronto's 'Little Jamaica," *Fader*, April 27, 2016, http://www.thefader.com/2016/04/27/little-jamaica-toronto -photographer-jon-blak.

88 Ebony Eye Beauty Supplies advertisement, *Contrast*, June 14, 1974, 14.

89 Eaton's Hairworks advertisement, *Contrast*, November 21, 1975, 3.

90 Eaton's Hairworks advertisement, *Contrast*, December 5, 1975, 16.

91 "Hairdressers Gather for Demonstration," *Contrast*, May 7, 1976, 3.

92 Logan Lessona, "Headwrapping Made Easy," *Contrast*, September 15, 1972, 14.

93 "Hair Relaxing and Mind-Blowing All in One Show," *Contrast*, May 12, 1977, 10.

94 Eaton's Fashion Fair advertisement, *Contrast*, May 19, 1977, 8.

95 Mulvey, "Visual Pleasure," 62–63.

96 Ibid., 59.

97 Gaines, "White Privilege," 295.

98 Pro-Line "Kiddie Kit" advertisement, *Contrast*, October 27, 1977, 14.

99 White, "Big Girl's Chair," 25.

100 Conrad, "Black-Owned Businesses," 241.

101 Willis and Williams, *Black Female Body*, 156.

102 Grayson Mitchell, "Battle of the Rouge," *Black Enterprise*, August 9, 1978, 25.

103 Ibid.

104 Weems, "Consumerism," 174.

105 Peter Scott, "Hairstylists Seek Opinion about Boycott," *Share*, November 13, 1986, 26.

106 Yla Eason, "Battle of the Beauticians," *Black Enterprise*, November 1980, 36.

107 Ibid.

108 Grayson Mitchell, "Battle of the Rouge," *Black* Enterprise, August 9, 1978, 29.

109 "Sta-Sof-Fro" advertisement, *Share*, April 8, 1978, 3.

110 Carson Products advertisement, *Share*, July 22, 1978, 2.

111 Cheryl Foggo, "Black Calgary Is Growing, Changing," *Contrast*, March 6, 1981, 10.

112 Ibid.

113 Multiculturalism advertisement, *Share*, February 24, 1979, 11.

114 Multiculturalism advertisement, *Share*, April 7, 1979, 11.

115 "What's Wrong with Her Natural Hair?" *Contrast*, September 29, 1969, 8.

116 Greene, "Black Women Can't," 413.

117 Daphne Estelle, "African Braids Are In This Summer," *Share*, March 29, 1980, 3.

118 Louise Sweeney, "Roberta Flack: A Viola in Her Voice," *Christian Science Monitor*, March 6, 1980, http://www.csmonitor.com/1980/0306/030653.html.

119 Byrd and Tharps, *Hair Story*, 102.

120 Ibid., 103.

121 Greene, "Black Women Can't," 413.

122 Bordo, *Unbearable Weight*, 254.

123 Byrd and Tharps, *Hair Story*, 105–6.

124 Ibid., 106.

125 Davis, "New Hair Freedom?" 33.

126 Jules Elder, "No Burns, Hair Product Claims," *Share*, September 2, 1978, 9.

127 Shopper's Drug Mart advertisement, *Contrast*, November 4, 1987, 22.

128 Dark & Lovely advertisement, *Share*, April 21, 1979, 2.

129 Dark & Lovely advertisement, *Share*, November 10, 1979, 8.

130 Jhally, *Codes of Advertising*, 106.

131 "Warning Issued on Hair Smoothing Products," CBC.ca, December 11, 2010, http://www.cbc.ca/news/canada/warning-issued-on-hair-smoothing-products-1.891091.

132 "Formaldehyde Found in More Hair Products," CBC.ca, April 12, 2011, http://www.cbc.ca/news/health/formaldehyde-found-in-more-hair-products-1.982602.

133 Nicole Catanese, "The Truth about Keratin," *Bazaar*, October 3, 2016, http://www.harpersbazaar.com/beauty/hair/advice/a1266/how-keratin-damages-hair/.

134 McMichael, "Hair and Scalp Disorders," 629–44.

135 Khumalo et al., "'Relaxers' Damage Hair," 402–8.

136 Wise et al. "Hair Relaxer Use," 432–40.

137 Anahad O'Connor, "Surgeon General Calls for Health Over Hair," *New York Times*, August 25, 2011, http://well.blogs.nytimes.com/2011/08/25/surgeon-general-calls-for-health-over-hair/?hp&_r=0.

138 Yemisi Dina, Ginette A. Okoye, and Crystal Aguh, "Association of Uterine Leiomyomas with Central Centrifugal Cicatricial Alopecia." *JAMA Dermatology* 154, no. 2 (February 2018): 213–214.

139 Angela Kyei et al., "Medical and Environmental," 909–14.

140 Inga Vesper, "Hair Products Popular with Black Women May Contain Harmful Chemicals," *Scientific American*, May 11, 2018, https://www.scientificamerican.com/article/hair-products-popular-with-black-women-may-contain-harmful-chemicals/.

141 Ibid.

142 Byrd and Tharps, *Hair Story*, 90.

143 "Johnson Company Unveils New Products at Sheraton Centre Next Weekend," *Contrast*, April 3, 1980, 9.

144 Ultra Sheen advertisement, *Contrast*, August 15, 1980, 12.

145 Davis, "New Hair Freedom?" 34.

146 Byrd and Tharps, *Hair Story*, 89.

147 Ibid.

148 Eaton's advertisement, *Share*, March 29, 1980, 5.

149 Walker, *Andre Talks Hair*, 98.

150 Shirley Lord, "Everybody's All-American," *Vogue*, February 1989, 312–19.

Chapter 4

1 Koehn, "Estée Lauder," 237.

2 Grayson Mitchell, "Battle of the Rouge," *Black* Enterprise, August 9, 1978, 23.

3 Ibid., 25.

4 Ibid.

5 Ibid., 23.

6 Ibid., 25.

7 Ibid., 23.

8 Kimberly Seals McDonald, "Hair Care Firms Get Ownership Makeover," *Black Enterprise*, September 1998, 19.

9 Elsevier Business Intelligence, "Revlon's African Pride Buy Offers A.P. Products International Opportunities," June 15, 1998, http://www.elsevierbi.com/publications/the-rose-sheet/19/024/revlons-african-pride-buy-offers-ap-products-international-opportunities.

10 See note 8 above.

11 Edward Tony Lloneau, "Mergers and Acquisitions," Black Owned Beauty Supply Association, July 19, 2013, http://bobsa.org/todays-post.

12 George White, "Black-Owned Hair Care Firm OKs Purchase," *Los Angeles Times*, June 15, 1993, http://articles.latimes.com/1993-06-15/business/fi-3370_1_johnson-products.

13 L'Oréal, "L'Oréal Signs Definitive Agreement to Acquire Carson," news release, February 28, 2000, http://www.loreal-finance.com/eng/news-release/loreal-signs-definitive-agreement-to-acquire-carson-72.htm.

14 Industry Today, "Pro-Line International," http://industrytoday.com/article_view.asp?ArticleID=1475.

15 Karen Bitz, "The Ethnic Hair Care Market," November 9, 2005, http://www.happi.com/contents/view_features/2005-11-09/the-ethnic-hair-care-market-84783/.

16 Ibid.

17 Clementine Fletcher, "Unilever to Buy Alberto Culver for $3.7 Billion," Bloomberg, September 27, 2010, http://www.bloomberg.com/news/2010-09-27/unilever-agrees-to-buy-chicago-based-alberto-culver-for-3-7-billion-cash.html.

18 Ni'kita Wilson, "Johnson Products Back in Black Hands," Grio.com, July 16, 2009, http://thegrio.com/2009/07/16/johnson-products-the-company-behind/.

19 Jack Neff, "P&G's $7 Bil Bid for Wella Seen as Wise," Ad Age, March 24, 2003, http://adage.com/article/news/p-g-s-7-bil-bid-wella-wise/49954/.

20 Andrew Ross Sorkin, "Procter & Gamble Agrees to Acquire Clairol for $4.95 Billion," New York Times, May 22, 2001, http://www.nytimes.com/2001/05/22/business/procter-gamble-agrees-to-acquire-clairol-for-4.95-billion.html.

21 "Procter & Gamble to Add Clairol to Hair-Care Lineup," Chicago Tribune, May 22, 2001, http://articles.chicagotribune.com/2001-05-22/business/0105220046_1_clairol-hair-coloring-hair-care.

22 Alfred Edmond, "Battle of the Vanities," Black Enterprise, March 1989, 46.

23 Ibid.

24 Caroline V. Clarke, "Redefining Beautiful: Black Cosmetics Companies and Industry Giants Vie for the Loyalty of Black Women," Black Enterprise, June 1993, 243–44.

25 Alfred Edmond, "Battle of the Vanities," Black Enterprise, March 1989, 51.

26 Peiss, Hope in a Jar, 263.

27 Caroline V. Clarke, "Redefining Beautiful: Black Cosmetics Companies and Industry Giants Vie for the Loyalty of Black Women," Black Enterprise, June 1993, 248.

28 Weems, "Consumerism," 175.

29 Caroline V. Clarke, "Redefining Beautiful: Black Cosmetics Companies and Industry Giants Vie for the Loyalty of Black Women," Black Enterprise, June 1993, 246.

30 Contrast, "Queen of Cosmetics Visits Toronto," 14 May 1982, 9.

31 Honest Ed's advertisement, Share, 18 April 1983, n.p.

32 Marina Strauss, "Rexall Takeover Shakes Up Canada's Drugstore Industry," Globe and Mail, March 2, 2016, http://www.theglobeandmail.com/report-on-business/mckesson-to-acquire-rexall-drugstore-chain-in-3-billion-deal/article28994105.

33 Grewal, Transnational America, 91.

34 Hae-Jung Hong and Yves Doz, "L'Oréal Masters Multiculturalism," Harvard Business Review, June 2013, https://hbr.org/2013/06/loreal-masters-multiculturalism.

35 Peiss, *Hope in a Jar*, 266.

36 bell hooks, cited in Ibid.

37 Caroline V. Clarke, "Redefining Beautiful: Black Cosmetics Companies and Industry Giants Vie for the Loyalty of Black Women," *Black Enterprise*, June 1993, 250.

38 Ibid., 248.

39 Archer-Straw, *Negrophilia*, 12.

40 Appadurai, *Social Life of Things*, 13.

41 Lancôme Rénergie Yeux advertisement, *Chatelaine*, April 1994, inside front cover.

42 L'Oréal Futur-e advertisement, *Chatelaine*, August 1998, n.p.

43 *About Face: Supermodels Then and Now*, directed by Timothy Greenfield-Sanders (Perth, Australia: Perfect Day Films, 2012).

44 Wek, *Alek*, 106.

45 Tate, *Black Beauty,*106.

46 Russell, Wilson, and Hall, *Color Complex*, 155.

47 Ibid., 156.

48 Ibid.

49 Charmaine Gooden, "Skin Color: Meet Your Match," *Chatelaine*, September 1992, 84.

50 Fleras, "Racializing Culture/Culturalizing Race," 441.

51 Bordo, "'Material Girl,'" 302.

52 Koehn, "Estée Lauder," 245.

53 James, *Beauty Imagined*, 2.

54 Ibid.

55 Ebony Onyxx, "Black Hair: Boomin' Billion Dollar Industry," Community Steeple, April 20, 2013, http://www.communitysteeple.com/urban-business/137-black-hair-boomin-billion-dollar-industry.html.

56 Elizabeth Dwoskin, "Startups, Target Go After the Multiracial Hair-Care Market," *Bloomberg*, June 20, 2013, https://www.bloomberg .com/news/articles/2013-06-20/startups-target-go-after-the-multiracial-hair-care-market.

57 Byrd and Tharps, *Hair Story*, 91.

58 Ibid.

59 Adrienne P. Samuels, "Guess Who Sells Your Weave? Koreans Capitalize on Black Beauty's Big Business," *Ebony*, May 2008, 176.

60 "Selling Black Cosmetics Proves a Tricky Business," *American Druggist* 176 (August 1977): 60.

61 Ibid.

62 Weems, "Consumerism," 172.

63 Phylis Johnson, "Plaza Drugs—The Only Black-Owned Drug Store in Western Canada," *Contrast*, June 1, 1988, 24.

64 "One of Toronto's First Black Hair Salons Still Going Strong after 52 Years," CityNews, February 28, 2014, http://www.citynews.ca/2014/02/28/one-of-torontos-first-black-hair-salons-still-going-strong-after-52-years-2/.

65 Lennox Grant, "Azan," *Contrast*, May 1978, 11.

66 SoftSheen-Carson advertisement for Hi Rez Hair Color, *Share*, November 6, 2003, 13.

67 Karen Bitz, "The Ethnic Hair Care Market," November 9, 2005, http://www.happi.com/contents/view_features/2005-11-09/the-ethnic-hair-care-market-84783/.

68 Veronica MacDonald, "Ethnic Hair Care: Options for Everyone," Happi, November 2005, https://www.happi.com/contents/view_features/2005-11-15/ethnic-hair-care-options-for-everyone/.

69 Matthew Fogel, "*Grey's Anatomy* Goes Colorblind," *New York Times*, May 8, 2005, http://www.nytimes.com/2005/05/08/arts/television/greys-anatomy-goes-colorblind.html.

70 Warner, "Racial Logic," 3.

71 Caldwell, "Look at Her Hair," 20.

72 Ibid.

73 Grayson, "Is It Fake?" 20.

74 Rooks, *Hair Raising*, 120.

75 Thompson, *An Eye for the Tropics*, 6.

76 Ibid., 301.

77 Tracy Clayton, "Sheryl Underwood Slams Natural Hair," Root.com, September 2, 2013, http://www.theroot.com/blog/the-grapevine/sheryl_underwood_slams_nappy_afro_hair/.

78 Rooks, *Hair Raising*, 118.

79 Ibid., 119.

80 Tananarive Due, "Thousands of Women Say Rio System Ruined Their Hair," *Free Lance-Star*, February 14, 1995, D6.

81 US Food and Drug Administration, "Does FDA Approve Cosmetics before They Go on the Market?" https://www.fda.gov/ForIndustry/FDABasicsfor Industry/ucm238793.htm.

82 Dario Balca, "Cosmetics Not Tested for Harmful Substances: Environment Commissioner," CTVNews.ca, May 31, 2016, http://www.ctvnews.ca/health/cosmetics-not-tested-for-harmful-substances-environment-commissioner-1.2924618.

83 "Recalls and Safety Alerts – Hair Care Products," Health Canada, http://www.healthycanadians.gc.ca/recall-alert-rappel-avis/hc-sc/2009/12632r-eng.php.

84 Grayson, "Is it Fake?" 22.

85 CoverGirl advertisement, *Essence*, December 2007, 26–27.

86 L'Oréal advertisement, *Essence*, August 2013, 24–25.

87 Nelson, *Representing the Black Female*, 78–79.

88 Ovalle, "Framing Jennifer Lopez," 167.

89 "L'Oréal Paris Debuts New True Match Campaign: Your Skin, Your Story," PR Newswire, January 7, 2017, http://www.prnewswire.com/news-releases/loreal-paris-debuts-new-true-match-campaign-your-skin-your-story-300387365.html.

90 Hunter, *Race, Gender*, 71.

91 Ruth La Ferla, "Generation E.A.: Ethnically Ambiguous," *New York Times*, December 28, 2003, http://www.nytimes.com/2003/12/28/style/generation-ea-ethnically-ambiguous.html?pagewanted=all&src=pm.

92 Shannon Proudfoot, "Number of Mixed-Race Couples on the Rise in Canada: StatsCan," *Canada.com*, April 23, 2010, http://www.canada.com/Number+mixed+race+couples+rise+Canada+StatsCan/2928592/story.html.

93 See note 91 above.

94 Sharpley-Whiting, *Pimps Up, Ho's Down*, 33.

95 Dunn, "*Baad Bitches*," 27.

96 Hobson, *Body as Evidence*, 41.

97 Baudrillard, *Simulacra and Simulation*, 81.

98 Angelique Chrisafis, "You're Worth It—If White: L'Oréal Guilty of Racism," *Guardian*, July 7, 2007, http://www.theguardian.com/world/2007/jul/07/france.angeliquechrisafis.

99 Ibid.

100 Alanah Eriksen, "White Out of Order! Beyoncé Is Looking Several Shades Lighter in Promo Shoot for Her New Album," *Daily Mail*, January 17, 2012, http://www.dailymail.co.uk/tvshowbiz/article-2087388/Beyonc-white-skin-row-Controversial-photo-shows-singer-looking-shades-lighter-usual-tone.html.

101 Alice Pfeiffer, "Explaining the Racist Response to the New Miss France," *Elle*, December 10, 2013, http://www.elle.com/news/culture/french-response-to-miss-france-reveals-racism.

102 Alexander Stille, "Can the French Talk about Race?" *New Yorker*, July 11, 2014, https://www.newyorker.com/news/news-desk/can-the-french-talk-about-race.

103 "Miss America Crowns 1st Winner of Indian Descent," CNN.com, September 17, 2013, http://www.cnn.com/2013/09/16/showbiz/miss-america-racist-reactions/.

104 Hobson, *Venus in the Dark*, 123.

105 Russell, Wilson and Hall, *Color Complex*, 151.

106 Ibid.

107 "Kerry Washington Fired for Not Being Black Enough," Stuff, June 9, 2016, http://www.stuff.co.nz/entertainment/tv-radio/80878082/kerry-washington-fired-for-not-being-black-enough.

108 Perry, "Who(se) Am I?" 138.

109 *Beauty: The Guide*, January/February 2014, http://beautytheguide.com.

Chapter 5

1 Charmaine Nelson, "Why Did a Cheerios Commercial Spark a Racist Meltdown?" *Huffington Post*, June 5, 2013, http://www.huffingtonpost.ca/charmaine-nelson/cheerios-commercial-racism_b_3387644.html.

2 Rooks, *Hair Raising*, 43.

3 Nicholas K. Geranios, "Rachel Dolezal Faces Uncertain Future after Race Scandal," *Toronto Star*, March 24, 2017, https://www.thestar.com/news/world/2017/03/24/rachel-dolezal-faces-uncertain-future-after-race-scandal.html.

4 Riss, *Race, Slavery, and Liberalism*, 97–98.

5 Ibid., 103–4.

6 Julee Wilson, "*Allure* Catches Hell for Teaching White Women How to Get an Afro," *Huffington Post*, August 3, 2015, http://www.huffingtonpost.com/entry/allure-afro-tutorial-outrage_us_55bf852ae4b06363d5a2b1ae.

7 Bordo, *Unbearable Weight*, 258.

8 Sperling, "Multiples and Reproductions," 296.

9 Willis and Williams, *Black Female Body*, 1.

10 Ehlers, *Racial Imperatives*, 35–36.

11 Mercer, *Welcome to the Jungle*, 102.

12 White and White, "Slave Hair," 50.

13 Byrd and Tharps, *Hair Story*, 13.

14 Russell, Wilson, and Hall, *Color Complex*, 15.

15 Hobbs, *Chosen Exile*, 29.

16 Russell, Wilson, and Hall, *Color Complex*, 16.

17 Buckridge, *Language of Dress*, 86.

18 Miller, *Slaves to Fashion*, 90.

19 Rediker, *Slave Ship*, 41–72.

20 Byrd and Tharps, *Hair Story*, 2–3.

21 Ibid., 3.

22 Ibid., 5–6.

23 Riss, *Race, Slavery, and Liberalism*, 98.

24 Willis and Williams, *Black Female Body*, 59–60.

25 Collins, "Historic Retrievals," 73.

26 Gilman, "Black Bodies," 219.

27 Bush, *Slave Women*, 15.

28 Smith, *Photography*, 6–7.

29 Ibid.

30 Williams, "Naked, Neutered, or Noble," 185.

31 Willis and Williams, *Black Female Body*, 22.

32 Ibid., 23.

33 Smith, *American Archives*, 118.

34 hooks, "In Our Glory," 46–47.

35 Wood, "Marketing the Slave Trade," 255.

36 Rooks, *Ladies' Pages*, 16.

37 Ibid., 17–18.

38 Ibid., 18.

39 Sheehan, "Face of Fashion," 182–83.

40 Ibid., 188.

41 "London 2012 Gymnastics: Gabby Douglas Says Focus on My Medals, Not My Hair," *Toronto Star*, August 6, 2012, https://www.thestar.com/sports/olympics/2012/08/06/london_2012_gymnastics_gabby_douglas_says_focus_on_my_medals_not_my_hair.html.

42 Sopan Deb, "After Apology, Bill O'Reilly Continues Attacks on Maxine Waters," *New York Times*, March 29, 2017, https://www.nytimes.com/2017/03/29/us/politics/bill-oreilly-maxine-waters-apology.html.

43 Charles, "Skin Bleachers' Representations," 163.

44 Candelario, *Black Behind the Ears*, 182.

45 Ibid.

46 Caldwell, "'Look at Her Hair,'" 20.

47 Ibid., 20. See also Gilliam, "Brazilian Mulata," 57–69.

48 Hunter, *Race, Gender*, 79.

49 Rudrapriya Rathore, "Many Shades of Invisible," *Walrus*, May 19, 2016, http://thewalrus.ca/many-shades-of-invisible/.

50 Thompson, "Black Women," 831–56.

51 Ibid., 840.

52 Jacobs-Huey, *From the Kitchen*, 72.

53 Kiini Ibura Salaam, "Hair Transgressions," November 18, 2003, http://goodhair.com, in Lara, "*Cimarronas, Ciguapas, Señoras*," 114.

54 "Singer's Dreadlocks Shorn, Vows Court Action," *Dominican Today*, January 23, 2013, https://dominicantoday.com/dr/local/2013/1/23/singers-dreadlocks-shorn-vows-court-action/.

55 Ed McCormack, "Bob Marley with a Bullet," *Rolling Stone*, August 12, 1976, http://www.rollingstone.com/music/news/bob-marley-with-a-bullet-19760812.

56 Dennis McLellan, "Perry Henzell, 70; His Movie *The Harder They Come* Brought Reggae to the World," *Los Angeles Times*, December 2, 2006, http://articles.latimes.com/2006/dec/02/local/me-henzell2.

57 King, "Co-optation," 78.

58 See Mastalia and Pagano, *Dreads*, 10–11, 14, 18, 20.

59 Mercer, *Welcome to the Jungle*, 108.

60 Ibid.

61 Alice Walker, introduction to *Dreads*, by Mastalia and Pagano, 8.

62 Russell, Wilson, and Hall, *Color Complex*, 86.

63 Ibid.

64 In Byrd and Tharps, *Hair Story*, 129–30.

65 Ashe, "Invisible Dread," 55.

66 Russell, Wilson, and Hall, *Color Complex*, 87–88.

67 Davis, "New Hair Freedom?" 34.

68 Byrd and Tharps, *Hair Story*, 130.

69 Philip Caulfield, "Zendaya Calls Out Giuliana Rancic for Saying Singer Looks Like She 'Smells like Weed' on Oscars Red Carpet," *New York Daily News*, February 24, 2015, http://www.nydailynews.com/entertainment/gossip/zendaya-slams-giuliana-rancic-smells-weed-comment-article-1.2127156.

70 Ashe, "'Why Don't He Like,'" 579–80.

71 Weekes, "Shades of Blackness," 115.

72 Rooks, *Hair Raising*, 35.

73 Mama, *Beyond the Masks*, 115.

74 Taylor, "Malcolm's Conk," 60; see also Rooks, *Hair Raising*, 132.

75 "Heritage Minutes: Underground Railroad" Historica Canada, https://www.historicacanada.ca/content/heritage-minutes/underground-railroad.

76 Glazer and Key, "Carry Me Back," 12.

77 Raimon, *"Tragic Mulatta" Revisited*, 93.

78 Ibid.

79 Murray, *Letters*, 83.

80 Ibid., 118.

81 Ibid., 198.

82 Stowe, *Uncle Tom's Cabin*, 351.

83 Ibid., 230.

84 Bernstein, *Racial Innocence*, 15.

85 Talty, *Mulatto America*, 53.

86 Ibid., 70.

87 Brody, *Impossible Purities*, 47.

88 Russell, Wilson, and Hall, *Color Complex*, 137.

89 Raimon, *"Tragic Mulatta" Revisited*, 13.

90 Tate, *Domestic Allegories*, 62.

91 Russell, Wilson, and Hall, *Color Complex*, 138–39.

92 Bogle, *Toms, Coons*, 13.

93 Ibid., 9.

94 Wald, *Crossing the Line*, 6.

95 Russell, Wilson, and Hall, *Color Complex*, 42.

96 Morrison, *Bluest Eye*, 46.

97 Walker, *Color Purple*, 46.

98 Ashe, "Why Don't He Like," 579–92.

99 Adichie, *Americanah*, 205.

100 Hobson, *Venus in the Dark*, 124.

101 Ibid., 127.

102 Johnson, "Newspaper Advertisements," 707.

103 Oak, *Negro Newspaper*, 119.

104 Sara Sidner, "Skin Whitener Advertisements Labeled Racist," CNN.com, September 9, 2009, http://www.cnn.com/2009/WORLD/asiapcf/09/09/india.skin/index.html.

105 "Hydroquinone Topical Side Effects – For the Consumer," Drugs.com, http://www.drugs.com/sfx/hydroquinone-side-effects.html.

106 "Global Skin Lighteners Market to Reach $10 Billion by 2015," *Skin Inc. Magazine*, June 23, 2009, http://www.skininc.com/spabusiness/global/48898927.html.

107 Ibid.

108 Hope, "From *Browning* to *Cake Soap*," 183.

109 Lauren Paxman, "So White It's Wrong: Skin Bleaching Products Unveiled for Men," *Daily Mail*, October 11, 2011, http://www.dailymail.co.uk/femail/article-2047898/So-white-wrong-Skin-bleaching-products-unveiled-FOR-MEN.html.

110 Bordo, "'Material Girl,'" 297.

111 Keller, Fiercely Real?" 147–64.

112 Bordo, "'Material Girl,'" 298.

113 Fanon, *Black Skin, White Masks*, 100.

114 Karl Marx, *Capital: A Critical Analysis of Capitalist Production: The Process of Capitalist Production* (New York: International Publishers, 1967), in Lury, *Consumer Culture*, 39.

115 Bordo, "'Material Girl,'" 297.

116 Wallis, preface, v.

117 Mercer, *Welcome to the Jungle*, 103.

118 Ibid.

119 "Who Invented the Weave," Thirsty Roots, March 20, 2010, http://thirstyroots.com/who-invented-the-weave.html.

120 Byrd and Tharps, *Hair Story*, 95.

121 Ibid., 122.

122 Luchina Fisher, "Naomi Campbell's Hair Weave Disaster," ABC News, August 9, 2012, https://abcnews.go.com/Entertainment/naomi-campbells-hair-weave-disaster/blogEntry?id=16969859.

123 Julee Wilson, "Countess Vaughn Reminds Us of the Dangers of Wigs and Weaves," *Huffington Post*, March 17, 2014, http://www.huffingtonpost.com/2014/03/17/countess-vaughn-hair-loss-lace-front-wigs_n_4980998.html?ir=Black+Voices.

124 Soul Cut Weave advertisement, *Share*, October 31, 1985, 19.

125 Sheer Advantage Hairstylists and Braiding Centre advertisement, *Contrast*, December 19, 1986, 17.

126 "Caring Your Weaves," *Contrast*, September 7, 1988, 26.

127 Armonie International advertisement, *Share*, April 26, 1990, 24.

128 Jones, "Hair Trade," 120.

129 Ibid., 121.

130 Ibid., 123.

131 Adrienne P. Samuels, "Guess Who Sells Your Weave? Koreans Capitalize on Black Beauty's Big Business," *Ebony*, May 2008, 141.

132 Ashante Infantry, "Documentary Weaves Hair into Laughter," *Toronto Star*, September 18, 2009, http://www.thestar.com/entertainment/movies/2009/09/18/documentary_weaves_hair_into_laughter.html.

133 Maria Puente, "Chris Rock's *Good Hair* Gets Tangled Up in Controversy," *USA Today*, October 25, 2009, http://usatoday30.usatoday.com/life/movies/news/2009-10-22-good-hair-main_N.htm.

134 Nedra Rhone, "Premium Human Hair Latest Target for Thieves," *Globe and Mail*, September 13, 2011, http://www.theglobeandmail.com/news/world/premium-human-hair-latest-target-for-thieves/article594162/.

135 Edward Tony Lloneau, "Hair, Hair, Hair: Human, Synthetic, Animal," *OTC Beauty Magazine*, November 2011, 68–70, http://issuu.com/otcbeautymagazine/docs/nov11.

136 Ibid.

137 Homa Khaleeli, "The Hair Trade's Dirty Secret," *Guardian*, October 28, 2012, http://www.theguardian.com/lifeandstyle/2012/oct/28/hair-extension-global-trade-secrets.

138 Ibid.

139 Edward Tony Lloneau, "Hair, Hair, Hair: Human, Synthetic, Animal," *OTC Beauty Magazine*, November 2011, 70, http://issuu.com/otcbeautymagazine/docs/nov11.

140 Fitzroy Greene, "New Concept for Beauty Supply Market," *Share*, October 26, 2000, 18.

141 Julee Wilson, "Tyra Banks Slaps Wig Companies with $10 Million Lawsuit," *Huffington Post*, October 2, 2013, http://www.huffingtonpost.com/2013/10/02/tyra-banks-wig-lawsuit-suing-companies-10-million_n_4030682.html.

142 Jones, "Hair Trade," 135.

143 Melissa Harris-Perry, "There's Big Business in Black Hair," MSNBC, June 9, 2012, https://www.msnbc.com/melissa-harris-perry/watch/harris-perry-theres-big-business-in-black-hair-44141123878?v=railb.

144 Kara Brown, "L'Oréal Buys Carol's Daughter following Bankruptcy," Jezebel.com, October 24, 2014, http://jezebel.com/loreal-buys-carols-daughter-following-bankruptcy-1650455109.

145 Deanna Utroske, "L'Oréal to Launch Multi-Cultural Division Starting with Carol's Daughter Acquisition," CosmeticsDesign.com, October 21, 2014, http://www.cosmeticsdesign.com/Business-Financial/L-Oreal-to-launch-multi-cultural-division-starting-with-Carol-s-Daughter-acquisition.

146 Ibid.

147 Ibid.

148 Davis, "New Hair Freedom?" 38.

149 "Cayman Islands: No Dreadlocks," *Share*, February 22, 1996, 13.

150 Stephania H. Davis and Jerry Thomas, "School's Hairdo Ban All Tangled: Some See It Clashing with Ethnic Culture," *Chicago Tribune*, November 12, 1996, http://articles.chicagotribune.com/1996-11-12/news/9611120106_1_gang-symbols-school-s-ban-hair.

151 "Dreadlocks," *Los Angeles Times*, November 27, 1998, http://articles.latimes.com/1998/nov/27/local/me-48232.

152 "Susan Taylor Protests School's No-Braids Policy," *Maynard Institute*, April 12, 2006, http://www.eurweb.com.

153 Patton, "'Hey Girl,'" 37–38.

154 Grayson, "Is It Fake?" 22.

155 Greene, "Black Women," 415.

156 Ferrell, *Let's Talk Hair*, 20.

157 Hannington Dia, "Woman Claims She Lost Job for Defending Black Co-Worker's 'Ghetto' Braids," NEWSONE.com, November 27, 2013, http://newsone.com/2792628/katherine-lemire-msa-lawsuit/.

158 Kate Dries, "Black Girl Threatened with Expulsion Over Hair Goes Back to School," December 2, 2013, Jezebel.com, http://jezebel.com/black-girl-threatened-with-expulsion-over-hair-goes-bac-1474934908.

159 Katie Mettler, "Boston-Area School Suspends Dress Code That Punished Girls for Wearing Braid Extensions," *Toronto Star*, May 22, 2017, https://www.thestar.com/news/world/2017/05/22/boston-area-school-suspends-dress-code-that-punished-girls-for-wearing-braid-extensions.html.

160 Greene, "Black Women," 411–12.

161 Ibid., 417.

162 Ibid.

163 Ibid., 421, 423–24.

164 Etcoff, *Survival of the Prettiest*, 126.

165 Anne Leclair, "Young Black Montrealer Claims She's Losing Work Over Her Hair," March 17, 2015, GlobalNew.ca, http://globalnews.ca/news/1888024/young-black-montrealer-claims-shes-losing-work-over-her-hair/.

166 See https://globalnews.ca/news/4732671/montreal-woman-wins-case-after-losing-job-at-madisons-because-of-her-hair/.

167 Verity Stevenson, "Demonstrators Declare: Black Hair Is Beautiful," *Toronto Star*, December 4, 2015, https://www.thestar.com/yourtoronto/education/2015/12/04/demonstrators-declare-black-hair-is-beautiful.html.

168 Makda Ghebreslassie, "Jack Astor's Waitress Claims She Was Sent Home Because Hair Was in a Bun," CBC.ca, March 9, 2016, http://www.cbc.ca/news/canada/toronto/jack-astors-hair-1.3484037.

169 Caldwell, "Hair Piece," 310.

170 Ibid., 314.

171 Ibid.

172 Noel Gutierrez-Morfin, "US Court Rules Dreadlock Ban during Hiring Process Is Legal," NBC News, September 21, 2016, http://www.nbcnews .com/news/nbcblk/u-s-court-rules-dreadlock-ban-during-hiring-process -legal-n652211.

173 Alexia Fernández Campbell, "A Black Woman Lost a Job Offer Because She Wouldn't Cut Her Dreadlocks. Now She Wants to Go to the Supreme Court, April 18, 2018, https://www.vox.com/2018/4/18/17242788/chastity -jones-dreadlock-job-discrimination.

174 Ibid.

175 "CBC Explores Black Hair," *Share*, January 28, 1999, 14.

Conclusion

1 Mensah, *Black Canadians*, 92.

2 "What Dolls Can Tell Us about Race in America," ABC News.com, October 11, 2006, http://abcnews.go.com/GMA/story?id=2553348.

3 "Study: White and Black Children Biased toward Lighter Skin," *CNN.com*, May 14, 2010, http://www.cnn.com/2010/US/05/13/doll.study/.

4 India Arie, "I Am Not My Hair," *Testimony: Vol. 1, Life & Relationship*, Motown, 2006.

5 Bordo, "Cassie's Hair," 404–5.

6 Sara Ilyas, "Did Dolce & Gabbana Send Racist Earrings Down the Catwalk?" *Guardian*, September 26, 2012, https://www.theguardian.com/ fashion/fashion-blog/2012/sep/26/dolce-gabbana-racist-earrings.

7 Julee Wilson, "*Garage* Magazine Editor-in-Chief Dasha Zhukova Sits on a 'Black Woman' Chair in Shocking Editorial," *Huffington Post*, January 20, 2014, http://www.huffingtonpost.com/2014/01/20/dasha-zhukova-black -woman-chair-buro-247-editorial_n_4633544.html.

8 Murray, "Branding 'Real' Social Change" 84.

9 Ibid. See also Nancy Etcoff, Susie Orbach, Jennifer Scott, and Heidi D'Agostino, "The Real Truth about Beauty: A Global Report: Findings of the Global Study on Women, Beauty and Well-Being," http://www.clubofam sterdam.com/contentarticles/52%20Beauty/dove_white_paper_final.pdf.

10 Murray, "Branding 'Real' Social Change," 84.

11 Cleve R. Wootson Jr. "Dove Sparks Backlash with Ad Slammed as 'Offensive,'" *Toronto Star*, October 8, 2017, https://www.thestar.com/news/ world/2017/10/08/dove-sparks-backlash-with-ad-slammed-as-offensive.html.

12 McClintock, *Imperial Leather*, 207.

13 Ibid., 208.

14 Hine, *Total Package*, 91–92.

15 Rifelj, *Coiffures*, 157.

16 My Black is Beautiful, https://www.facebook.com/mbib/.

17 "Hair Relaxer Sales Decline 26% over the Past Five Years," Mintel, September 4, 2013, http://www.mintel.com/press-centre/beauty-and-personal -care/ hairstyle-trends-hair-relaxer-sales-decline.

18 Nana Ekua Brew-Hammond, "Natural Hair Care's Next Wave," Grio .com, November 6, 2013, http://thegrio.com/2013/11/06/natural-hair-cares -next-wave/.

19 "Natural Hair Movement Drives Sales of Styling Products in US Black Hair-care Market," Mintel, December 17, 2015, http://www.mintel.com/press -centre/beauty-and-personal-care/natural-hair-movement-drives-sales-of -styling-products-in-us-black-haircare-market.

20 Kayla Greaves, "Gabrielle Union to Launch Natural Hair Care Line for Black Women," February 2, 2017, *Huffington Post*, http://www.huffington post.ca/2017/02/02/gabrielle-union-natural-hair-line_n_14574702.html.

21 Kimberly Walker, "Loc'd Out: Has the Style Lost Its Luster?" *Ebony*, January 30, 2012, http://www.ebony.com/style/locs-out-style-lost-luster.

22 See note 19 above.

23 Dani-Elle Dubé, "Hair Dyes, Relaxers Linked to Increased Risk of Breast Cancer: Study," GlobalNews.ca, June 19, 2017, https://globalnews.ca/news/ 3539250/hair-dyes-relaxers-linked-to-increased-risk-of-breast-cancer-study/.

24 Ibid.

25 Julee Wilson, "'You Can Touch My Hair' Explores Fascination with Black Hair, Sparks Debate," *Huffington Post*, June 7, 2013, http://www.huffington post.com/2013/06/07/you-can-touch-my-hair-exhibit-black-women-hair_ n_3401692.html?utm_hp_ref=hair-beauty.

26 Gill, "Postfeminist Media Culture," 153.

27 "Hair Extravaganza!" *O, the Oprah Magazine*, September 2013, 142.

28 Ibid., 147.

29 Hobson, *Venus in the Dark*, 115.

30 Ibid., 115–16.

31 Bailey, "Redefining Representation," 73.

32 Some of these sites include Around the Way Curls (Philadelphia), Black Girl With Long Hair (Chicago), Black Hair Kitchen (Washington, DC), Black Naps (New Jersey), Natural Hair Love Affair (Brooklyn), Coily Hair (New York), Curly Nikki (Pennsylvania), Going Natural (Brooklyn), Hair Milk (Baltimore), Hairscapades (Randolph, New Jersey), Naturally Curly (Austin, Texas), Natural Hair Rules (Las Vegas), Just Grow Already (Massachusetts), Kinky-Curly (Los Angeles), K is for Kinky (Los Angeles), Mixed Chicks (New Jersey), Motown Girl (Detroit), Les Curls (Montreal), 83 To Infinity (Toronto), Toni Daley (Toronto), Natural Hair Congress Canada (Canada), Natural Neiicey (Canada), My Fro and I (Johannesburg), and Natural Belle (England).

33 See note 19 above.

34 Sandra Stevenson, "Our Tangled World of Hair," *New York Times*, April 9, 2017, https://www.nytimes.com/2017/04/09/us/our-tangled-world-of -hair.html.

35 Sara Barnes, "Baroque-Inspired Portraits Celebrate the Beauty of Black Girls' Natural Hair," MyModernMet.com, November 14, 2017, https:// mymodernmet.com/afro-art-creativesoul-photography/.

36 Afua Hirsch, "Nivea's Latest 'White Is Right' Advert Is the Tip of a Reprehensible Iceberg," *Guardian*, October 22, 2017, https://www .theguardian.com/media/media-blog/2017/oct/22/niveas-latest-white-is-right-advert-is-the-tip-of-a-reprehensible-iceberg.

37 Ibid.

38 Tiffany Onyejiaka, "Hollywood's Colorism Problem Can't Be Ignored Any Longer," *TeenVogue*, August 22, 2017, https://www.teenvogue.com/story/hollywoods-colorism-problem-cant-be-ignored.

39 Cameron Glover, "Why *Wonder Woman* Is Bittersweet for Black Women," *Harper's Bazaar*, June 9, 2017, http://www.harpersbazaar.com/culture/film-tv/a9992873/wonder-woman-black-women-erasure/.

40 Mary-Rose Abraham, "Dark Is Beautiful: The Battle to End the World's Obsession with Lighter Skin," *Guardian*, September 4, 2017, https://www .theguardian.com/inequality/2017/sep/04/dark-is-beautiful-battle-to-end-worlds-obsession-with-lighter-skin.

41 Ibid.

42 Kristina Rodulfo, "Hijabi Beauty Vlogger Nura Afia Is CoverGirl's New Brand Ambassador," *Elle*, November 3, 2016, http://www.elle.com/beauty/makeup-skin-care/news/a40454/muslim-beauty-vlogger-nura-afia -covergirl-ambassador/.

43 Alicia Androich, "*Sway* Magazine Ceases Publication amidst Weak Ad Revenues," *Marketing*, August 7, 2012, http://www.marketingmag.ca/news/media-news/sway-magazine-ceases-publication-amidst-weak-ad -revenues-58883.

SELECTED BIBLIOGRAPHY

Adams, Tracey. "Making a Living: African-Canadian Workers in London, Ontario, 1861–1901." *Labour/Le Travail* 67 (Spring 2011): 9–44.

Adichie, Chimamanda Ngozi. *Americanah*. New York: Alfred A. Knoff, 2013.

Alexander, Ken, and Avis Glaze. *Towards Freedom: The African-Canadian Experience*. Toronto: Umbrella Press, 1996.

Appadurai, Arjun. *The Social Life of Things: Commodities in Cultural Perspective*. Cambridge: Cambridge University Press, 1988.

Archer-Straw, Petrine. *Negrophilia: Avant-Garde Paris and Black Culture in the 1920s*. New York: Thames & Hudson, 2000.

Aronczyk, Melissa. *Branding the Nation: Global Business of National Identity*. New York: Oxford University Press, 2013.

Arvidsson, Adam. "Brands: A Critical Perspective." *Journal of Consumer Culture* 5, no. 2 (2005): 235–58.

Ashe, Bertram D. "Invisible Dread: From *Twisted: The Dreadlock Chronicles*." In *Blackberries and Redbones: Critical Articulations of Black Hair/Body Politics in Africana Communities*, edited by Regina E. Spellers and Kimberly R. Moffat, 53–66. Cresskill, NJ: Hampton Press, 2010.

———. "'Why Don't He Like My Hair?': Constructing African-American Standards of Beauty in Toni Morrison's *Song of Solomon* and Zora Neale Hurston's *Their Eyes Were Watching God*." *African American Review* 29, no. 4 (Winter 1995): 579–92.

Austin, David. "All Roads Led to Montreal: Black Power and the Black Radical Tradition in Canada." In *Ebony Roots, Northern Soil: Perspectives on Blackness in Canada*, edited by Charmaine A. Nelson, 206–35. Newcastle upon Tyne, UK: Cambridge Scholars, 2010.

Backhouse, Constance. *Colour-Coded: A Legal History of Racism in Canada 1900–1950*. Toronto: University of Toronto Press, 1999.

Bailey, Moya. "Redefining Representation: Black Trans and Queer Women's Digital Media Production." *Screen Bodies* 1, no. 1 (Spring 2016): 71–86. https://doi.org/10.3167/screen.2016.010105.

Banks, Ingrid. *Hair Matters: Beauty, Power, and Black Women's Consciousness.* New York: New York University Press, 2000.

Barnes, Natasha. *Cultural Conundrums: Gender, Race, Nation, and the Making of Caribbean Cultural Politics.* Ann Arbor: University of Michigan Press, 2006.

———. "Face of the Nation: Race, Nationalism and Identities in Jamaican Beauty Pageants." *Massachusetts Review* 35, no. 2 3/4 (Autumn 1994): 471–92.

Basten, Fred E. *Max Factor: The Man Who Changed the Faces of the World.* New York: Arcade Publishing, 2008.

Baudrillard, Jean. *Simulacra and Simulation.* Trans. Sheila Faria Glaser. Ann Arbor: University of Michigan Press, [1981] 1994.

Belisle, Donica. *Retail Nation: Department Stores and the Making of Modern Canada.* Vancouver: UBC Press, 2011.

Bennett, Lerone Jr. *The Shaping of Black America: The Struggles and Triumphs of African-Americans, 1619 to the 1990s.* Middlesex, UK: Penguin Books, 1993.

Berger, Martin. "Race, Visuality, and History." *American Art* 24, no. 2 (2010): 94–99.

Berlant, Lauren. *The Female Complaint: The Unfinished Business of Sentimentality in American Culture.* Durham, NC: Duke University Press, 2008.

Bernstein, Robin. *Racial Innocence: Performing American Childhood from Slavery to Civil Rights.* New York: New York University Press, 2011.

Blackwelder, Julia K. *Styling Jim Crow: African American Beauty Training during Segregation.* College Station: Texas A&M University Press, 2003.

Bogle, Donald. *Toms, Coons, Mulattoes, Mammies, and Bucks: An Interpretive History of Blacks in American Films.* New York: Continuum, 2000.

Bordo, Susan. "Cassie's Hair." In *Material Feminisms*, edited by Stacy Alaimo and Susan Hekman, 400–424. Bloomington: Indiana University Press, 2008.

———. "'Material Girl': The Effacements of Postmodern Culture." In *Negotiating at the Margins: The Gendered Discourses of Power and Resistance*, edited by Sue Fisher and Kathy Davis, 295–316. New Brunswick, NJ: Rutgers University Press, 1993.

———. *Unbearable Weight: Feminism, Western Culture, and the Body.* Berkeley: University of California Press, 1995.

Braithwaite, Rella. *The Black Woman in Canada.* Unknown, 1976.

Brand, Dionne. *No Burden to Carry: Narratives of Black Working Women in Ontario, 1920s–1950s.* Toronto: Women's Press, 1991.

———. "'We Weren't Allowed to Go into Factory Work until Hitler Started the War': The 1920s to the 1940s." In *We're Rooted Here and They Can't Pull Us Up: Essays in African Canadian Women's History*, edited by Peggy Bristow, 171–91. Toronto: University of Toronto Press, 1994.

Bristol, Douglas Walter, Jr. *Knights of the Razor: Black Barbers in Slavery and Freedom.* Baltimore: Johns Hopkins University Press, 2009.

Brody, Jennifer DeVere. *Impossible Purities: Blackness, Femininity, and Victorian Culture.* Durham, NC: Duke University Press, 1998.

Buckridge, Steeve O. *The Language of Dress: Resistance and Accommodation in Jamaica, 1760–1890.* Kingston, Jamaica: University of the West Indies Press, 2004.

Burman, Jenny. *Transnational Yearnings: Tourism, Migration, and the Diasporic City.* Vancouver: UBC Press, 2010.

Bush, Barbara. *Slave Women in Caribbean Society 1650–1838.* Indiana: Indiana University Press, 1990.

Byrd, Ayana D., and Lori L. Tharps. *Hair Story: Untangling the Roots of Black Hair in America.* New York: St. Martin's Press, 2001.

Caldwell, Kia Lilly. "'Look at Her Hair': The Body Politics of Black Womanhood in Brazil." *Transforming Anthropology* 11, no. 2 (2004): 18–29. https://doi.org/10.1525/tran.2003.11.2.18.

Caldwell, Paulette. "A Hair Piece: Perspectives on the Intersection of Race and Gender." In *Critical Race Feminism: A Reader,* edited by Adrien Katherine Wing, 309–17. New York: New York University Press, 2003.

Candelario, Ginetta. *Black Behind the Ears: Dominican Racial Identity from Museums to Beauty Shops.* Durham, NC: Duke University Press, 2007.

Carby, Hazel. *Reconstructing Womanhood: The Emergence of Afro-American Woman Novelist.* New York: Oxford University Press, 1987.

Charles, Christopher A. D. "Skin Bleachers' Representations of Skin Color in Jamaica." *Journal of Black Studies* 40, no. 2 (November 2009): 153–70.

Clark, Danae. "Commodity Lesbianism." In *Out in Culture: Gay, Lesbian, and Queer Essays on Popular Culture,* edited by Corey Creekmur and Alexander Doty Durham, 484–500. Durham, NC: Duke University Press, 1995.

Collins, Lisa Gail. "Historic Retrievals: Confronting Visual Evidence and the Imaging of Truth." In *Black Venus 2010: They Called Her "Hottentot,"* edited by Deborah Willis, 71–86. Philadelphia: Temple University Press, 2010.

Collins, Patricia Hill. *Black Feminist Thought: Knowledge, Consciousness and the Politics of Empowerment.* Boston: Unwin Hyman, 1990.

The Colour of Beauty. Directed by Elizabeth St. Philip. CAN: NFB, 2010.

Conor, Liz. *The Spectacular Modern Woman: Feminine Visibility in the 1920s.* Bloomington: Indiana University Press, 2004.

Conrad, Cecelia A. "Black-Owned Businesses: Trends and Prospects." In *African Americans in the U.S. Economy,* edited by Cecilia A. Conrad, John Whitehead, Patrick L. Mason, and James Stewart, 237–45. New York: Rowman & Littlefield, 2005.

Cooper, Afua. "The Search for Mary Bibb, Black Woman Teacher in Nineteenth-Century Canada West." In *"We Specialize in the Wholly Impossible:*

A Reader in Black Women's History," edited by Darlene Clark Hine, Linda Reed, and Wilma King, 171–85. Brooklyn, NY: Carlson, 1995.

Craig, Maxine Leeds. *Ain't I a Beauty Queen? Black Women, Beauty, and the Politics of Race.* Oxford: Oxford University Press, 2002.

Davis, Judy Foster. "New Hair Freedom? 1990s Hair Care Marketing and the African-American Woman." In *Milestones in Marketing History,* edited by Terrance H. Witkowski, 31–40. Long Beach, CA: Association for Historical Research in Marketing, 2001.

Detweiler, Frederick G. *The Negro Press in the United States.* Chicago: University of Chicago Press, 1922.

Dowbiggin, Ian Robert. *Keeping America Sane: Psychiatry and Eugenics in the United States and Canada, 1880–1940.* Ithaca, NY: Cornell University Press, 1997.

Ducille, Anne. "Dyes and Dolls: Multicultural Barbie and the Merchandising of Difference." *differences: A Journal of Feminist Cultural Studies* 6, no. 1 (1994): 47–68.

Dunn, Stephanie. *"Baad Bitches" and Sassy Supermamas: Black Power Action Films.* Champaign: University of Illinois Press, 2008.

Ehlers, Nadine. *Racial Imperatives: Discipline, Performativity, and Struggles Against Subjection.* Bloomington: Indiana University Press, 2012.

Etcoff, Nancy. *Survival of the Prettiest: The Science of Beauty.* New York: Anchor Books, 1999.

Fanon, Frantz. *Black Skin, White Masks.* Translated by Charles Lam Markmann. New York: Grove Press, 1967.

Farrington, Lisa A. *Creating Their Own Image: The History of African-American Women Artists.* New York: Oxford University Press, 2005.

Ferrell, Pamela. *Let's Talk Hair.* Washington, DC: Cornrows, 1996.

Fleras, Augie. "Racializing Culture/Culturalizing Race: Multicultural Racism in Multicultural Canada." In *Racism, Eh? A Critical Inter-Disciplinary Anthology of Race and Racism in Canada,* edited by Camille A. Nelson and Charmaine A. Nelson, 429–43. Concord, ON: Captus Press, 2004.

Francis, Daniel. *National Dreams: Myth, Memory, and Canadian History.* Vancouver: Arsenal Pulp Press, 2011.

Freeman, Barbara. "From No Go to No Logo: Lesbian Lives and Rights in *Chatelaine.*" *Canadian Journal of Communication* 31 (2006): 815–41.

Gaines, Jane. "White Privilege and Looking Relations: Race and Gender in Feminist Film Theory." In *Feminist Film Theory: A Reader,* edited by Sue Thornham, 293–306. New York: New York University Press, 2006.

Glazer, Lee, and Susan Key. "Carry Me Back: Nostalgia for the Old South in Nineteenth-Century Popular Culture." *Journal of American Studies* 30, no. 1 (April 1996): 1–24.

Gill, Rosalind. "Postfeminist Media Culture: Elements of Sensibility." *European Journal of Cultural Studies* 10, no. 2 (May 2007): 147–66. https://doi.org/10.1177/1367549407075898.

Gill, Tiffany Melissa. "I Had My Own Business…So I Didn't Have to Worry": Beauty Salons, Beauty Culturists, and the Politics of African-American Female Entrepreneurship." In *Beauty and Business: Commerce, Gender, and Culture in Modern America*, edited by Philip Scranton, 169–94. New York: Routledge, 2001.

Gilliam, Angela. "The Brazilian Mulata: Images in the Global Economy." *Race & Class* 40, no.1 (July 1998): 57–69. https://doi.org/10.1177/030639689804000105.

Gilman, Sander. "Black Bodies, White Bodies: Toward an Iconography of Female Sexuality in Late Nineteenth-Century Art, Medicine, and Literature." *Critical Inquiry* 12, no. 1 (Autumn 1985): 204–42.

Goldberg, David Theo. *The Racial State*. Hoboken, NJ: Wiley-Blackwell, 2001.

Grayson, Deborah R. "Is It Fake? Black Women's Hair as Spectacle and Spec(tac)ular." *Camera Obscura Collective* 36, no. 3 (36) (September 1995): 13–31.

Greene, D. Wendy. "Black Women Can't Have Blonde Hair…in the Workplace." *Journal of Gender, Race and Justice* 14, no. 2 (Spring 2011): 405–30.

Grewal, Inderpal. *Transnational America: Feminisms, Diasporas, Neoliberalism*. Durham, NC: Duke University Press, 2005.

Grove, Jaleen. "A Castle of One's Own: Interactivity in *Chatelaine Magazine*, 1928–35." *Journal of Canadian Studies* 45, no. 3 (Fall 2011): 166–93. https://doi.org/10.3138/jcs.45.3.167.

Haidarali, Laila. "Polishing Brown Diamonds: African American Women, Popular Magazines, and the Advent of Modeling in Early Postwar America." *Journal of Women's History* 17, no. 1 (Spring 2005): 10–37.

Harrison, Bonnie Claudia. "'Shining in the Sun': Remembering Gladys M. James and The Poro School of Beauty." *Transforming Anthropology* 11, no. 2 (July 2003): 43–50. https://doi.org/10.1525/tran.2003.11.2.43.

Henry, Keith S. *Black Politics in Toronto Since World War I*. Toronto: Multicultural History Society of Ontario, 1981.

Higginbotham, Evelyn Brooks. *Righteous Discontent: The Women's Movement in the Black Baptist Church 1880–1920*. Cambridge, MA: Harvard University Press, 1993.

Hill, Lawrence. *Women of Vision: The Story of the Canadian Negro Women's Association 1951–1976*. Toronto: Umbrella Press, 1996.

Hine, Thomas. *The Total Package: The Evolution and Secret Meanings of Boxes, Bottles, Cans, and Tubes*. Boston: Little, Brown, 1995.

Hobbs, Allyson. *A Chosen Exile: A History of Racial Passing in American Life*. Cambridge, MA: Harvard University Press, 2014.

Hobson, Janell. *Body as Evidence: Mediating Race, Globalizing Gender*. Albany, NY: State University of New York Press, 2012.

———. *Venus in the Dark: Blackness and Beauty in Popular Culture*. New York: Routledge, 2005.

hooks, bell. *Black Looks: Race and Representation.* Boston: South End Press, 1992.

———. "In Our Glory: Photography and Black Life." In *Picturing Us: African American Identity in Photography,* edited by Deborah Willis, 43–53. New York: New Press, 1994.

Hope, Donna. "From *Browning* to *Cake Soap*: Popular Debates on Skin Bleaching in the Jamaican Dancehall." *Journal of Pan African Studies* 4, no. 4 (June 2011): 165–94.

Horne, Gerald. *The Rise & Fall of the Associated Negro Press: Claude Barnett's Pan-African News and the Jim Crow Paradox.* Chicago: University of Illinois Press, 2017.

Hunter, Margaret. *Race, Gender and the Politics of Skin Tone.* New York: Routledge, 2005.

Jacobs-Huey, Lanita. *From the Kitchen to the Parlor: Language and Becoming in African American Women's Hair Care.* New York: Oxford University Press, 2006.

James, Geoffrey. *Beauty Imagined: A History of the Global Beauty Industry.* Oxford: Oxford University Press, 2010.

Jhally, Sut. *The Codes of Advertising: Fetishism and the Political Economy of Meaning in the Consumer Society.* New York: Routledge, 1990.

Johnson, Guy B. "Newspaper Advertisements and Negro Culture." *Journal of Social Forces* 3 (May 1925): 706–9.

Jones, Lisa. "The Hair Trade." In *Talking Visions: Multicultural Feminism in a Transnational Age,* edited by Ella Shotat, 119–36. New York: MIT Press, 1998.

Keller, Jessalynn Marie. "Fiercely Real? Tyra Banks and the Making of New Media Celebrity." *Feminist Media Studies* 14, no. 1 (2014): 147–64. DOI: 10.1080/14680777.2012.740490.

Kelley, Robin D. G. *Yo' Mama's Disfunktional! Fighting the Culture Wars in Urban America.* Boston: Beacon Press, 1997.

Khumalo, Nonhlanhla P., Janet Stone, Freedom Gumedze, Emily McGrath, Mzudumile R. Ngwanya, and David de Berker. "'Relaxers' Damage Hair: Evidence from Amino Acid Analysis." *Journal of the American Academy of Dermatology* 62, no. 3 (March 2010): 402–8. https://doi.org/10.1016/j.jaad.2009.04.061.

Kibler, Alison M. *Rank Ladies: Gender and Cultural Hierarchy in American Vaudeville.* Chapel Hill: University of North Carolina Press, 1999.

King, Stephen A. "The Co-optation of a 'Revolution': Rastafari, Reggae, and the Rhetoric of Social Control." *Howard Journal of Communication* 10, no. 2 (1999): 77–95. https://doi.org/10.1080/106461799246834.

King, Toni C. "'Who's That Lady?': *Ebony* Magazine and Black Professional Women." In *Disco Divas: Women and Popular Culture in the 1970s,* edited by Sherrie A. Inness, 87–102. Philadelphia: University of Pennsylvania Press, 2003.

Koehn, Nancy. "Estée Lauder: Self-Definition and the Modern Cosmetics Market." In *Beauty and Business: Commerce, Gender, and Culture in Modern America*, edited by Philip Scranton, 217–53. New York: Routledge, 2001.

Korinek, Valerie J. *Roughing It in the Suburbs: Reading* Chatelaine *Magazine in the Fifties and Sixties*. Toronto: University of Toronto Press, 2000.

Kyei, Angela, Wilma Fowler Bergfeld, Melissa Piliang, and Pamela Summers. "Medical and Environmental Risk Factors for the Development of Central Centrifugal Cicatricial Alopecia: A Population Study." *JAMA Dermatology* 147, no. 8 (August 2011): 909–14. https://doi.org/10.1001/archdermatol.2011.66.

Lara, Ana-Maurine. "*Cimarronas, Ciguapas, Señoras*: Hair, Beauty, Race, and Class in the Dominican Republic." In *Blackberries and Redbones: Critical Articulations of Black Hair/Body Politics in Africana Communities*, edited by Regina E. Spellers and Kimberly R. Moffat, 113–28. Cresskill, NJ: Hampton Press, 2010.

Lorinc, John. Introduction to *The Ward: The Life and Loss of Toronto's First Immigrant Neighbourhood*. Edited by John Lorinc, Michael McClelland, Ellen Scheinberg, and Tatum Taylor. Toronto: Coach House Books, 2015.

Lury, Celia. *Consumer Culture*. 2nd ed. New Brunswick, NJ: Rutgers University Press, 2011.

Mama, Amina. *Beyond the Masks: Race, Gender and Subjectivity*. London: Routledge, 1995.

Marano, Carla. "'Rising Strongly and Rapidly': The Universal Negro Improvement Association of Canada, 1919–1940." *Canadian Historical Review* 91, no. 2 (June 2010): 233–59.

Mastalia, Francesco, and Alfonse Pagano. *Dreads*. New York: Artisan, 1999.

Mathieu, Sarah-Jane. *North of the Color Line: Migration and Black Resistance in Canada, 1870–1955*. Chapel Hill: University of North Carolina Press, 2010.

Matthews, Mary Catherine. "Working for Family, Nation and God: Paternalism and the Dupuis Frères Department Store, Montreal, 1926–1952." MA thesis, McGill University, 1997.

Maynard, Robyn. *Policing Black Lives: State Violence in Canada from Slavery to the Present*. Halifax: Fernwood, 2017.

Maynard, Rona. Introduction to *Chatelaine, A Woman's Place: Seventy Years in the Lives of Canadian Women*, 7–10. Edited by Sylvia Fraser. Toronto: Key Porter Books, 1997.

McAndrew, Malia. "A Twentieth-Century Triangle Trade: Selling Black Beauty at Home and Abroad, 1945–1965." *Enterprise & Society* 11, no. 4 (December 2010): 784–810.

McClintock, Anne. *Imperial Leather: Race, Gender and Sexuality in the Colonial Conquest*. New York: Routledge, 1995.

McCracken, Grant. *Big Hair: A Journey into the Transformation of Self*. Toronto: Penguin Books, 1996.

McFarquhar, Colin. "The Black Occupational Structure in Late-Nineteenth-Century Ontario: Evidence from the Census." In *Racism, Eh? A Critical Inter-Disicplinary Anthology of Race and Racism in Canada*, edited by Camille A. Nelson and Charmaine A. Nelson, 50–62. Concord, ON: Captus Press, 2004.

McLaren, Angus. *Our Own Master Race: Eugenics in Canada, 1885–1945.* Toronto: McClelland & Stewart, 1990.

McMichael, Amy. "Hair and Scalp Disorders in Ethnic Populations." *Dermatologic Clinics* 21, no. 4 (October 2003): 629–44.

Mensah, Joseph. *Black Canadians: History, Experiences, Social Conditions.* Halifax: Fernwood, 2002.

Mercer, Kobena. *Welcome to the Jungle: New Positions in Black Cultural Studies.* New York: Routledge, 1994.

Meyerowitz, Joanne. "Women, Cheesecake, and Borderline Material: Responses to Girlie Pictures in the Mid-Twentieth-Century U.S." *Journal of Women's History* 8, no. 3 (Fall 1996): 9–35.

Miller, Monica. *Slaves to Fashion: Black Dandyism and the Styling of Black Diasporic Identity.* Durham, NC: Duke University Press, 2009.

Morrison, Toni. *The Bluest Eye.* New York: Plume Printing, 1994.

Mulvey, Laura. "Visual Pleasure and Narrative Cinema." In *Feminist Film Theory: A Reader*, edited by Sue Thornham, 58–69. New York: New York University Press, 2006.

Murray, Amelia M. *Letters from the United States, Cuba and Canada.* New York: G. P. Putnam, 1856.

Murray, Dara Persis. "Branding 'Real' Social Change in Dove's Campaign for Real Beauty." *Feminist Media Studies* 13, no. 1 (January 2012): 83–101. https://doi.org/10.1080/14680777.2011.647963.

Neal, Mark Anthony. "Sold Out on Soul: The Corporate Annexation of Black Popular Music." *Popular Music & Society* 21, no. 3 (1997): 117–36.

Nelson, Charmaine. "The 'Hottentot Venus' in Canada: Modernism, Censorship and the Racial Limits of Female Sexuality." In *Black Venus 2010: They Called Her "Hottentot,"* edited by Deborah Willis, 112–25. Philadelphia: Temple University Press, 2010.

———. *Representing the Black Female Subject in Western Art.* New York: Routledge, 2010.

Nicholas, Jane. "Gendering the Jubilee: Gender and Modernity in the Diamond Jubilee of Confederation Celebrations, 1927." *Canadian Historical Review* 90, no. 2 (June 2009): 247–74. https://doi.org/10.3138/chr.90.2.247.

Oak, Vishnu V. *The Negro Newspaper.* Westport, CT: Negro Universities Press, 1948.

O'Donnell, Lorraine. "Visualizing the History of Women at Eaton's, 1869 to 1976." PhD diss., McGill University, 2003.

Ovalle, Priscilla Peña. "Framing Jennifer Lopez: Mobilizing Race from the Wide Shot to the Close-Up." In *The Persistence of Whiteness: Race and Con-*

temporary Hollywood Cinema, edited by Daniel Bernardi, 165–84. London: Routledge, 2007.

Pachai, Bridglal, and Henry Bishop. *Historic Black Nova Scotia*. Halifax: Nimbus, 2006.

Patton, Tracey Owens. "'Hey Girl, Am I More Than My Hair?': African American Women and Their Struggles with Beauty, Body Image, and Hair." *NWSA Journal* 18, no. 2 (Summer 2006): 24–51.

Peiss, Kathy. *Hope in a Jar: The Making of America's Beauty Culture*. New York: Metropolitan Books, 1998.

———. "Making Up, Making Over: Cosmetics, Consumer Culture, and Women's Identity." In *The Sex of Things: Gender and Consumption in Historical Perspective*, edited by Victoria de Grazia and Ellen Furlough, 311–36. Berkeley: University of California Press, 1996.

Perry, Imani. "Who(se) Am I? The Identity and Image of Women in Hip-Hop." In *Gender, Race, Class in Media: A Text-Reader*, edited by Gail Dines and Jean M. Humez, 136–48. London: Sage Publications, 2003.

Plitt, Jane R. *Martha Matilda Harper and the American Dream: How One Woman Changed the Face of Modern Business*. Syracuse, NY: Syracuse University Press, 2000.

Polykoff, Shirley. *Does She... or Doesn't She? And How She Did It*. New York: Doubleday, 1975.

Prince, Althea. *The Politics of Black Women's Hair*. Toronto: Insomnia Press, 2009.

Raimon, Eve Allegra. *The "Tragic Mulatta" Revisted: Race and Nationalism in Nineteenth-Century Antislavery Fiction*. New Brunswick, NJ: Rutgers University Press, 2004.

Rediker, Marcus. *The Slave Ship: A Human History*. New York: Penguin Books, 2007.

Reynolds, Graham. *Viola Desmond's Canada: A History of Blacks and Racial Segregation in the Promised Land*. Halifax: Fernwood, 2016.

Rifelj, Carol. *Coiffures: Hair in Nineteenth-Century French Literature and Culture*. Newark: University of Delaware Press, 2010.

Riss, Arthur. *Race, Slavery, and Liberalism in Nineteenth-Century American Literature*. New York: Cambridge University Press, 2006.

Roberts, Cynthia. *Barbie: Thirty Years of America's Doll*. Chicago: Contemporary, 1989.

Robson, Wanda. *Sister to Courage: Stories from the World of Viola Desmond, Canada's Rosa Parks*. Wreck Cove, NS: Breton Books, 2010.

Rooks, Noliwe M. *Hair Raising: Beauty, Culture, and African American Women*. New Brunswick, NJ: Rutgers University Press, 1996.

———. *Ladies' Pages: African American Women's Magazines and the Culture That Made Them*. New Brunswick, NJ: Rutgers University Press, 2004.

Roseman, Michele Tapp. *Hairlooms: The Untangled Truth about Loving Your Natural Hair and Beauty*. Deerfield Beach, FL: HCI Books, 2017.

Rowe, Rochelle. "'Glorifying the Jamaican Girl': The 'Ten Types One People' Beauty Contest, Racialized Femininities, and Jamaican Nationalism." *Radical History Review* 103 (Winter 2009): 36–58.

Ruck, Calvin. *Canada's Black Battalion: No. 2 Construction 1916–1920.* Halifax: Society for the Protection and Preservation of Black Culture in Nova Scotia, 1986.

Russell, Kathy, Midge Wilson, and Ronald Hall. *The Color Complex: The Politics of Skin Color among African Americans.* New York: Anchor Books, 1992.

Rymell, Heather. "Images of Women in the Magazines of the '30s and '40s." *Canadian Women Studies* 3, no. 2 (1981): 96–99.

Shadd, Adrienne. *The Journey from Tollgate to Parkway: African Canadians in Hamilton.* Toronto: Natural Heritage Books, 2010.

Sharpley-Whiting, T. Denean. *Pimps Up, Ho's Down: Hip Hop's Hold on Young Black Women.* New York: New York University Press, 2007.

Shaw, Andrea. *The Embodiment of Disobedience: Fat Black Women's Unruly Political Bodies.* Lanham, MD: Rowman & Littlefield, 2006.

Shaw, Melissa N. "'Most Anxious to Serve Their King and Country': Black Canadians' Fight to Enlist in WWI and Emerging Race Consciousness in Ontario, 1914–1919." *Histoire sociale/Social History* 49, no. 100 (2016): 543–80.

Sheehan, Elizabeth M. "The Face of Fashion: Race and Fantasy in James VanDerZee's Photography and Jessie Fauset's Fiction." In *Cultures of Femininity in Modern Fashion,* edited by Ilya Parkins and Elizabeth M. Sheehan, 180–202. Durham, NH: University of New Hampshire Press, 2011.

Sherrow, Victoria. *Encyclopedia of Hair: A Cultural History.* Westport, CT: Greenwood Press, 2006.

Silva, Fred. Introduction to *Focus on The Birth of a Nation,* 1–15. Edited by Fred Silva. Englewood Cliffs, NJ: Prentice-Hall, 1971.

Smith, Shawn Michelle. *American Archives: Gender, Race, and Class in Visual Culture.* Princeton, NJ: Princeton University Press, 1999.

———. *Photography on the Color Line: W.E.B. Du Bois, Race, and Visual Culture.* Durham, NC: Duke University Press, 2004.

Spencer, Emily. *Lipstick and High Heels: War, Gender and Popular Culture.* Kingston, ON: Canadian Defence Academy Press, 2007.

Sperling, Joy. "Multiples and Reproductions: Prints and Photographs in Nineteenth-Century England—Visual Communities, Cultures, and Class." In *A History of Visual Culture: Western Civilization from the 18th to the 21st Century,* edited by Jane Kromm and Susan Benforado Bakewell, 296–308. New York: Berg, 2010.

Spray, W.A. *The Blacks in New Brunswick.* Fredericton, NB: Brunswick Press, 1972.

Stowe, Harriet Beecher. *Uncle Tom's Cabin; or, Life among the Lowly.* Boston, 1852. Reprint, edited by Ann Douglas. New York: Penguin Books, 1981.

Sutherland, Fraser. *The Monthly Epic: A History of Canadian Magazines 1789–1989.* Markham, ON: Fitzhenry & Whiteside, 1989.

Talty, Stephan. *Mulatto America: At the Crossroads of Black and White Culture: A Social History*. New York: HarperCollins, 2003.

Tate, Claudia. *Domestic Allegories of Political Desire: The Black Heroine's Text at the Turn of the Century*. New York: Oxford University Press, 1992.

Tate, Shirley. *Black Beauty: Aesthetics, Stylization, Politics*. Surrey, UK: Ashgate, 2009.

Taylor, Paul C. "Malcolm's Conk and Danto's Colors; or, Four Logical Petitions Concerning Race, Beauty, and Aesthetics." In *Beauty Matters*, edited by Peg Zeglin Brand, 57–64. Bloomington: Indiana University Press, 2000.

Thomas, Owen. "Cultural Tourism, Commemorative Plaques, and African-Canadian Historiography: Challenging Historical Marginality." *Social History / Histoire Sociale* 29 (1996): 431–39.

Thompson, Cheryl. "Black Women, Beauty, and Hair as a Matter of *Being*." *Women's Studies: An Interdisciplinary Journal* 38, no. 8 (October 2009): 831–56. https://doi.org/10.1080/00497870903238463.

———. "Cultivating Narratives of Race, Faith, and Community: *The Dawn of Tomorrow*, 1923–1971." *Canadian Journal of History* 50, no. 1 (Spring-Summer/printemps-été 2015): 30–67.

———. "'I'se in Town, Honey': Reading Aunt Jemima Advertising in Canadian Print Media, 1919 to 1962." *Journal of Canadian Studies* 49, no. 1 (Winter/hiver 2015): 205–37.

Thompson, Krista. *An Eye for the Tropics: Tourism, Photography, and Framing the Caribbean Picturesque*. Durham, NC: Duke University Press, 2006.

Tobias, Andrew. *Fire and Ice: The Story of Charles Revson—The Man Who Built the Revlon Empire*. New York: William Morrow, 1976.

Toney, Jared G. "Locating Diaspora: Afro-Caribbean Narratives of Migration and Settlement in Toronto, 1914–1929." *Urban History Review* 38, no. 2 (Spring 2010): 75–87.

Trotman, David V. "Transforming Caribbean and Canadian Identity: Contesting Claims for Toronto's Caribana." *Atlantic Studies* 2, no. 2 (August 2005): 177–98. https://doi.org/10.1080/10494820500224392.

Trotz, D. Alissa. "Rethinking Caribbean Transnational Connections: Conceptual Itineraries." *Global Networks* 6, no. 1 (February 2006): 41–59. https://doi.org/10.1111/j.1471-0374.2006.00132.x.

Ulysee, Gina. "Uptown Ladies and Downtown Women: Female Representations of Class and Color in Jamaica." In *Representations of Blackness and the Performance of Identities*, edited by Jean Muteba Rahier 147–72. Westport, CT: Bergin & Garvey, 1999.

Van Deburg, William L. *New Day in Babylon: The Black Power Movement and American Culture, 1965–1975*. Chicago: University of Chicago Press, 1992.

Wald, Gayle. *Crossing the Line: Racial Passing in Twentieth-Century US Literature and Culture*. Durham, NC: Duke University Press, 2000.

Walker, Alice. *The Color Purple*. Orlando, FL: Harcourt, 1982.

Walker, Andre. *Andre Talks Hair*. New York: Simon and Schuster, 1997.

Walker, Barrington. Introduction to *The History of Immigration and Racism in Canada*, 11–13. Edited by Barrington Walker. Toronto: Canadian Scholars' Press, 2008.

Walker, James St.G. *The West Indians in Canada*. Ottawa: Canadian Historical Association, 1984.

Walker, James W. *Racial Discrimination in Canada: The Black Experience*. Ottawa: Canadian Historical Association Historical Booklet, 1985.

Walker, Susannah. "Black Is Profitable: The Commodification of the Afro, 1960–1975." In *Beauty and Business: Commerce, Gender, and Culture in Modern America*, edited by Philip Scranton, 254–77. New York: Routledge, 2001.

———. *Style and Status: Selling Beauty to African American Women, 1920–1975*. Lexington: University Press of Kentucky, 2007.

Wallace-Sanders, Kimberly. *Mammy: A Century of Race, Gender, and Southern Memory*. Ann Arbor: University of Michigan Press, 2008.

Wallis, Maria. Preface to *The Politics of Race in Canada*, v–ix. Edited by Maria Wallis and Augie Fleras. Don Mills, ON: Oxford University Press, 2009.

Warner, Kristen. "The Racial Logic of *Grey's Anatomy*: Shonda Rhimes and Her 'Post-Civil Rights, Post-Feminist' Series." *Television & New Media* (2014): 1–17.

Weekes, Debbie. "Shades of Blackness: Young Black Female Constructions of Beauty." In *Black British Feminism: A Reader*, edited by Heidi Safia Mirza, 113–26. London: Routledge, 1997.

Weems, Robert E., Jr. "Consumerism and the Construction of Black Female Identity in Twentieth-Century America." In *The Gender and Consumer Cultural Reader*, edited by Jennifer Scanlon, 166–77. New York: New York University Press, 2000.

Wek, Alek. *Alek: Sudanese Refugee to International Supermodel*. London: Virago Press, 2007.

White, Shane, and Graham White. "Slave Hair and African American Culture in the Eighteenth and Nineteenth Centuries." *Journal of Southern History* 61, no. 1 (February 1995): 45–76.

———. *Stylin': African American Expressive Culture from Its Beginnings to the Zoot Suit*. Ithaca, NY: Cornell University Press, 1998.

White, Shauntae Brown. "The Big Girl's Chair: A Rhetorical Analysis of How Motions for Kids Markets Relaxers to African American Girls." In *Blackberries and Redbones: Critical Articulations of Black Hair/Body Politics in Africana Communities*, edited by Regina E. Spellers and Kimberly R. Moffitt, 17–28. Cresskill, NJ: Hampton Press, 2010.

Williams, Carla. "Naked, Neutered, or Noble: The Black Female Body in America and the Problem of Photographic History." In *Skin Deep, Spirit Strong: The Black Female Body in American Culture*, edited by Kimberly Wallace-Sanders, 182–200. Ann Arbor: University of Michigan Press, 2002.

Williams, Dorothy. *The Road to Now: A History of Blacks in Montreal.* Montreal: Véhicule Press, 1997.

Willis, Deborah. *Reflections in Black: A History of Black Photographers 1840 to the Present.* New York: W. W. Norton, 2000.

Willis, Deborah, and Carla Williams. *The Black Female Body: A Photographic History.* Philadelphia: Temple University Press, 2002.

Winks, Robin W. *The Blacks in Canada: A History.* 2nd ed. Montreal: McGill-Queen's University Press, [1971] 1997.

————. "The Canadian Negro: A Historical Assessment: The Negro in the Canadian-American Relationship: Part I." *Journal of Negro History* 53, no. 4 (October 1968): 283–300.

Wise, Lauren A., Julie R. Palmer, David Reich, Yvette C. Cozier, and Lynn Rosenberg. "Hair Relaxer Use and Risk of Uterine Leiomyomata in African-American Women." *American Journal of Epidemiology* 175, no. 5 (March 1, 2012): 432–40. https://doi.org/10.1093/aje/kwr351.

Witt, Doris. *Black Hunger: Food and the Politics of US Identity.* New York: Oxford University Press, 1999.

Wolf, Naomi. *The Beauty Myth.* Toronto: Random House, 1997.

Wood, Marcus. "Marketing the Slave Trade: Slavery, Photography, and Emancipation: Time and Freedom in 'The Life of the Picture.'" In *A History of Visual Culture: Western Civilization from the 18th to the 21st Century*, edited by Jane Kromm and Susan Benforado Bakewell, 255–66. New York: Berg, 2010.

Young, Lola. *Fear of the Dark: 'Race,' Gender and Sexuality in the Cinema.* New York: Routledge, 1996.

INDEX

French Perm No-Base Creme Relaxer, 142, 149; Rio, De Classe Cosmetics, 183–86; Ultra Sheen Permanent Creme Relaxer, 104, 118, 136–37, 149, 157, 161; Ultra Sheen Precise TM Conditioning, 160; Ultra Wave Hair Culture, 29, 104, 118

hair trade: in Canada, 231; global, 32, 93, 225, 227–32. *See also* Korean hair merchants

Half-Century Magazine for the Colored Home and Homemaker, 53

Hamilton, Alfred, 30, 125. *See also Contrast*

Harlem Renaissance, 16, 36

Harper, Martha Matilda, 52

Health Canada, testing of cosmetics, 186

Heritage Minutes, 213–14

Hispanic women, in advertising, 188

Imagine a Future (2013), 250

Imitation of Life (1934, 1959), 218

immigration: and anti-black sentiment, 40–41; assimilation of white Anglo-Saxons, 11–12; exclusionary policies, 17, 40, 79–80; and multiculturalism, 18–19, 121; points system, 79–80. *See also* multiculturalism

immigration, of black migrants: early black immigration (1890–1940), 36, 40; to Maritimes, 44; mid-century black immigration (1940–1970), 79–80, 84–85, 123

Jenkins, James F., 39, 57. *See also Dawn of Tomorrow*

Johnson, George E., 29, 104–5, 177

Johnson, John H., 65, 137

Jungle Fever (1991), 220

Klu Klux Klan, in Canada, 77–78

Korean hair merchants, 225, 228, 231

Lauder, Estée, 100–101, 135, 165, 169

Lil' Kim (Kimberly Jones), 191

Little Black Sambo, 7, 81, 90

makeup: development of modern industry, 98–100; expansion of market to black women, 169–70, 187–88; and feminine identity, 98

Malone, Annie Turnbo, 59–61

Mammy, stereotype, 10–11, 41–43, 66

Marley, Bob, 208, 225

Martina Big, 258–59

Mascoll, Beverly, 31, 136

Mattel dolls, 129

middle class, emergence of, 48–49

Middle Passage, the, 200–202

miscegenation, 216

modernity: in black women's magazines, 48; and womanhood, 9, 43

Montreal, black community in, 46

mulatto, in literature, 215–18

multiculturalism: as Canadian brand, 18, 31, 121, 152, 194; Canadian national mythmaking, 19, 121–22; erasure of black Canadian history, 19, 31, 73, 152–53, 213; as marketing tool, 31–32, 163, 171, 175–76, 233, 249–50; as policy, 18

"My Black is Beautiful" (MBIB), 250

National Association for the Advancement of Colored People (NAACP), 15–16, 39, 46, 112

Negro Dolls Clubs, 71–72

negrophilia, 8

Neith, 50

New Negro: Canadian New Negro, 38; and consumerism, 45–46, 49; history of, 16, 203; impact on Canadian communities, 45–46

New Negro Woman: and beauty culturists, 52–53; history of, 29; light-skinned, 53; spread through newspapers, 16, 29, 48, 51, 57